The Acupuncture Handbook

The Acupuncture Handbook

Editor: Ophelia Burnett

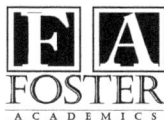

FA FOSTER
ACADEMICS

www.fosteracademics.com

www.fosteracademics.com

F A
FOSTER
ACADEMICS

Cataloging-in-Publication Data

The acupuncture handbook / edited by Ophelia Burnett.
   p. cm.
Includes bibliographical references and index.
ISBN 978-1-63242-857-8
1. Acupuncture. 2. Acupuncture points. 3. Alternative medicine. I. Burnett, Ophelia.
RM184 .A284 2019
615.892--dc23

© Foster Academics, 2019

Foster Academics,
118-35 Queens Blvd., Suite 400,
Forest Hills, NY 11375, USA

ISBN 978-1-63242-857-8 (Hardback)

Contents

Preface

Acupuncture is an important type of alternative medicine, involving the insertion of thin needles into the body. It is of utmost significance in traditional Chinese medicine (TCM). It is most commonly used for the purpose of relieving pain. It is often used as a complementary medicine, i.e., with other forms of treatment. The benefits of acupuncture are short-lived. It is primarily used to treat cases of musculoskeletal problems, including knee pain, lower back pain and shoulder stiffness. Some of the common therapeutic procedures associated with it include cupping therapy, electroacupuncture, moxibustion and fire needle acupuncture. This book traces the progress of acupuncture and highlights some of its key concepts and applications. This book is a collective contribution of a renowned group of international experts. A number of latest researches have been included to keep the readers up-to-date.

This book unites the global concepts and researches in an organized manner for a comprehensive understanding of the subject. It is a ripe text for all researchers, students, scientists or anyone else who is interested in acquiring a better knowledge of this dynamic field.

I extend my sincere thanks to the contributors for such eloquent research chapters. Finally, I thank my family for being a source of support and help.

Editor

Primary care physicians, acupuncture and chiropractic clinicians, and chronic pain patients: a qualitative analysis of communication and care coordination patterns

Lauren S. Penney[1], Cheryl Ritenbaugh[2], Charles Elder[3], Jennifer Schneider[3], Richard A. Deyo[4] and Lynn L. DeBar[3*]

Abstract

Background: A variety of people, with multiple perspectives, make up the system comprising chronic musculoskeletal pain (CMP) treatment. While there are frequently problems in communication and coordination of care within conventional health systems, more opportunities for communicative disruptions seem possible when providers use different explanatory models and are not within the same health management system. We sought to describe the communication system surrounding the management of chronic pain from the perspectives of allopathic providers, acupuncture and chiropractor (A/C) providers, and CMP patients.

Methods: We collected qualitative data from CMP patients (n = 90) and primary care physicians (PCPs) (n = 25) in a managed care system, and community acupuncture and chiropractic care providers (n = 14) who received high levels of referrals from the system, in the context of a longitudinal study of CMP patients' experience.

Results: Multiple points of divergence and communicative barriers were identified among the main stakeholders in the system. Those that were most frequently mentioned included issues surrounding the referral process (requesting, approving) and lack of consistent information flow back to providers that impairs overall management of patient care. We found that because of these problems, CMP patients were frequently tasked and sometimes overwhelmed with integrating and coordinating their own care, with little help from the system.

Conclusions: Patients, PCPs, and A/C providers desire more communication; thus systems need to be created to facilitate more open communication which could positively benefit patient outcomes.

Keywords: Chronic musculoskeletal pain, Complementary and alternative medicine, Managed care system, Interprofessional communication, Chronic care, Acupuncture, Chiropractic

Background

While estimates of chronic musculoskeletal pain (CMP) prevalence vary, CMP is both common and costly [1–4], and difficult to manage with conventional treatments. Indeed, CMP symptoms are among the top five reasons that patients visit clinics and emergency departments [4, 5]. People with CMP frequently utilize both conventional and complementary and alternative medicine (CAM) therapies [6]. Acupuncture and chiropractic (A/C) care are considered the most highly accepted by physician groups [7, 8] with the best evidence to support their use [9–12].

Although progress is being made, poor integration of care remains a challenge across the US health care system [13]. As more insurers offer alternative treatment benefits [14] and as more physicians support the use of CAM treatments for pain management [15], additional potential coordination difficulties arise. Research suggests little communication occurs directly between

* Correspondence: lynn.debar@kpchr.org
[3]Kaiser Permanente-Center for Health Research, 3800 N. Interstate Avenue, Portland, OR 97227-1098, USA
Full list of author information is available at the end of the article

allopathic providers and their CAM counterparts [16, 17], making this an important place to study communication within a patient care management network.

Thus far, most research on coordination within this care network in non-integrative medicine settings has focused the perspectives of patients [18–20], allopathic providers [21], CAM providers [22], or care dyads, such as patients and allopathic providers [23–25] or allopathic and CAM providers [26–29]. This work has identified areas that frequently inhibit better care coordination, such as lack of disclosure of CAM use by patients [18, 24], poor interprofessional communication [22, 28], and providers working from different explanatory models and utilizing distinct sets of jargon [21]. However, researchers have generally not examined how treatment coordination is simultaneously viewed by patients, allopathic providers, and CAM providers. With few exceptions [30, 31], they have also not looked at these groups within the contexts of systems in which providers are working for the same insurer system but are not co-located or within an integrative medicine program.

This paper presents qualitative data collected as part of a large mixed methods study of the impact of acupuncture and chiropractic as implemented in usual care of CMP [32]. The goal of the qualitative data analysis presented here is to describe the communication system surrounding the management of chronic pain from the perspectives of allopathic providers, A/C providers, and CMP patients. We identify points of divergence and communicative barriers among the main stakeholders in the system. Rather than only pointing to problems within any one of the dyadic relationships, we discern how communication systems occur within a managed care program, and where opportunities exist for more fluid care coordination.

Methods
Design
This paper draws on data gathered during the second phase of a multi-phase, mixed-method study to evaluate the outcomes of real-world acupuncture and chiropractic (A/C) services for CMP (see [32] for a full description of the study). Qualitative methods were employed during phase two to gain a better understanding of the characteristics of A/C services received by users and the decision-making processes patients and allopathic providers used when choosing A/C services. This information was used in the design of the third phase's prospective cohort study. Additionally, during analysis, two consistent themes manifested across participant groups: communication and access challenges, and use of opioid drugs. This paper is a result of an exploration of the former theme as it emerged within our data. Systemic communication and access issues were not a focus of the study, rather a complication we uncovered in the use of A/C because of qualitative data gathering.

Setting
Kaiser Permanente Northwest is an HMO providing medical care to approximately 530,000 members in Oregon and Washington. Nearly all members have a chiropractic care benefit, and most (with the exception of Medicare patients) have an acupuncture benefit. These two clinical services represent the overwhelming majority of complementary and integrative care provided to members, and are thus the focus of this analysis. Kaiser Permanente Northwest contracts with Complementary Health Plans, which is a network of acupuncturists, chiropractors, and other clinicians, to provide clinical acupuncture and chiropractic care. All credentialing and quality of care monitoring for acupuncturists and chiropractors is performed by the Complementary Health Plan network. Patients with musculoskeletal pain can be referred by an HMO primary care or specialty physician to a Complementary Health Plan acupuncturists or chiropractor for a limited number of visits when clinically indicated. Referrals are first vetted by the Kaiser Permanente Northwest referral office for appropriateness, and after approval, the patient can select and appoint with a Complementary Health Plan clinician.

Participants
This paper draws on data gathered through interviews and focus groups with managed care system CMP plan members who had and had not used acupuncture and/or chiropractic therapies ($n = 90$), allopathic PCPs with low to high referral rates to A/C care ($n = 25$), and contracted community A/C providers who treated a high volume of managed care CMP patients ($n = 14$). More detailed discussion of the overall project methods can be found in the design paper [32]; the Phase 2 methods described there closely match the methods used here. All interviews and focus groups were audio-recorded and transcribed for analysis and quality assurance. The Institutional Review Board of Kaiser Permanente Northwest approved all procedures. Consent forms were reviewed and signed by participants at the beginning of focus groups or interviews. All interviews were conducted by trained interview staff from the Kaiser Permanente Northwest Center for Health Research, which has a long track record of careful and responsive research within the health plan.

A total of 90 CMP health plan members participated in either a focus group ($n = 80$) or an individual interview ($n = 10$). Participants were identified from among those who endorsed a willingness to participate and consented to outreach at the end of a large-scale survey of Kaiser Permanente Northwest members that queried information about patterns of chiropractic and acupuncture utilization. (For complete results of that survey, see [33]) The survey provided information on participants' use of acupuncture and chiropractic that allowed for stratification of focus group composition (managed care plan referral or self-pay; acupuncture or chiropractic). Our 11 focus groups were composed of the following: we held two focus groups for patients with an HMO referral to acupuncture, two for patients with an HMO referral to chiropractic care, two for patients who had received other acupuncture (e.g., self-referred and out-of-plan care), two for patients who had other chiropractic care (e.g., self-referred and out-of-plan care), and three for comparable CMP patients who have not received either acupuncture or chiropractic care. Each focus group contained between six and 10 individuals.

Overall, letters were sent to 480 eligible survey respondents; 63 actively refused, 90 participated in 11 focus group sessions ($n = 80$) or interviews ($n = 10$), and the remainder did not return messages or were not pursued once focus groups were filled. Because Portland has few individuals of minority race/ethnicity, and because of concerns that their experiences might differ in unknown ways, individuals who further endorsed a minority race on the survey were selected from each of the focus group pools to be specifically invited for individual interviews using the same interview guide as the focus groups. Individual interviews allowed greater flexibility in timing and location of interviews to enhance participation. Thirty-seven (of the 480) letters were mailed to these individuals, and 10 participants were interviewed. Demographic data for patients were collected as part of that survey [33]. Patient participants were 67.7 years of age on average and 70 % were female. The racial/ethnic breakdown was 76 % white, 8 % African American, 2 % Native American, 6 % other, and 8 % unknown/refused to state. As noted above, ethnic minorities were specifically oversampled to increase their representation in the study.

We also conducted 25 PCP interviews, distributed nearly evenly among PCPs (internal and family medicine) who were high, medium and low for acupuncture and/or chiropractic referrals (four to five PCPs/cell) according to plan referral records for both types of services. Level of referral was determined by comparing individual PCP referral frequency to their HMO colleagues from January 1, 2008 to June 30, 2010. High referrers were defined as those at the 80th to 100th percentile of referrals, with at least 15 patients referred to A/C. Moderate referrers were at the 40th to 60th percentile of referrals, with five to 10 referrals to A/C. Low referrers were those at the 0 to 20th percentile, with two to three patient referrals to A/C.

We sent invitation emails to 86 PCPs; 13 actively declined, and the remainder were in some stage of establishing contact when the study cells were filled.

We similarly recruited acupuncturists and chiropractors, who saw a high volume of CMP patients from the health plan based on health plan referral records, from community settings in Oregon and Southwest Washington. A recruitment list for A/C providers was generated in two ways. Primarily we asked Complementary Health Plan administrators to identify a list of providers who received a high volume of referrals for HMO patients. Additionally, several PCPs who participated in the study suggested A/Cs they were aware of from their patients' experiences. Interviews were completed with eight acupuncturists (out of 27 recruited) and six chiropractors (out of 21 recruited).

Analysis

Qualitative coding was conducted using Atlas.ti software. Using the interview guide as a basis, an initial code book was created with five broad thematic areas and related sub-codes. For example, under the thematic code Decision Making and Referral Journey were child codes such as Beliefs about CAM and Referral Process. Codes were further refined after initial coding was completed and emerging themes identified. An informal reliability coding process was used to ensure conceptual clarity. Coder reliability was determined through duplicate coding of one out of every six interviews and focus groups. The coders compared how each transcript was coded and discussed discrepancies. In some cases these conversations led to refinement of code definitions in the code book and, in a few cases, the recoding of transcripts.

For this paper, we analyzed codes related to communication between patients and providers, communication between CAM and allopathic providers, the referral process, and treatment barriers. Although acupuncture and chiropractic are quite different therapies, we have combined them here because (1) referrals for both utilize exactly the same procedures in the health plan, and these are the only CAM therapies with frequent referrals for pain; (2) PCPs rarely make clear distinctions between them; and (3) the issues raised in the focus groups and patient interviews regarding referral and communication with the health plan were virtually identical. For the purposes of this paper, the similarities in situations (i.e. they were all dealing with the same communication issues, under similar referral guidelines) vastly outweigh the minor differences between them. For a similar reason in our analysis we have combined all PCP's responses, regardless of referral level, because we found they talked about communication issues in the same way due to working under the same system conditions.

Results

Acupuncture and chiropractic referral

Frequently, a patient is referred to A/C after he or she makes a personal request. Figure 1, developed from the interview data, provides a schematic of the communication pathways. PCPs generally did not initiate discussions about A/C with their CMP patients. Patients who asked for referral often had previous or current experience with CAM modalities, knew someone who had success with those treatments, or had heard they were services available through the insurer. However, not all CMP patients had knowledge of or exposure to CAM, or knew that they could receive that care under their insurance benefits.

Both PCPs and patients described physicians as having a variety of responses to patient requests for A/C: from immediate assent, to recommendations to try more conventional therapies first, to denial. Some PCPs reported they might also selectively refer patients who had previous positive A/C experience. According to PCPs, they would usually only outright deny a request for referral if the patient's medical condition contraindicated acupuncture or chiropractic treatment according to the benefit guidelines. However, some admitted that they would sometimes submit referrals even when they knew they would be denied because they wanted to appease the patient, were anxious to help the patient, and/or did not have time to personally deny the patient.

Occasionally patients had A/C proposed by their PCPs. Physicians were selective about which patients they recommended to A/C; it was not a possibility they opened to all their patients. They might discuss these therapies with patients with conditions they believed would be most responsive (e.g. did not want to take opioids), or patients who seemed more open to or had previous experience with CAM treatments. Many expressed the belief that A/C care was largely successful because of placebo, and would be less effective if the patient was not open to or believing in them. When physicians held such views, referrals to A/C were often deemed to be unproductive if the patient was perceived to not believe in CAM . However, in focus groups, patients who were naïve to CAM said they would be open to trying A/C if their physicians, who they trusted, suggested it. Notably, many PCPs stated they did not know enough about A/C, nor about the practitioners who were treating the patients, to feel qualified to make decisions about referrals.

For patients granted a referral, the next step was choosing from a list of A/C providers. Almost all of the Health Maintenance Organization (HMO) providers reported that, because of lack of familiarity, they were not able to refer patients to any particular provider. The process of selecting a provider could be daunting for patients, particularly those who were used to the HMO system in which they faced few similar provider choices. Patients made selections based, for example, on word of mouth, office location, and random selection from the list of available providers. In some cases, patients used friends, family, and personal experiences to guide them. Less frequently, PCPs might have a community provider

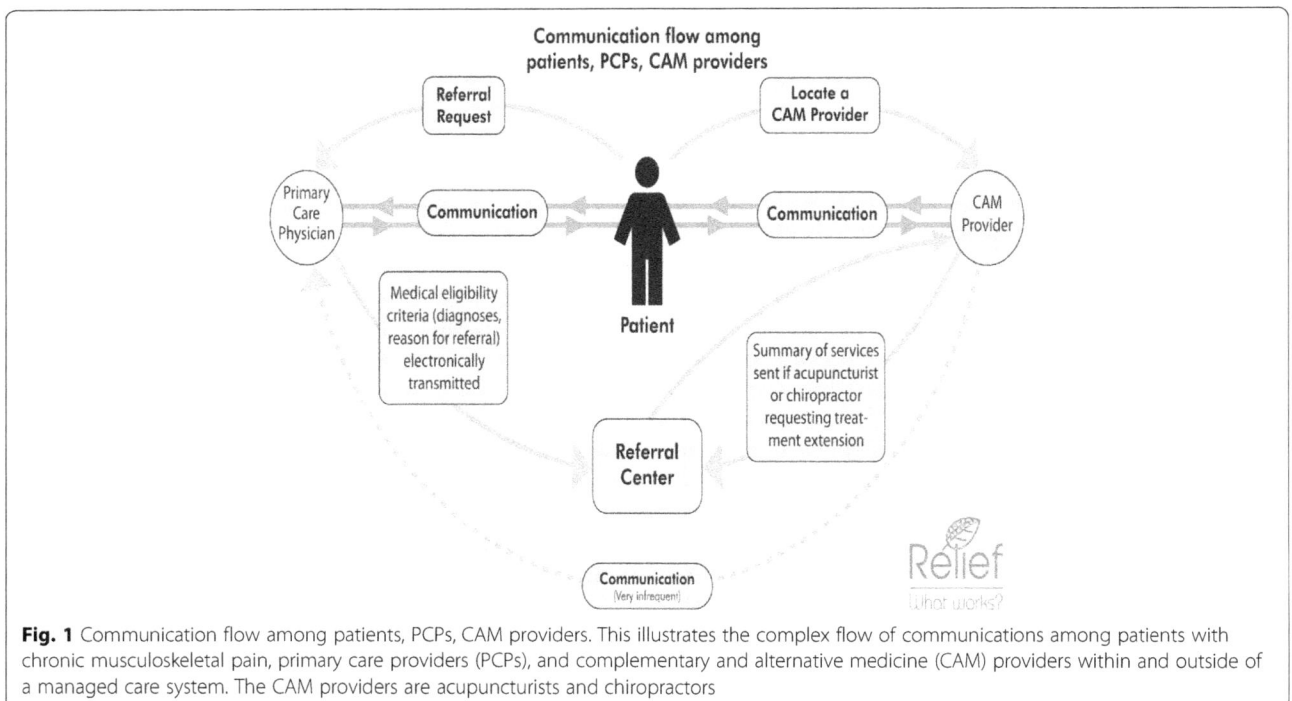

Fig. 1 Communication flow among patients, PCPs, CAM providers. This illustrates the complex flow of communications among patients with chronic musculoskeletal pain, primary care providers (PCPs), and complementary and alternative medicine (CAM) providers within and outside of a managed care system. The CAM providers are acupuncturists and chiropractors

they could recommend, often based on personal or other patients' experiences. When lacking other guidance, many patients selected a provider based on ease of access (e.g., proximity to home), provider credentials (e.g., medical degree), or arbitrarily chose from the list.

Physicians expressed concern over not being able to provide patients more guidance, seemed anxious about the lack of oversight, and questioned the quality controls for ensuring patient treatment. PCPs, patients, acupuncturists and chiropractors all described variability among A/C provider practices and quality, which made choosing from a list of providers with no other context somewhat risky. Given the lack of feedback in the communication system to PCPs, there were not opportunities for them to learn about differences among various A/C treatments and providers, or to be better informed when referring patients to the community for A/C treatment.

Communication among PCPs, acupuncturists, and chiropractors

Direct communication channels between PCPs and A/C providers were almost non-existent (see Fig. 1). Table 1 provides illustrative quotes from physicians and A/C providers on this issue. Because A/C providers were external to the HMO system, there were no systematic or institutionalized ways for sharing information or even knowing the names of other providers. A/C providers submitted some treatment paperwork to the HMO's referral center, but this information was not routinely shared with PCPs. Lack of time and interest on the part of PCPs, as well as A/C provider uncertainty about receptivity of allopathic physicians to interaction, were additional barriers. Patients were relied upon to communicate with their providers and share information; however this was neither consistent nor complete.

Table 1 Communication between PCPs and A/C providers

	PCPs	A/C providers
No effective communication	"We do not get any written documentation of what they've done."	"There's no effective communication here." "I don't know if I'm supposed to [communicate with PCPs]. I don't know if they're open to it, if they want to hear back how these patients are doing."
Spotty communication	"I've had a few [chiropractors] who have actually have sent me like their note or this improved. And that's great. That's wonderful. And I actually wish there was a little bit more of that"	"It's rare, very rare [to interact with HMO clinician]. Usually, I'm communicating through the client. A couple of times through e-mail"
Contrasting attitudes toward communication	"I think if I were getting reports from acupuncturists, I think that would just annoy me. So I'm kind of glad there's not a lot of back and forth. I feel like, like getting a report from the dentist, I kind of don't care."	"I want to be working in conjunction with a primary care doctor."
	"Frankly, I don't have time to call any other providers or anything like that, unless they contact me with a problem. You know, I have way too many things to do…"	"I think it would be wonderful to have an open channel of communication with whatever the doctor is seeing, you know."
	"I mean, I'm certainly open to it, if someone has something they feel it's important for me to know. But, the discipline is so very different from Western medicine, that I'm not certain how the information it would provide me would add to what would be familiar enough or make sense to me, to really add anything to what I'm already doing or what I already know."	"We do our chart notes. And I suppose, yeah, just sending chart notes back and forth. […] all doctors who have a full practice are very busy. And so are acupuncturists. […] would the doctor get the chart note or even want the time to review the chart note. I really don't know in a perfect world how it could work. But I'm thinking e-mail with just something really quick, back and forth, might reassure the doctor too. I mean, I'm sure doctors worry. What the heck is going on? I haven't seen this person. And they haven't been back. And what are they doing? You know, that happens for us too. And we always like when people come back and say, oh, I didn't keep coming because I got better, so… But there are people that you don't really know where they stand, you know, how things finished with them or what ended up happening."
	"I think it [feedback from these providers] would be really helpful. I mean, I think that they probably have insight in terms of the pain…you know, the etiology, the non-physical etiology of the pain."	"He [PCP] doesn't know if the patient got better, got worse, who they even went to. I want to use that place again because it seems like they have a pretty good success rate. Doesn't happen."

Given lack of feedback in the referral system, PCPs often did not know whether patients had received or utilized their A/C referrals, where they had gone for treatment, what treatment they received, or what outcomes they experienced. A/C providers on occasion might call a physician or send a note, but this was not systematic. In many cases, A/C providers reached out to PCPs, rather than vice versa. Sometimes those efforts were responded to, and other times not. Some A/C providers were dubious as to the openness or desire of PCPs for communication (see Table 1).

A/C providers expressed openness to providing feedback to PCPs about patient treatment, but were unsure whether such information would be welcomed. Some assumed that physicians were gleaning patient outcomes from direct evaluation of patients and a few encouraged patients to talk to their physicians about positive outcomes. However, patient reports back to PCPs were inconsistent, making many PCPs unaware of outcomes. A/C providers also described how lack of communication of outcomes, particularly positive ones (see Table 3 below about negative bias in outcomes reporting), negatively impacted their ability to demonstrate and advertise their skill and success in treating chronic pain. As one acupuncturist described, more feedback would also ease PCP worries about sending patients out for treatment of which they had no oversight or access.

A number of PCPs indicated that while they might like the system to have more oversight of A/C care, they did not necessarily want, value, or understand the type of treatment feedback from these providers (see Table 1). Coupled with difficulty interpreting A/C notes, time pressures left little time for PCPs to communicate with these providers. Some PCPs also expressed doubt in the veracity of the information, particularly on outcomes, that A/C providers (chiropractors in particular) might claim. In such cases, the patient was the preferred purveyor of treatment information (see below). In rare instances, physicians indicated they would find clinical value in the type of information they might receive from

A/C providers. Almost everyone agreed that more communication would be preferable, even, in the case of PCPs, if the information they received from the other provider was not seen as clinically relevant.

The near consensus from both PCPs and A/C providers was there was no effective communication. This, coupled with the negative bias in the occasional reports from patients (see below Table 4), further eroded PCP confidence in these modalities:

"I've actually had less happiness with chiropractors the longer I've been in practice, just because of what I hear back from patients. [...] part of it is I don't know who I'm referring to. Because it's this sort of contract, people that we contract with. [...] I also don't get notes back from them. So I have no feedback as to what they're doing. Whereas, all the Kaiser physical therapists put a note in [the chart]... And I can review what they've done, and how many times the patient has gone and the progress they've made or not made."

Patient communication with PCP about acupuncture and chiropractic

Given the lack of communication between A/C providers and PCPs, patients are relied upon to ferry information back and forth (see Fig. 1). However, patients varied in the degree to which they discussed their treatments or outcomes with their PCPs. Additionally, in part due to feedback problems in the referral process and access to treatments, PCPs did not have prompts to ask patients about their experience.

As with requesting referral for A/C, patients were often left to initiate discussions about their A/C treatment (see Table 2). While most physicians were not systematic about inquiring about patient experiences, some PCPs asked patients to report back by phone or email after several weeks of A/C. At other times, patients took an active part in ensuring that their PCP was informed

Table 2 Communication between patients and PCPs about A/C treatment

	Patients	PCPs
PCP initiated communication	"I had gone to the doctor and he was amazed [...] He asked me so many questions in regards to acupuncture and what [the acupuncturist had] done"	"I do follow-ups on the telephone within four to six weeks, or have them follow-up in the office"
Patient initiated communication	"I just always think it's very good, especially when you're doing things that are considered complementary or outside their system [...] We have to let [doctors] know what we're doing, what works and what doesn't work."	"There's the outgoing type of patient who's open to anything. [...] they'll go ahead and describe their experience in great detail, for as long as I'm willing to listen."
Little communication	"And I don't volunteer [information]. I mean, I guess I just don't think of it."	"It is probably the minority of people that report consistently." "I can't remember very much in the way of feedback [on acupuncture]."

of their treatment progress and outcomes. Many patients said it was important that their providers know about the treatments they were using and their experiences with them. This was especially true if an aspect of the treatment might interact with their allopathic treatment, or if they wanted the PCP to know that the treatment was effective so that the PCP would be willing to refer again in the future.

Overall, feedback from patients to physicians was spotty and inconsistent. PCPs and patients described several issues that interfere with patient feedback to PCPs about A/C treatment (see Table 3). Physicians especially noted the problem of negative bias in reporting, which can skew their overall impression of the effectiveness of A/C treatment. PCPs said if patients return for another appointment soon after referral, it is often because the treatment was ineffective, or for another purpose and thus the A/C treatment does not come up. Indeed, patients expressed that because of time barriers, they would selectively utilize doctors' office visits to bring up issues of current import. For those with successful reduction in pain, too, it might be months before they are back to see the PCP, and several PCPs noted that this would cause them to question whether time or the treatment had caused the improvement. In addition, because doctors do not receive direct feedback about referrals, unless the patient mentions treatment, there is no prompt to facilitate the PCP inquiries.

Patients described a number of reasons why they might not initiate discussions about their treatment (see Table 3). Many said that the degree to which they discussed their A/C treatment depended, in part, on their physicians' receptivity and understanding of it. Other times, patients did not think the treatment information was relevant to their allopathic doctors. Many noted that

because their PCP had never asked them about it, they never volunteered the information.

Discrepancies between allopathic and CAM explanatory models, transmitted via patients, were described as causing problems for PCPs in particular. Patients would sometimes be sent back to PCPs with new diagnoses or requests for additional investigation that did not always make sense from a biomedical model (see Table 4). Some patients expressed concern about the lack of communication between their PCPs and A/C providers, and articulated desires that there be more communication between them. Barriers to communication between providers placed patients, often uncomfortably, in the middle.

Patients as care managers

While both HMO providers and A/C providers continually pointed to and deferred to PCPs as the responsible party in patient care, it was implicit, and sometimes explicit, that ultimate responsibility for accessing, coordinating, and managing care fell on the patient (see Table 5). This is particularly the case when patients are using allopathic and CAM treatments, and providers both inside and outside the HMO.

As the above discussions illustrate, the lack of feedback and communication results in patients being charged with channeling communications that are using different languages and explanatory models, which are not mutually intelligible. Often CAM providers use the same words as PCPs, but the meaning and intentions behind the words are different. Patients must work very hard to use conventional and CAM therapies. Patients are aware that in order to have their needs met, they have to work the system to access care. As one patient reflected, "I had to be vigilant. And I had to stay on task.

Table 3 Barriers to and challenges for patient-PCP communication

Patients	PCPs
"I guess it just didn't really cross my mind to discuss it with [my PCP]. I guess he never said, well…Probably if he'd said well, [Name], you know, give me a call or come in and discuss it"	"I get no records, and have no chart information, I don't have anything to look at or review, it's not like there's something that's going to trigger me asking it. Because, you know, if they go see the physical therapist there's a note. And I can review the note. And I can see that their last three visits were with the therapist. And so I'm much more likely to say, oh, how did it go with the physical therapist? Whereas with the chiropractor, there's nothing. It's just a big blank."
"I never did [talk to my PCP about seeing an A/C]. [...] I paid for it. They didn't ask. They didn't have any interest in any of that."	
"[Interaction with PCP has changed] In that, when I go to see my primary care physician, I don't tell her anything about if I've had chiropractic or massage therapy or acupuncture, or anything, because her attitude was not one that seemed like it was…would be received well."	"It's like most of medicine, and what we hear about is failures. Okay? If they get better, nobody bothers calling us back. We only get called back if somebody says, oh, I didn't get better. Well, if they're better, they don't come back and I don't know."
"I just figure that I'll talk about things that they [PCPs] will help with. And it's only fifteen minutes. So, I will talk about the other things."	"If they get the referral, I may not see them again for six months, or nine months, or whatever. And so, no, they don't make that feedback loop to me that, yeah, it was great benefit. You know, was it the chiropractic, or was it the time that it had actually gotten better.
"Fifteen minutes is not enough time when you're there for a sore throat or for something else. You can't talk about everything. And I just figure, he really told me he didn't believe in it. So I just go, forget it. You don't need to know, I guess."	Who knows. But, no, I don't normally get short term feedback from patients who have gone to chiropractors."

Table 4 Three-way communication issues: A/C provider to patient to PCP

A/C providers	Patients	PCPs
"I tell the patient, you know, your headaches aren't because of your musculoskeletal system is off or your mechanics is off. Your function is congested. It's because your pain medication has side effects. So let's talk about that. And then give them information that they can take back to their primary, and they can change their meds up."	"Everything is on an electronic record and I'm supposed to get my medical record so I can give it a chiropractor, and then tell my doctor what the chiropractor…It's like going out on this totally different area. When kind of the allure, at least for me with [HMO], is this kind of big, managed plan. But then I'm encouraged to go off on my own to go do something, without any…You know, it's not like a chiropractor can look at my MRI. [Someone agreeing] I'm going to have to request my record, you know. And then is my [HMO] provider really going to trust what this chiropractor, who they don't even know, is going to recommend for my care?"	"Usually what happens is the acupuncturist will tell the patient, this is a weird lump. Get back in to your doctor and have them check it out. And so then they'll just come back in on their own and say, hey, they told me to come back and get this checked out. I rarely see any…There's no back and forth otherwise."
"The patient should always go back to evaluate with their doctors, right? So I would think that the doctor would see the progress, from their patients, their firsthand report. Yeah?" "And, of course, I always tell the patient, especially if they get really good results […] I'll say, you know, your doc needs to hear about this."		"And it annoys me when someone comes back with a wrong diagnosis having to do with their leg or their shoulder. It's completely wrong. And yet they're like, well, the chiropractor…You know, as if the chiropractor is qualified to diagnose that. […] it irritates me."

And I had to find help […] You know, I have a vested interest in taking care of myself." However, not all patients have the knowledge of the system, or the capacities and resources necessary to communicate across it, to hold everything together and access available care.

Discussion

Our analyses of the main players in the CAM health care triad highlight deficiencies of communication between PCPs and A/C providers, with patients being left to manage the information and communication. In line with previous research [16, 17, 28], we found that the two clinicians, PCP and A/C, manage the patient not as a team, but in parallel. They do not have a relationship with one another, so there is no basis for communication and mutual understanding. Indeed, there was very little person-to-person exchange of information from A/C providers to PCPs, and essentially none from PCPs to A/C providers. As a result, there is little learning that takes place for either type of practitioner. As noted above, feedback would be mutually beneficial to PCPs and A/C providers, as it might be able to facilitate referrals to proven, successful providers.

In these respects the issues that are highlighted may be similar to some deficiencies in communication between PCPs and subspecialists [34, 35]. Within the HMO, there are the usual care integration problems, such as practitioners not fully reviewing incoming charts and care being provisioned at different sites. However, in comparison to CAM treatments, allopathic care was discussed by our participants as integrated through the patient medical record and through the housing of providers within HMO facilities. In addition to the HMO providing structure for integration, allopathic care was integrated through documenting treatment in a language based on common assumptions about human physiology and pathology. In the case of CAM, the two clinicians, PCP and CAM provider, may be operating from different paradigms, with different explanatory models, different diagnoses, and different expectations for outcomes (see also [21, 36, 37]), a concern expressed more by the PCPs above than by the A/C providers. In our setting, while the A/C providers were reimbursed by the HMO, their practices were largely outside the HMO network. They maintained separate patient medical records from the PCPs, and could not easily provide patient updates to the patient's HMO medical record. While the A/C providers expressed a desire to share information, the PCPs were skeptical of the potential clinical value of such sharing, even while complaining that they did not know about how their patients were being treated and wanted more information about it.

Table 5 Patients as care coordinators

Patients	Pain clinic providers
"I had to be vigilant. And I had to stay on task. And I had to find help […] You know, I have a vested interest in taking care of myself."	"So when you think about how to integrate the care and how to have it run smoothly, I think that works best if they're a pretty motivated patient. They can communicate across systems."
"I'm taking a more active role. I didn't know, really, what to expect or how to get the train to go the way I wanted it to go, so I kind of let them do the thinking and the planning. And this time, I made it clear from the very first visit that I wanted to look at maintenance."	"So, for the patient who wants to integrate both into one, I think it then falls on the patient to be carrying […] the information from the acupuncturist to their primary care provider. So it falls on the patient to become that coordinator. And I think, for the most part, patients struggle with that, especially if they're already dealing with, you know, lots of different health conditions […] it essentially stays un-integrated, unless the patient actively makes that happen."

The only communication bridge between these parallel worlds is the patient. Often the patient's first task is to raise the issue of A/C treatment in order to obtain a referral, a conversation that may be a difficult one to initiate. Once referred and receiving A/C treatment, all communication between practitioners has to occur via the patient, who attempts to ferry critical information back and forth (for similar examples from breast cancer and gynecology see [38, 39]). This requires that a successful patient be resourceful, savvy, and persistent. On top of that, from the perspective of both allopathic and CAM providers, patients must "do their part" by actively engaging in self-care. Programs such as the pain management group provide training ground for patients to learn about care options and make, apparently, informed decisions about treatment. These groups, along with self care advice given by all providers, educate patients in order to empower them and make them invested and "active" parties to their treatment. It also reinforces the construction of patient as both treatment coordinator and care manager. However the task is far too complex for most patients to have much chance of success when they are not sure what their roles are or the PCP reception of what they have to say, and when they might not share any or all of the information related to their CAM treatment [24, 25, 33, 40, 41].

The current study is limited by several methodological factors. First, the study was conducted within an HMO and many of the communication issues, especially between A/C and allopathic providers, were influenced by particularities of the HMO's structure and processes. This possibly limits the generalizability of our findings. Future research should examine the triad in other managed care or non-managed care settings. Second, we rely on patient and provider self-report. We were unable to observe and document actual interactions between members of the triad. Future research might incorporate an observational component of patient office visits, as well as examine written communications, to study first-hand the communicative exchanges. Third, our community A/C provider sample size was narrow because of pragmatic recruitment considerations. This was not a free-standing qualitative study, but rather embedded as Phase 2 in a larger mixed-methods study of outcomes associated with acupuncture and chiropractic care (see [32] for an overview of all components of the study.) Additional research might broaden the sample to include providers receiving some, but not a lot of referrals from the HMO to see how their experiences differ or are similar to those with high rates of referrals. Finally, in our analyses we considered acupuncturists and chiropractors as a single group of clinicians. We took this approach as representing the vantage point of the managed care network and the primary care physicians who, from the standpoint of policy and clinical integration, may likely view interactions these 2 groups as raising similar categories of issues. Future research might focus on exploring the distinctions between acupuncture and chiropractic clinicians in terms of their relationships with the conventional healthcare providers.

Conclusions
The communication hiatus identified in our research may be viewed as a major contributing factor to the ongoing chronic pain management/chronic opioid therapy conundrum. CAM plays a major role in the management of chronic pain for many patients [6]. Thus the inefficiencies and quality of care deficiencies inherent in such a dysfunctional communication system may be contributing materially to suboptimal outcomes. Improvements in PCP/CAM provider communication could contribute to improved care for individual patients, and improved patient management algorithms with properly coordinated care. How might such improvements in communication be achieved? One important step wherever feasible would be to include progress notes from CAM visits in the electronic medical record, while likewise providing some type of access to the electronic medical record to CAM practitioners (cf. [42, 43]), such as would occur if the health plan included A/C on staff. This would allow for at least some exchange of clinical data. On the other hand, we know that PCPs and subspecialists share the same electronic medical record access, and between those two groups many of the same communication challenges exist. In any case, further research and policy initiatives are needed to delineate mechanisms for improving communication and understanding among the various classes of clinicians caring for patients with chronic pain. Finally, the system does not make explicit to patients their important role in communication between providers. Short of other solutions, it may be reasonable to identify strategies for more clearly empowering patients to step into the void.

Finally, the results of the study may be viewed as strongly arguing for the use of integrative medicine clinicians within established biomedical health system, as a mechanism for providing, and integrating this type of care. However, such a strategy cannot stand alone at this time, because it cannot be fully scaled. That is to say, the number of integrative medicine practitioners is still relatively small, while the volume of acupuncture and chiropractic use is high.

Competing interests
The authors declare that they have no competing interests.

Authors' contributions
CR, LD, CE, JS, and RD participated in the conception and design of the study. LP conducted the qualitative analysis. LP, CR, LD, and CE contributed to the interpretation of the data. LP drafted the main manuscript, and CR, LD, JS, and CE provided substantial supplementary text. All authors (LP, CR, LD, CE, JS, and RD) provided editorial feedback and approved of the final manuscript.

Acknowledgements
The authors gratefully acknowledge that our study received funding support from the National Institutes of Health, National Center for Complementary and Alternative Medicine Grant (R01 AT005896).

Author details
[1]South Texas Veterans Health Care System, 7400 Merton Minter Blvd, San Antonio, TX 78229, USA. [2]The University of Arizona-Department of Family and Community Medicine, 1450 N Cherry Ave, Tucson, AZ 85719, USA. [3]Kaiser Permanente-Center for Health Research, 3800 N. Interstate Avenue, Portland, OR 97227-1098, USA. [4]Oregon Health and Science University-Department of Family Medicine, Oregon Health and Science University, Mail Code FM, 3181 SW Sam Jackson Park Road, Portland, OR 97239, USA.

References
1. Gerdle B, Björk J, Cöster L, Henriksson K, Henriksson C, Bengtsson A. Prevalence of widespread pain and associations with work status: a population study. BMC Musculoskelet Disord. 2008;9:102.
2. Goldenberg DL, Burckhardt C, Crofford L. Management of fibromyalgia syndrome. JAMA. 2004;292:2388–95.
3. Maetzel A, Li L. The economic burden of low back pain: a review of studies published between 1996 and 2001. Best Pract Res Clin Rheumatol. 2002;16:23–30.
4. Manek NJ, MacGregor AJ. Epidemiology of back disorders: prevalence, risk factors, and prognosis. Curr Opin Rheumatol. 2005;17:134–40.
5. Kaiser Permanente Northwest Clinical Practice Guidelines. Low back problems and lumbar radiculopathy. An Evidence-Based Clinical Practice Guideline. 2004.
6. Barnes PM, Bloom B, Nahin RL. Complementary and alternative medicine use among adults and children: United States, 2007. Hyattsville: National Health Statistics Reports; No 12; 2008.
7. Berman BM, Singh BB, Hartnoll SM, Singh BK, Reilly D. Primary care physicians and complementary-alternative medicine: training, attitudes, and practice patterns. J Am Board Fam Pract. 1998;11:272–81.
8. Levine SM, Weber-Levine ML, Mayberry RM. Complementary and alternative medical practices: training, experience, and attitudes of a primary care medical school faculty. J Am Board Fam Pract. 2003;16:318–26.
9. Cherkin DC, Deyo RA, Battié M, Street J, Barlow W. A comparison of physical therapy, chiropractic manipulation, and provision of an educational booklet for the treatment of patients with low back pain. N Engl J Med. 1998;339:1021–9.
10. Cherkin DC, Sherman KJ, Avins AL, Erro JH, Ichikawa L, Barlow WE, et al. A randomized trial comparing acupuncture, simulated acupuncture, and usual care for chronic low back pain. Arch Intern Med. 2009;169:858–66.
11. Hurwitz EL, Morgenstern H, Harber P, Kominski GF, Yu F, Adams AH. A randomized trial of chiropractic manipulation and mobilization for patients with neck pain: clinical outcomes from the UCLA neck-pain study. Am J Public Health. 2002;92:1634–41.
12. Sherman KJ, Cherkin DC, Ichikawa L, Avins AL, Barlow WE, Khalsa PS, et al. Characteristics of patients with chronic back pain who benefit from acupuncture. BMC Musculoskelet Disord. 2009;10:114.
13. Bodenheimer T. Coordinating care–a perilous journey through the health care system. N Engl J Med. 2008;358:1064–71.
14. Pelletier KR, Astin JA. Integration and reimbursement of complementary and alternative medicine by managed care and insurance providers: 2000 update and cohort analysis. Altern Ther Health Med. 2002;8:38–9. 42, 44 passim.
15. Chen PW. Doctor and patient - when the patient can't afford the care. The New York Times Well Blog 2010. http://well.blogs.nytimes.com/2010/02/04/when-patients-cant-afford-their-care/?_r=0.
16. Cherkin DC, Deyo RA, Sherman KJ, Hart LG, Street JH, Hrbek A, et al. Characteristics of visits to licensed acupuncturists, chiropractors, massage therapists, and naturopathic physicians. J Am Board Fam Med. 2002;15:463–72.
17. Weigel PAM, Hockenberry JM, Bentler SE, Kaskie B, Wolinsky FD. Chiropractic episodes and the co-occurrence of chiropractic and health services use among older Medicare beneficiaries. J Manipulative Physiol Ther. 2012;35:168–75.
18. Elder NC, Gillcrist A, Minz R. Use of alternative health care by family practice patients. Arch Fam Med. 2009;6:181–4.
19. Emmerton L, Fejzic J, Tett SE. Consumers' experiences and values in conventional and alternative medicine paradigms: a problem detection study (PDS). BMC Complement Altern Med. 2012;12:39.
20. Jong MC, van de Vijver L, Busch M, Fritsma J, Seldenrijk R. Integration of complementary and alternative medicine in primary care: what do patients want? Patient Educ Couns. 2012;89:417–22.
21. Breen A, Carrington M, Collier R, Vogel S. Communication between general and manipulative practitioners: a survey. Complement Ther Med. 2000;8:8–14.
22. Casey M, Adams J, Sibbritt D. An examination of the clinical practices and perceptions of professional herbalists providing patient care concurrently with conventional medical practice in Australia. Complement Ther Med. 2008;16:228–32.
23. Chao MT, Handley MA, Quan J, Sarkar U, Ratanawongsa N, Schillinger D. Disclosure of complementary health approaches among low income and racially diverse safety net patients with diabetes. Patient Educ Couns. 2015. doi:10.1016/j.pec.2015.06.011.
24. Koenig CJ, Ho EY, Yadegar V, Tarn DM. Negotiating complementary and alternative medicine use in primary care visits with older patients. Patient Educ Couns. 2012;89:368–73.
25. Shelley BM, Sussman AL, Williams RL, Segal AR, Crabtree BF. 'They don't ask me so I don't tell them': patient-clinician communication about traditional, complementary, and alternative medicine. Ann Fam Med. 2003;7:139–47.
26. Allareddy V, Greene BR, Smith M, Haas M, Liao J. Facilitators and barriers to improving interprofessional referral relationships between primary care physicians and chiropractors. J Ambul Care Manage. 2007;30:347–54.
27. Ben-Arye E, Scharf M, Frenkel M. How should complementary practitioners and physicians communicate? A cross-sectional study from Israel. J Am Board Fam Med. 2007;20:565–71.
28. Mainous AG, Gill JM, Zoller JS, Wolman MG. Fragmentation of patient care between chiropractors and family physicians. Arch Fam Med. 2000;9:446–50.
29. Schiff E, Frenkel M, Shilo M, Levy M, Schachter L, Freifeld Y, et al. Bridging the physician and CAM practitioner communication gap: suggested framework for communication between physicians and CAM practitioners based on a cross professional survey from Israel. Patient Educ Couns. 2011;85:188–93.
30. Ben-Arye E, Frenkel M, Klein A, Scharf M. Attitudes toward integration of complementary and alternative medicine in primary care: perspectives of patients, physicians and complementary practitioners. Patient Educ Couns. 2008;70(3):395–402.
31. Mior S, Barnsley J, Boon H, Ashbury FD, Haig R. Designing a framework for the delivery of collaborative musculoskeletal care involving chiropractors and physicians in community-based primary care. J Interprof Care. 2010;24:678–89.
32. DeBar LL, Elder C, Ritenbaugh C, Aickin M, Deyo R, Meenan R, et al. Acupuncture and chiropractic care for chronic pain in an integrated health plan: a mixed methods study. BMC Complement Altern Med. 2011;11:118.
33. Elder C, DeBar LL, Ritenbaugh C, Vollmer W, Deyo RA, Dickerson J, et al. Acupuncture and chiropractic care: utilization and electronic medical record capture. Am J Manag Care. 2015;21:e414–21.
34. Durbin J, Barnsley J, Finlayson J, Jaakkimainen B, Lin L, Berta E, et al. Quality of communication between primary health care and mental health care: an examination of referral and discharge letters. J Behav Health Serv Res. 2012;39:445–61.
35. Garåsen H, Johnsen R. The quality of communication about older patients between hospital physicians and general practitioners: a panel study assessment. BMC Health Serv Res. 2007;7:133.
36. Caspi O, Bell IR, Rychener D, Gaudet TW, Weil AT. The tower of Babel: communication and medicine. Arch Intern Med. 2000;160:3193–5.
37. Konefal J. The challenge of educating physicians about complementary and alternative medicine. Acad Med. 2002;77:847–50.
38. Adler SR, Wrubel J, Hughes E, Beinfield H. Patients' interactions with physicians and complementary and alternative medicine practitioners: older women with breast cancer and self-managed health care. Integr Cancer Ther. 2009;8:63–70.

39. Chez RA, Jonas WB. The challenge of complementary and alternative medicine. Am J Obstet Gynecol. 1997;177:1156–61.
40. Rao JK, Mihaliak K, Kroenke K, Bradley J, Tierney WM, Weinberger M. Use of complementary therapies for arthritis among patients of rheumatologists. Ann Intern Med. 1999;131:409–16.
41. Verhoef MJ, Scott CM, Hilsden RL. A multimethod research study on the use of complementary therapies among patients with inflammatory bowel disease. Altern Ther Health Med. 1998;4:68–72.
42. Keshet Y, Ben-Arye E, Schiff E. The use of boundary objects to enhance interprofessional collaboration: integrating complementary medicine in a hospital setting. Sociol Health Illn. 2013;35:666–81.
43. Maizes V, Rakel D, Niemiec C. Integrative medicine and patient-centered care. Explor J Sci Heal. 2009;5:277–89.

2

Comparison of the placebo effect between different non-penetrating acupuncture devices and real acupuncture in healthy subjects

Leonardo Yung dos Santos Maciel[1], Paula Michele dos Santos Leite[1], Mauricio Lima Poderoso Neto[1], Andreza Carvalho Rabelo Mendonça[1], Carla Carolina Alves de Araujo[2], Jersica da Hora Santos Souza[2] and Josimari Melo DeSantana[3]*

Abstract

Background: Several studies have used placebo acupuncture methods in recent years as a way for blinding therapeutic effect of acupuncture, however placebo method selection has not followed enough methodological criteria to the point of stabilishing a consensus of what should be the best method to be used. This study aimed to evaluate the effectiveness of three different placebo acupuncture methods for blinding applied in healthy subjects.

Methods: This study was approved by the Ethics Committee of the Federal University of Sergipe with the number 47193015.5.0000.5546 and all individuals participating in the study signed a free and informed consent. For this study, 321 healthy volunteers were randomly divided into seven groups using the abdominal point stomach (ST) 25 and seven groups using the lumbar point bladder (Bl) 52 for stimulation. For real acupuncture procedure, three different methods of placebo acupuncture plus a mix between real acupuncture and placebo applied in the same individual, totaling fourteen groups in this study. Outcome assessments were performed before and immediately after applying the technique. Investigator who assessed variables had no knowledgement about the method was applied. Identification, weight and height were measured before puncture by using. At the end, subjects were asked if they believed they were receiving real or placebo acupuncture.

Results: There was no significant difference between groups for the perception about the type o stimulation (wheter real or placebo puncture). Percentage of subjects who reported to have received real acupuncture in the abdominal point was 69.56% in real group, 86.95% in group Park Sham, 82.60% in needle + foam, 91.30% in insertion and removal, 78.26% in real + Park Sham, 86.36% in real + needle and foam, 86.95% in real + insertion and removal, and for the lumbar point was 86.36% in real group, 86.95% in group Park Sham, 69.56% in needle + foam, 72% in insertion and removal, 86.95% in real + Park Sham, 81.81% in real + needle and foam and 78.26% in real + insertion and removal.

Conclusion: All placebo acupuncture methods proposed in this study were equally effective for bliding the study participants using either abdominal or lumbar acupoints, and none of the placebo methods presented benefit compared to the other to be used in future clinical trials.

(Continued on next page)

* Correspondence: desantana@pq.cnpq.br
[3]Professor of the Department of Physical Therapy and Post Graduate Programs in Health Sciences and Physiological Sciences, Federal University of Sergipe, Rua Cláudio Batista, s/n. Bairro Santo Antônio, CEP 49060-100 Aracaju, Sergipe, Brasil
Full list of author information is available at the end of the article

(Continued from previous page)

Ethics Committee: Federal University of Sergipe (UFS), number of approval: 47193015.5.0000.5546

Trial registration: ensaiosclinicos.gov.br RBR-3w2p32 Registered in 28th January 2016.

Keywords: Acupuncture, Placebo, Acupuncture Points, Healthy Volunteers

Background

In the last decades, acupuncture treatment became popular in the Western world because of its therapeutic effects. However, studies have reported conflicting results when using a control group in research to test the true effectiveness of real acupuncture [1]. Some studies have consistently shown that both real and placebo acupuncture had advantages over untreated control groups [2, 3], while some studies have suggested that real acupuncture is more effective than placebo [4–6]; others have failed to show benefits of real acupuncture over placebo one [7–10].

Although the reasons for such contradictory results are not fully clarified, they call attention to a further investigation about placebo-controlled groups in researches in acupuncture field [1, 11, 12]. Randomized clinical trials double blinded serve as gold standard when comparing the effects of an active against placebo-controlled group. [13]. In clinical trials with acupuncture or any other type of device or drug, the ideal is that the control device used is physiologically inert and indistinguishable from real treatment to not produce therapeutic effects and to provide comparison with real treatment group [1].

Clinical trials that incorporate these controls by using placebo gained notoriety because they tried to follow the concept of control as ideal in literature. Patients must not detect the type of treatment they are receiving [14, 15]. In some cases, the investigator who applies acupuncture also has no knowledgement if the application was real or placebo [16].

The lack of a consensus led to the development and use of various placebo acupuncture devices used in the scientific setting, such as the Streitberger device [17], Park Sham device [16], devices using adhesive foam on the skin to prevent the needle penetration into the skin [1, 18, 19], application with toothpick [20, 21] or pressure at the point only with the guide tube [22]. Some authors develop their own placebo acupuncture strategies, but these are not always visually similar to real acupuncture, which does not allow the application in visible regions of patients [1].

To minimize this gap in the literature, this study selected three distinct placebo acupuncture techniques widely used in clinical trials such as 1) Park sham device, 2) insertion and removal of the needle and 3) needle and foam. Only the Park Sham can be used as a double blinded. Our study aimed to investigate whether the placebo acupuncture techniques are indistinguishable from each other and also to the real acupuncture. Moreover one wanted to identify which placebo device is more effective for bliding the subjects when applied to both abdominal and lumbar points.

Methods

Type of Study

This is a randomized, double-blinded, placebo-controlled clinical trial. Random distribution was performed by using sequentially numbered, opaque and sealed envelopes, containing numbers from 1 to 14, corresponding to 14 study groups. Randomization was blocked in a proportion of 1:1, in order to assure proportionality of the number of subjects allocated in 14 groups.

Two types of investigators participated in the study: investigator 1 and investigator 2. Investigator 1 was responsible for the evaluation of subjects and measurement of all variables, before and after treatment. Investigator 2 held the administration of treatment, applying the technique of acupuncture. Investigator 1 didn't know which treatment patient was receiving. This procedure ensured that the study was double-blinded, since the subjects evaluated were instructed to not look at the needles during the procedure and only investigator 2 had knowledgement of the technique used.

Sample

Only healthy subjects with no pain or discomfort in the region selected for the puncture, aging 18 years or more who have never received treatment by acupuncture were recruited to this study.

Exclusion criteria included: 1) pregnant or who have recently given birth with birth in the last 3 months; 2) cutaneous lesions in the puncture site; 3) active infectious processes; 4) nerve tissue or disease affecting the region of dermal puncture; 5) inability to understand the instructions or consent to the study; 6) psychiatric disorders; 7) presence of auditory, visual or communication disturbance; or 8) moderate or severe cognitive or psychiatric disorder.

Recruitment of subjects occurred at the buildings of the Federal University of Sergipe, and after acceptation to be included they got through the screening room and were considered fit to participate in the survey, then they were conducted to carry out the initial steps. Only after these measures subjects were taken to the room where the investigator 2 was to indicate in which group the subject would be allocated, and performed the procedure holding the person lying on the stretcher for the same length of time that the accomplished in all groups, to send it back to the room, where all measures were carried out with the investigator 1.

For the calculation of sample size, intensity of discomfort was considered as the main outcome from the pilot study. Assuming standard deviation = 1.7, difference to be detected = 2 (from 0 to 10), significance level = 5%, power test = 95%, obtaining a minimum sample size of 21 subjects in each group.

Ethical Aspects

This study was approved by the Ethics Committee for Research with Humans at the Federal University of Sergipe (UFS), with CAAE number: 47193015.5.0000.5546 and Report number 1275651. Also, it was recorded in the Brazilian Plataform of Clinical Trials, with registration number RBR-3w2p32. All subjects included in the study signed the informed consent form prior to the evaluation.

Study Groups

Subjects were randomly allocated into 14 study groups in accordance with the Table 1 below.

Points selected for this study were BL52 and ST25, with only one of these points investigated in each group and punctures occurred bilaterally in all groups.

Point ST25 is located on the upper abdomen region, 2 cun lateral to the center of umbilicus and BL52 point located in the lumbar region, at the same level as the inferior border of the spinous process of the second lumbar vertebra (L2), 3 cun lateral to the posterior median line [23]. These points were selected because they are part of the meridians widely considered to apply acupuncture in the clinical practice to treat back pain, intestinal and abdominal disorders, in addition to the use in both researches with animal [24, 25] and humans [26–31] (Fig. 1).

In the real acupuncture group, standard procedures were performed by expert acupuncturist, inserting the needle bilaterally to a depth of 10 mm [5] at the point corresponding to the group (BL52 or ST25) that was randomly selected, the needles remained in place for 30 min.

Group Park Sham (PS) used the device developed by Park et al. [16], in which the equipment is very similar to the real needle, but it has a guide tube inside another larger one, which is held together by adhesive perpendicular to the skin. When it is pressed, the smaller guide tube containing the needle inside, slides inside the larger tube; if the needle is conventional, it penetrates the skin, but if it is unconventional (blunt needle), just press the skin without penetrating, we use the second type of needle, because we want to use only the placebo park sham

Table 1 Groups investigated, demographic, anthropometric and distribution of the sample. Values expressed as mean ± standard deviation. Kruskal Wallis, $p = 0.015$

Group	Acupoint	Age (years)	BMI (kg/m^2)	Sex Fem.(%)	Sex Men.(%)	Subject (n)
Real	St25	24,3 ± 8,8	21,7 ± 2,7	78,25	21,75	23
Park Sham	St25	25,3 ± 5,4	23,8 ± 2,1	52,17	47,83	23
Needle + Foam	St25	26,6 ± 7,8	25,8 ± 3,8	52,17	47,83	23
Insertion and Removal	St25	24,7 ± 7,0	22,5 ± 3,5	86,95	13,05	23
Real + Park Sham	St25	28,3 ± 8,8	24,7 ± 4,7	86,95	13,05	23
Real + Needle and foam	St25	24,3 ± 5,5	23,8 ± 4,2	95,45	4,55	22
Real + insertion and remo.	St25	21,6 ± 3,4	22,9 ± 3,7	82,60	17,4	23
Real	Bl52	24,3 ± 7,1	24,1 ± 6,9	81,81	18,19	22
Park Sham	Bl52	25,1 ± 7,7	23,0 ± 3,9	86,95	13,05	23
Needle + foam	Bl52	29,2 ± 8,0	24,0 ± 5,1	69,56	30,44	23
Insertion and Removal	Bl52	24,6 ± 6,5	22,8 ± 5,7	76	24	25
Real + Park Sham	Bl52	30,8 ± 7,6	23,7 ± 3,1	52,17	47,83	23
Real + Needle and foam	Bl52	27,0 ± 8,3	24,2 ± 4,8	77,27	22,73	22
Real + insertion and remo.	Bl52	25,4 ± 6,7	22,7 ± 3,1	78,26	21,74	23
General:		25,8 ± 7,0	23,5 ± 4,1	75,46	24,54	321
P value				$p = 0.015$		

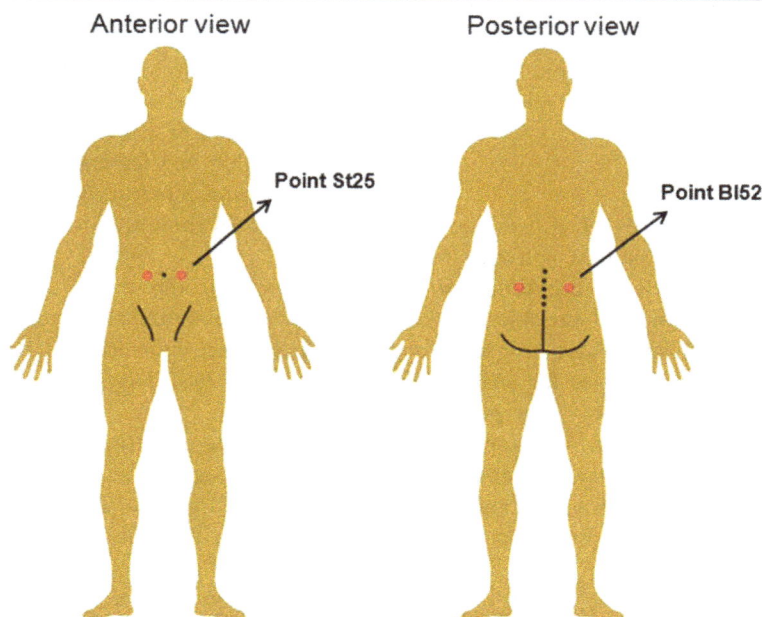

Fig. 1 Acupuncture points: dorsal and ventral. Created by the author

mode. Guide tube stuck by adhesive remained on the local of the puncture for 30 min, holding position similar to real needle after penetrate the skin.

The group Needle + foam used a self adhesive foam adhered to the skin, which was applied in order that the needle penetrated just the foam and not the skin, and then it remained vertically fixed for 30 min. In the group insertion and removal, real needles were used and inserted into acupuncture points, repeating the procedure such as in the real acupuncture group. However, they were removed immediately after insertion. Subjects remained 30 min without the needles inserted and at the end, the acupuncturist simulated the removal of needles with guide tube.

Groups that associated real acupuncture with some placebo techinique (Real + PS, real + Needle and foam, real + insertion and removal) performed the insertion of the real needle in a body side and one of the placebo techiniques on the contralateral side, so the same subjects could experience two procedures in their body, allowing a sensitivity comparison.

All subjects remained 30 min with needles or placebo device, applied by experienced and trained acupuncturist to perform all placebo methods, and the subjects were informed to not look at the local of needles insertion. After the performance of the technique, they all received a sticker where the application was made and were directed to the evaluation room to respond to the questionnaire applied by the researcher 1.

The volunteers were initially told that the aim of this study was to analyze the sensation promoted by different types of puncture, acupuncture techniques and only after participating of all stages of research, they had been told their real purpose. That was done to not influence the response of the questionnaire, which contained the following questions: 1) Was acupuncture a pleasant therapy for you?, 2) Do you felt some discomfort at the time of puncture?, 3) What was the intensity of discomfort on a scale of 0 until 10?, 4) Was the feeling located at the point stimulated?, 5) How long was this feeling?, 6) Do you think that your treatment was real or placebo?, just before the sixth question the researcher explained to volunteer the difference between a placebo and real therapy, after the explanation the subject could answer the question.

Measurement of discomfort caused by cupuncture

The intensity of discomfort caused by puncture was investigated to evaluate the perception of this variable by the research subjects at the moment of puncture. For that, the 11-point numerical scale, ranging from 0 to 10, with zero indicating "no discomfort" and 10 indicating the "worst discomfort imaginable" was used, and the evaluator requested the subject to verbally classify its discomfort in this range [32].

Study Procedures

Initially, a screening of healthy subjects that showed no discomfort in any region chosen for puncture was performed. Subjects who met the inclusion criteria were evaluated individually. In the evaluation sheet, demographic data such as age, height, weight, body mass index (BMI), educational level, marital status, occupation and questions about the use of alcohol, cigarettes and physical activity were recorded. Measurement of discomfort and the questionnaire was done only after the end of technique (Fig. 2).

Statistical analysis

Research data were taken to an Excel data sheet for Windows 2007 and then to the Bioestat software, version 6.1, for the following analyzes: Shapiro-Wilk test to analyze the normality of the numerical variables, which indicated the need of the use of non-parametric tests for all variables. Kruskal Wallis test was used for analysis of body mass index, intensity of discomfort of the puncture and duration of the needling sensation. Post hoc test of Dunn was used for multiple comparisons when necessary. Chi square test was used for analysis of categorical variables. Data value of $p < 0.05$ were considered statistically significant.

Results

Volunteers

Three hundred and fifty subjects were recruited and evaluated to participate in. Of these, eight volunteers were excluded in the initial phase of data collection, because they fit into one or more exclusion criteria, 21 subjects did not appear to the reassessmet stage, and were therefore excluded, totaling 29 exclusions as described in Fig. 3. Thus the survey had 321 participants allocated in the 14 groups whose demographic and anthropometric characteristics are shown in Table 1.

General perception of acupuncture

There was no significant difference in the presence of prick sensation promoted by different placebo methods investigated ($p > 0.05$). The values of this response are presented in absolute frequency in Fig. 4 for all the groups that used the ST25 or BL52 points.

Discomfort at the moment of puncture

Presence of discomfort from the puncture did not differ significantly between study groups ($p > 0.05$), as shown in Fig. 5.

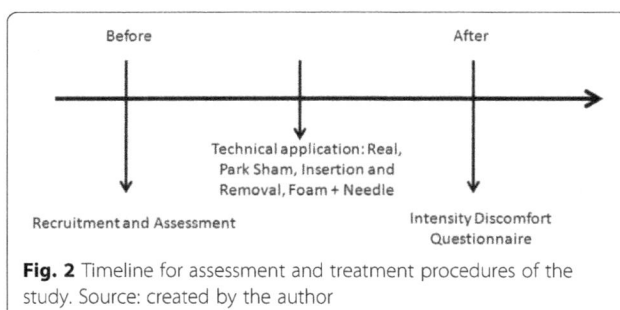

Fig. 2 Timeline for assessment and treatment procedures of the study. Source: created by the author

Location of the feeling of puncture

Comparing the responses of all investigated groups there was no statistically significant difference in this variable.

Figure 6 represents both ST25 and BL52 points for the question posed at the time of reassessment that wondered whether the feeling percived by the volunteer at the moment of puncture was located or not in the stimulated point. Values are presented in absolute frequency.

Intensity of discomfort

There was no significant statistical difference in the intensity of discomfort caused by the puncture between groups ($p = 0.768$) (Fig. 7).

Duration of the puncture sensation

There was a significant higher value for the duration of sensation in Real BL52 point compared with Foam + Needle ST25, Park Sham BL52 and Real + Needle and foam on BL52 groups ($p < 0.05$). Also, real group + insertion and removal on ST25 showed a significant higher needling sensation duration than the Real group + foam and needle in BL52 ($p < 0.05$). The duration of the puncture sensation for ST25 and BL52 groups is shown in Fig. 8.

Placebo vs. Real

There was no significant difference between the groups when the subjects were asked whether they thought they were getting real acupuncture or placebo (Fig. 9 for all the groups).

Discussion

The present study showed that all placebo acupuncture groups had similar results to the group that received real acupuncture for masking the patients, both at the ST25 BL52 points, suggesting that any of these placebo methods can be used in future research to simulate real acupuncture.

With regard to the occurrence of discomfort at the moment of puncture, no difference was found between subjects receiving placebo or real puncture, in both acupoints analyzed. This may not be considered as a key determinant aspect for the choice of placebo method, therefore besides analyzing the presence or absence of discomfort, respondents who reported discomfort were questioned about its intensity, which did not differ between groups.

The location for the needling sensation, also known as "Qi", had its occurrence in puncture point in all groups investigated, and was not diffuse as reported in some studies [1, 33, 34], but when analyzing the duration of this sensation in each subject, the real group BL52 and Real group + insertion and removal ST25, showed a greater sensation period of needling than the others,

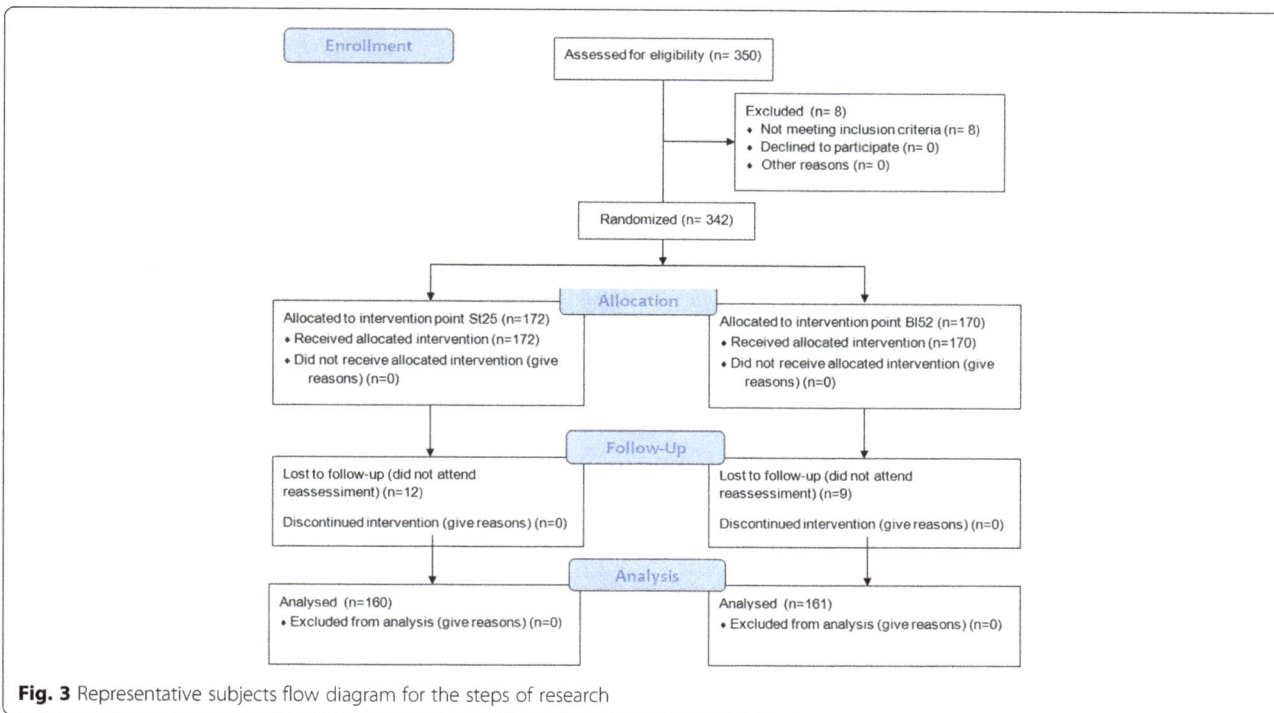

Fig. 3 Representative subjects flow diagram for the steps of research

corroborating with work. Similarly, Junnila [35] observed chronic pain patients also had a needling sensation for longer periods than 2 min.

In contrast, Park Sham BL52 group and Real group + needle and foam BL52 showed shorter duration for the needling sensation, and this sensation is one of the main events in individuals who receive real acupuncture therapy [34]. To our knowledge, this study is the first clinical trial to evaluate the efficacy of masking procedure of three methods of placebo acupuncture versus real acupuncture in healthy subjects.

The coping strategy of pain has an important role regarding to reduce pain intensity. Patient who undergoes to therapy and conveys confidence about its effectiveness, even if the subject feels to having control, or to being part of driving this therapy, it has been shown to be a catalyzing factor that results for pain relief [36], once that this one is one of the main reasons for

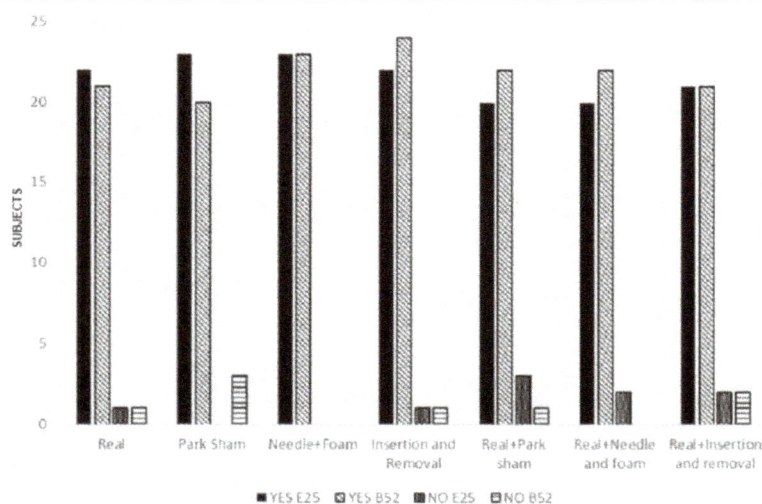

Fig. 4 Presence of puncture sensation at the point ST25 or BL52. Values obtained from a questionnaire applied in the reassessment phase in all study groups. Values were presented as absolute frequency. Chi-Square test ($p = 0.48$)

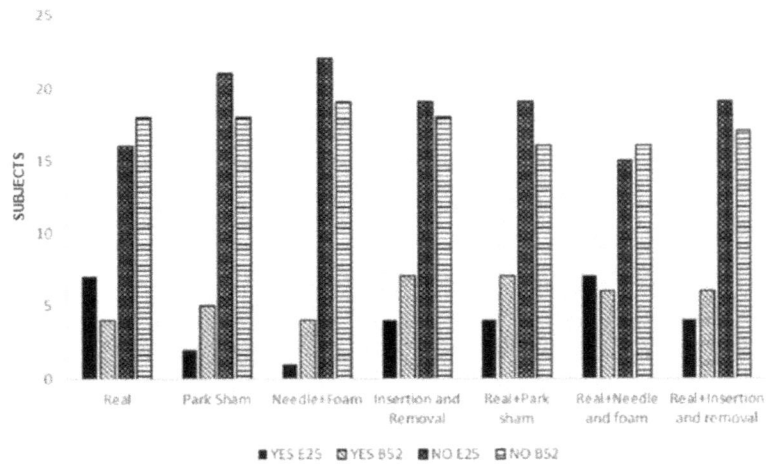

Fig. 5 Presence of discomfort at the time of puncture at points ST25 and BL52. Values obtained from a questionnaire applied in the revaluation phase in all study groups. Values were presented as absolute frequency. Chi-Square Test ($p = 0.5$)

seeking placebo acupuncture techniques that adeuately simulates as much as possible the feeling promoted by real acupuncture.

One of the main challenges faced by non-penetrating placebo acupuncture methods is to simulate the senation usually promoted by the puncture, since some studies reported that this sensation is directly related to the depth of needle penetration [33, 37]. According our findings, since the real group BL52 and real + foam and needle BL52 group, both of them using invasive procedures for stimulation, produced a greater time period for the puncture sensation than in noninvasive technique Park Sham BL52 group, which so the feeling sensation may be a determining factor to the volunteer research believes in the veracity of the technique.

The literature provides a large amount of placebo acupuncture techniques, such as Park Sham device,

developed by Park et al., [16], which aims to serve as a masking to both patient and acupuncturist. In the research setting, for validation purposes, this device was firstly used in healthy subjects and then in patients who had suffered stroke, and, in both cases, the placebo device was not detected as placebo or not penetrating by the volunteers. These data confirm our findings, because the placebo acupuncture devices showed results similar to real acupuncture at both ST25 and BL52 points, when individuals were asked if they believed they had received real placebo treatment. Similar results were also found in other studies with healthy subjects [38–42].

Some placebo acupuncture devices that intended to mask both acupuncturist and patient were not effective to do it as acupuncturists found that it was a fake device, while the volunteers believed it was real acupuncture [43, 44]. Other studies have shown that placebo

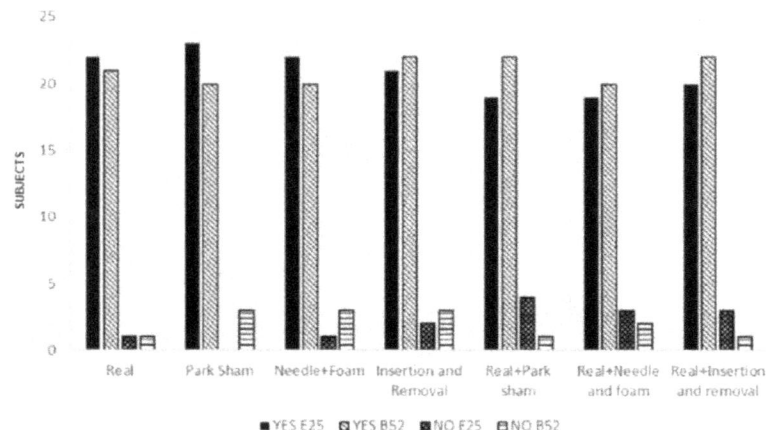

Fig. 6 Sensation in the puncture points ST25 and BL52. Values obtained through a questionnaire applied in the reassessment in all study groups. Values were presented as absolute frequency. Chi-square test ($p = 0.719$)

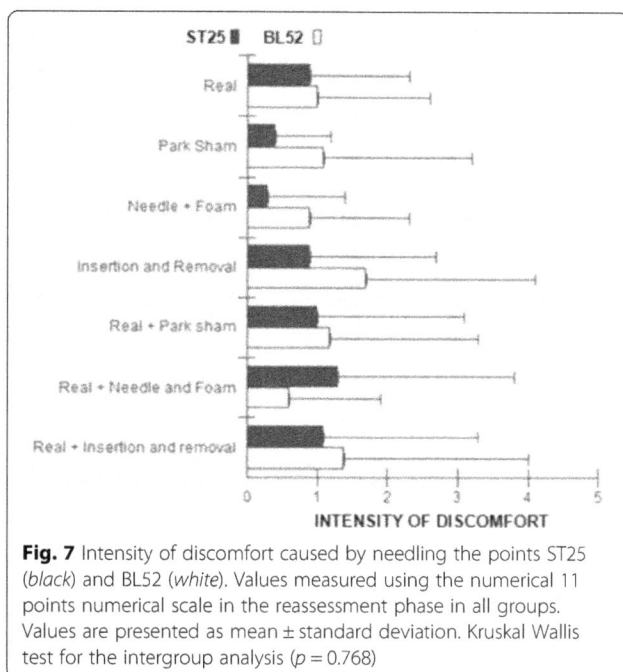

Fig. 7 Intensity of discomfort caused by needling the points ST25 (*black*) and BL52 (*white*). Values measured using the numerical 11 points numerical scale in the reassessment phase in all groups. Values are presented as mean ± standard deviation. Kruskal Wallis test for the intergroup analysis ($p = 0.768$)

acupuncture technique is not effective to mask even the patient [1, 45]. Mechanical changes were measured by using computerized system, and showed that, at the moment of insertion and removal of needles, professional modifies the forces of application and removal when using placebo methods compared to real acupuncture [46], which is always a possibility of perception for the patient who has previous experience with acupuncture,

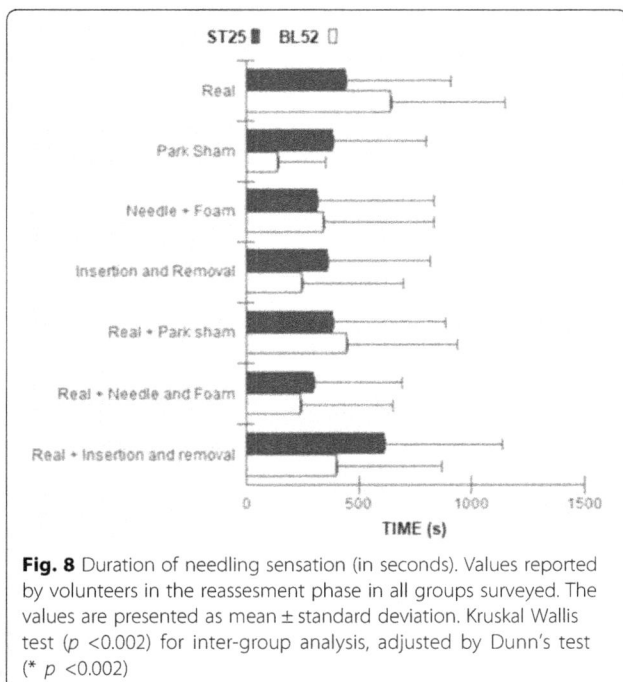

Fig. 8 Duration of needling sensation (in seconds). Values reported by volunteers in the reassessment phase in all groups surveyed. The values are presented as mean ± standard deviation. Kruskal Wallis test ($p < 0.002$) for inter-group analysis, adjusted by Dunn's test (* $p < 0.002$)

to identify the difference on the technique, which was not observed in our study because we measured a high credibility index.

In our study, we had groups that used real acupuncture in a body area and a placebo method in another one in the same subject, in order to simulate the occurrence of individuals who had previous experience with acupuncture. Interestingly, the result for masking the participants was similar to the groups receiving real acupuncture or placebo device. In a study with eight experienced acupuncturists in order to develop a regulation for usig a method of non-invasive sham acupuncture, it became clear that to maintain an appropriate standard is required frequent contact between all professionals who will apply the placebo technique [47].

Studies with real acupuncture and sham acupuncture showed similar therapeutic results to increase muscle strength in the quadriceps [38], treatment of low back pain [8] and for pain relief in knee [48], suggesting that the therapeutic results of this study has a strong relationship with the placebo effect. However, studies in which acupuncture was applied in patients with muscle pain in the upper trapezius [49] or with nonspecific low back pain [21] pointed out that the real acupuncture therapy was more effective than placebo acupuncture for pain relief.

Our findings indicated a low level of discomfort at the moment of puncture in subjects treated with all the methods investigated in both acupuncture points, however, this intensity was not different between groups; this suggests that the intensity of discomfort can not be considered a determining factor for the choice of placebo method to be used in clinical trials investigating the effects of acupuncture. These data corroborate findings by Hübscher et al. [38] that evaluated the effect of acupuncture and placebo group with no intervention in muscle soreness, noting that no difference in the intensity of discomfort was observed in the first 48 h between study groups. Whereas after 72 h, only the acupuncture group showed a significant reduction in the intensity of discomfort.

Subjects were asked if acupuncture was pleasant or not. Most of them in all groups said that acupuncture had been nice and no differences were found between the methods, showing once again that all placebo and real acupuncture techniques were similar to each other for the pleasantness factor, which should be regarded as a decisive factor for the choice of the placebo method to be used in the clinical research setting, whether in the abdominal point ST25 or lumbar point BL52.

Our findings contribute to modern science that seeks to avoid erroneous conclusions in no placebo-controlled studies, which provides differences in results between

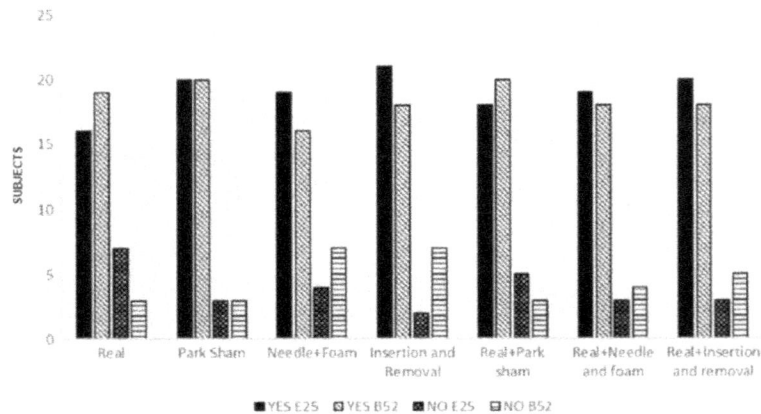

Fig. 9 Response of the subject indicating whether they thought had received real or placebo procedure in point ST25 or BL52. Values obtained through questionnaire applied in the reassessment in all study groups. The values were presented as absolute frequency. Teste Chi-Square ($p = 0.677$)

the groups investigated, regardless of the odds and potential that the belief of healing provides these improvements [50]. A systematic review with 250 random clinical trials demonstrated superior therapeutic effect, around 17%, for the groups that did not use masking in comparison to the groups who performed [51].

Our clinical trial occurred with random distribution and volunteer was unaware about the acupuncture technique that would be received, researchers responsible for the assessment also had no knowledge about allocation, and were trained to conduct the survey question about the subjects' belief if they received placebo or real admnisration of needle, characterizing it as a double-blinded study. Studies that mask the volunteers as the evaluators have fundamental importance, because the person who is aware that a real treatment method was not performed will be less prone to follow the protocol of the test, search for additional treatment and making the data less reliable, as well as blind investigators are less likely to transfer expectations to volunteers ensuring more impartial data [52, 53].

Conclusion
The results allow to state that all the placebo groups were similarly effective to promote appropriate masking of the study subjectsand therefore all of them are reliable alternatives to characterize a placebo-controlled group in the research setting using acupuncture at either abdominal or lumbar points. All groups showed low intensity of sensory discomfort, which was similar between the methods studied. Furthermore, the puncture sensation was reported as located by most individuals in all groups for the ST25 and BL52 points. The groups that

had a higher maintenance puncture sensation time were those stimulated with real acupuncture at acupoint BL52 and real acupuncture + insertion and removal in acupoint ST25. Most individuals of all groups have reported that the acupuncture treatment was a pleasant therapy received.

Acknowledgment
Thanks to those who helped in the recruitment and running of the collection, Emanuelle Lais Santos Passos, Maria Morgana Lima Silva, Carlos Roberto Xavier Santos Filho, Wendell Medeiros Cardoso, Erika Thatyana Nascimento Santana.

Funding
We would like to thank FAPITEC, Sergipe organ which funded our research.

Authors' contributions
LYSM was responsible for study design, collection and analysis of data and writing of the manuscript. PMSL, ACRM, MLPN, CCAA and JHSS They were responsible for study design and data collection. JMD responsible for study design, interpretation of data and manuscript review. All authors participated in the discussion of the results of the study. All authors read and approved the final manuscript.

Competing interests
The authors declare that they have no competing interests.

Declarations
This study is part of an attempt to elucidate and contribute to research on acupuncture, and a second part of this work is being developed to add sham acupuncture devices that could not get to use in this research, in addition to wanting to uncover the possible belief that this receiving real acupuncture treatment can cause superficial or deep sensory changes when compared to the placebo acupuncture group with real acupuncture group.

Author details
[1]Post Graduate Program in Health Sciences, Federal University of Sergipe, Rua Cláudio Batista, s/n, Santo Antônio, 49060-100 Aracaju, SE, Brasil. [2]Department of Physical Therapy, Federal University of Sergipe, Rua Cláudio Batista, s/n. Bairro Santo Antônio, CEP 49060-100 Aracaju, Sergipe, Brasil. [3]Professor of the Department of Physical Therapy and Post Graduate Programs in Health Sciences and Physiological Sciences, Federal University of Sergipe, Rua Cláudio Batista, s/n. Bairro Santo Antônio, CEP 49060-100 Aracaju, Sergipe, Brasil.

Comparison of the placebo effect between different non-penetrating acupuncture devices and real...

21

References

1. Zhu D, Gao Y, Chang J, Kong J. Placebo acupuncture devices: considerations for acupuncture research. Evid Based Complement Alternat Med. 2013. doi:10.1155/2013/628907.
2. Ballegaard S, Muteki T, Harada H, et al. Modulatory effect of acupuncture on the cardiovascular system: a crossover study. Acupuncture and ElectroTherapeutics Research. 1993;18(2):103–15.
3. Coan RM, Wong G, Liang Ku S. The acupuncture treatment of low back pain: a randomized controlled study. American Journal of Chinese Medicine. 1980;8(12):181–9.
4. Berman BM, Lao L, Langenberg P, Lee WL, Gilpin AMK, Hochberg MC. Effectiveness of acupuncture as adjunctive therapy in osteoarthritis of the knee. A randomized, controlled trial. Ann Intern Med. 2004;141(12):901–10.
5. Itoh K, Katsumi Y, Hirota S, Kitakoji H. Effects of trigger point acupuncture on chronic low back pain in elderly patients—a shamcontrolled randomised trial. Acupunct Med. 2006;24(1):5–12.
6. Vickers AJ, Cronin AM, Maschino AC, et al. Acupuncture for chronic pain: individual patient data metaanalysis. Arch Intern Med. 2012;172(19):1444–53.
7. Assefi NP, Sherman KJ, Jacobsen C, Goldberg J, Smith WR, Buchwald D. A randomized clinical trial of acupuncture compared with sham acupuncture in fibromyalgia. Ann Intern Med. 2005;143(1):10–9.
8. Cherkin DC, Sherman KJ, Avins AL, Erro JH, Ichikawa L, Barlow WE, Delaney K, Hawkes R, Hamilton L, Pressman A, Khalsa PS, Deyo RA. A randomized trial comparing acupuncture, simulated acupuncture, and usual care for chronic low back pain. Arch Intern Med. 2009;169(9):85866. doi:10.1001/archinternmed.2009.65.
9. Haake M, Müller H, SchadeBrittinger C, et al. German Acupuncture Trials (GERAC) for chronic low back pain: randomized, multicenter, bl inded, parallelgroup trial with 3 groups. Arch Intern Med. 2007;167(17):1892–8.
10. White AR, Resch KL, Chan JCK, et al. Acupuncture for episodic tensi ontype headache: a multi centre randomized controlled trial. Cephalalgia. 2000; 20(7):632–7.
11. Kaptchuk TJ. Powerful placebo: the dark side of randomised controlled trial. Lancet. 1998;351:1722–5.
12. Sharpe L, Ryan B, Albard S, Sensky T. Testing for the integrity of blinding in clinical trials: how valid are forced choice paradigms? Psychother Psychosom. 2003;72:128–31.
13. Irnich D, Salih N, Offenbacher M, et al. Is sham laser a valid control for acupuncture trials? Evid Based Complement Altern Med. 2011;2011(8):485945.
14. Appleyard I, Lundeberg T, Robinson N. Should systematic reviews assess the risk of bias from sham-placebo acupuncture control procedure? Eur J Integr Med. 2014;6:234–43.
15. Streitberger K, Diefenbacher M, Bauer A, et al. Acupuncture compared to placeboacupuncture for postoperative nausea and vomiting prophylaxis: a randomised placebocontrolled patient and observer blind trial. Anaesthesia. 2004;59(2):142–9.
16. Park J, White A, Stevinson C, Ernst E, James M. Validating a new non¬penetrating sham acupuncture device: two randomised controlled trials. Acupunct Med. 2002;20(4):168–74.
17. Streitberger K, Kleinhenz J. Introducing a placebo needle into acupuncture research. Lancet. 1998;352(9125):364–5.
18. Kreiner M, Zaffaroni A, Alvarez R, Clark G. Validation of a simplified sham acupuncture technique for its use in clinical research: a randomised, single blind, crossover study. Acupunct Med. 2010;28(1):33–6.
19. Tam L, Leung P, Li TK, Zhang L, Li EK. Acupuncture in the treatment of rheumatoid arthritis: a doubleblind controlled pilot study. BMC Complement Altern Med. 2007;7:article 35.
20. Lao L, Bergman S, Hamilton GR, Langenberg P, Berman B. Evaluation of acupuncture for pain control after oral surgery: a placebocontrolled trial. Arch Otolaryngol. 1999;125(5):567–72.
21. Sherman KJ, Hogeboom CJ, Cherkin DC, Deyo RA. Description and validation of a noninvasive placebo acupuncture procedure. J Altern Complement Med. 2002;8(1):11–9.
22. Inoue M, Kitakoji H, Ishizaki N, Tawa M, Yano T, Katsumi Y, Kawakita K. Relief of low back pain immediately after acupuncture treatment–a randomised, placebo controlled trial. Acupunct Med. 2006;24(3):103–8.
23. Lian YL, Chen CY, Hammes M, Kolster BC. Atlas gráfico de acupuntura-Um manual ilustrativo dos pontos de acupuntuta. Marburg: Editora Konemann; 2005.
24. Lai A, Chow DH, Siu WS, et al. Effects of electroacupuncture on a degenerated intervertebral disc using an in-vivo rat-tail model. Proc Inst Mech Eng H. 2008;222(2):241–8.

25. Pontes MC, Heck LC, Coelho JC. Behavioral and biochemical effects of pharmacopuncture (ST 36 and ST 25) in obese rats. BMC Complement Altern Med. 2015;15:297.
26. Hao C, Zhang T, Qi J, Ji L. Acupuncture at Zhibian (BL 54) through Shuidao (ST 28) for polycystic ovary syndrome. Zhongguo Zhen Jiu. 2015;35(5):461–4.
27. Liu J, Zhou W, Lv H, Feng Y, Yu X, Fu X, He Y, Zhao JP. Law of the meridian abnormality based on the effectiveness of electroacupuncture for severe functional constipation. Zhongguo Zhen Jiu. 2015;35(8):785–90.
28. Ma Y, Li X, Li F, Yu W, Wang Z. Clinical research of chronic pelvic cavity pain syndrome treated with acupoint catgut embedding therapy. Zhongguo Zhen Jiu. 2015;35(6):561–6.
29. Molsberger AF, Zhou J, Arndt D, Teske W. Chinese acupuncture for chronic low back pain: an international expert survey. J Altern Complement Med. 2008;14(9):1089–95.
30. Ren Z, Wu QM, Li DD, Liu WA, Li XR, Lin XM. Post-stroke constipation treated with acupuncture therapy of regulating qi circulation of fu-organ. Zhongguo Zhen Jiu. 2013;33(10):893–6.
31. Xue QM, Pan H, Huang L, Li N. Effects of acupuncture at ST25 on inflammatory mediators and nuclear factor κB activation in a rat model of severe acute pancreatitis. Acupunct Med. 2015;33(4):299–304. doi:10.1136/acupmed-2014-010609.
32. Corrêa JB, Costa LOP, DeOliveira NTB, A Sluka KA, Liebano RE. Effects of the carrier frequency of interferential current on pain modulation in patients with chronic nonspecific low back pain: a protocol of a randomised controlled trial. BMC Musculoskelet Disord. 2013;14:195.
33. Choi YJ, Lee JE, Moon WK, Cho SH. Does the effect of acupuncture depend on needling sensation and manipulation? Complement Ther Med. 2013; 21(3):207–14. doi:10.1016/j.ctim.2012.12.009.
34. Itoh K, Minakawa Y, Kitakoji H. Effect of acupuncture depth on muscle pain. Chin Med. 2011;6(1):24. doi:10.1186/1749-8546-6-24.
35. Junnila SY. Long-term treatment of chronic pain with acupuncture. Acupunct Electrother Res. 1987;12:23–36.
36. Lee J, Napadow V, Park K. Pain and sensory detection threshold response to acupuncture is modulated by coping strategy and acupuncture sensation. BMC Complement Altern Med. 2014;14:324. doi:10.1186/1472-6882-14-324.
37. Lin JG, Chou PC, Chu HY. An Exploration of the Needling Depth in Acupuncture: The Safe Needling Depth and the Needling Depth of Clinical Efficacy. Evid Based Complement Altern Med. 2013;2013:740508. doi:10.1155/2013/740508.
38. Hübscher M, Vogt L, Bernhörster M, Rosenhagen A, Banzer W. Effects of acupuncture on symptoms and muscle function in delayed-onset muscle soreness. J Altern Complement Med. 2008;14(8):1011–6. doi:10.1089/acm.2008.0173.
39. Kim S, Lee S, Choi S, Park J, Kim S. Discrimination accuracy between real and sham press needles in the hands. Acupunct Med. 2015;33(4):2938. doi:10.1136/acupmed2014010678.
40. Lee H, Bang H, Kim Y, Park J, Lee S, Lee H, Park HJ. Nonpenetrating sham needle, is it an adequate sham control in acupuncture research? Complement Ther Med. 2011;19 Suppl 1:S418. doi:10.1016/j.ctim.2010.12.002.
41. Liu B, Xu H, Ma R, Mo Q, Yan S, Liu Z. Effect of blinding with a new pragmatic placebo needle: a randomized controlled crossover study. Medicine (Baltimore). 2014;93(27):e200. doi:10.1097/MD.0000000000000200.
42. Tough EA, White AR, Richards SH, Lord B, Campbell JL. Developing and validating a sham acupuncture needle. Acupunct Med. 2009;27(3):11822. doi:10.1136/aim.2009.000737.
43. To M, Alexander C. The effects of Park sham needles: a pilot study. J Integr Med. 2015;13(1):204. doi:10.1016/S20954964(15)601534.
44. Vase L, Baram S, Takakura N, Takayama M, Yajima H, Kawase A, Schuster L, Kaptchuk TJ, Schou S, Jensen TS, Zachariae R, Svensson P. Can acupuncture treatment be doubleblinded? An evaluation of doubleblind acupuncture treatment of postoperative pain. PLoS One. 2015;10(3):e0119612. doi:10.1371/journal.pone.0119612. eCollection 2015.
45. Tsukayama H, Yamashita H, Kimura T, Otsuki K. Factors that influence the applicability of sham needle in acupuncture trials: two randomized, singleblind, crossover trials with acupunctureexperienced subjects. Clin J Pain. 2006;22(4):3469.
46. Chae Y, Um SI, Yi SH, Lee H, Chang DS, Yin CS, Park HJ. Comparison of biomechanical properties between acupuncture and nonpenetrating sham needle. Complement Ther Med. 2011;19 Suppl 1:S8S12. doi:10.1016/j.ctim.2010.09.002. Epub 2010 Oct 14.

47. McManus CA, Kaptchuk TJ, Schnyer RN, Goldman R, Kerr CE, Nguyen LT, Stason WB. Experiences of acupuncturists in a placebocontrolled, randomized clinical trial. J Altern Complement Med. 2007;13(5):5338.

48. White P, Lewith G, Hopwood V, Prescott P. The placebo needle, is it a valid and convincing placebo for use in acupuncture trials? A randomised, single-blind, cross-over pilot trial. Pain. 2003;106(3):401–9.

49. Couto C, de Souza IC, Torres IL, Fregni F, Caumo W. Paraspinal stimulation combined with trigger point needling and Needle rotation for the treatment of myofascial pain: a randomized shamcontrolled clinical trial. Clin J Pain. 2014;30(3):21423. doi:10.1097/AJP.0b013e3182934b8d.

50. Karanicolas PJ, Farrokhyar F, Bhandari M. Blinding:Who, what, when, why, how? Can J Surg. 2010;53:6–16.

51. Schulz KF, Chalmers I, Hayes RJ, et al. Empirical evidence of bias. Dimensions of methodological quality associated with estimates of treatment effects in controlled trials. JAMA. 1995;273:408–12.

52. Balk EM, Bonis PA, Moskowitz H, et al. Correlation of quality measures with estimates of treatment effect in meta-analyses of randomized controlled trials. JAMA. 2002;287:2973–82.

53. Schulz KF, Grimes DA. Blinding in randomised trials: hiding who got what. Lancet. 2002;359:696–700.

3

Eye exercises of acupoints: their impact on myopia and visual symptoms in Chinese rural children

Zhong Lin[1], Balamurali Vasudevan[2], Su Jie Fang[3], Vishal Jhanji[5], Guang Yun Mao[1,4], Wei Han[3], Tie Ying Gao[3], Kenneth J. Ciuffreda[6] and Yuan Bo Liang[1*]

Abstract

Background: Chinese traditional "eye exercises of acupoints" have been advocated as a compulsory measure to reduce visual symptoms, as well as to retard the development of refractive error, among Chinese students for decades. The exercises are comprised of a 5-min, bilateral eye acupoint self-massage. This study evaluated the possible effect of these eye exercises among Chinese rural students.

Methods: Eight hundred thirty-six students (437 males, 52.3 %), aged 10.6 ± 2.5 (range 6–17) years from the Handan Offspring Myopia Study (HOMS) who completed the eye exercises and vision questionnaire, the convergence insufficiency symptom survey (CISS) questionnaire, and had a cycloplegic refraction were included in this study.

Results: 121 (14.5 %) students (64 males, 52.9 %) performed the eye exercises of acupoints in school. The multiple odds ratio (OR) and 95 % confidence interval (CI) for those having a "serious attitude" towards performing the eye exercises (0.12, 0.03–0.49) demonstrated a protective effect for myopia, after adjusting for the children's age, gender, average parental refractive error, and the time spent on near work and outdoor activity. The more frequently, and the more seriously, the students performed the eye exercises each week, the less likely was their chance of being myopic (OR, 95 % CI: 0.17, 0.03–0.99), after adjusting for the same confounders. However, neither the "seriousness of attitude" of performing the eye exercises (multiple β coefficients: -1.58, $p = 0.23$), nor other related aspects of these eye exercises, were found to be associated with the CISS score in this sample.

Conclusions: The traditional eye exercises of acupoints appeared to have a modest protective effect on myopia among these Chinese rural students aged 6–17 years. However, no association between the eye exercises and near vision symptoms was found.

Keywords: Eye exercises, Acupoints, Myopia, Near vision symptoms, CISS

Abbreviations: BMPS, The Beijing Myopia Progression Study; CI, Confidence interval; CISS, Convergence insufficiency symptom survey; HES, The Handan Eye Study; HOMS, The Handan Offspring Myopia Study; OR, Odds ratio

Background

The traditional Chinese "eye exercises of acupoints" have been a compulsory measure performed by school children twice a day (5 min each morning and afternoon) for the purpose of relieving visual symptoms and reduction of myopia since the early 1960s. As

* Correspondence: yuanboliang@126.com
[1]The Eye Hospital, School of Ophthalmology and Optometry, Wenzhou Medical University, No. 270 West College Road, Wenzhou, Zhejiang 325027, China
Full list of author information is available at the end of the article

described in detail previously in the Beijing Myopia Progression Study (BMPS), [1] they comprise bilateral acupoint self-massage that includes: (1) knead Tianying (Ashi) point, (2) press and squeeze Jingming (BL1), (3) press and knead Sibai (ST2), and (4) press Taiyang (EX-HN5) and scrape Cuanzhu (BL2), Yuyao (EX-HN4), Sizhukong (TE23), Tongziliao (GB1), Chengqi (ST1). Despite insisting on performing this intervention for overhalfa century, the prevalence of myopia and myopia-related visual impairment is on the rise in both urban and rural Chinese children [2–4]. Our previous study from BMPS found that the urban students who performed the eye exercises seriously, followed the instruction when performing the eye exercises, and were acquainted with these eye exercises, tended to have a lower convergence insufficiency symptom survey (CISS) score, e.g., less ocular-based, near fatigue symptoms [1]. However, the exercises appeared to have no measurable effect on the refractive error [1]. This could be related to the greater myopic refraction and apparent myopigenic environment among the urban students [1]. Hence, it would be interesting to determine if these eye exercises have an effect on myopia reduction in a parallel rural population with its less myopigenic environment.

The Handan Offspring Myopia Study (HOMS) was designed to determine the prevalence of myopia among rural children, namely the offspring of the Handan Eye Study (HES) population [5, 6]. It is noteworthy that the children from HOMS were in a similar age range (6–17 years), and had several vision examinations (e.g., visual acuity, ocular biometry, cycloplegic autorefraction) and questionnaires in common with the BMPS [6, 7]. Hence, the present study aimed to evaluate the impact of the eye exercises of acupoints among Chinese *rural* students, and furthermore to compare them to Chinese *urban* students.

Methods
Subjects
Details of the study design, sample size estimation, and baseline characteristics of HOMS were reported elsewhere [6]. Briefly, between October 2006 and October 2007, a population-based eye study in adults aged 30 years and older in Handan (Handan Eye Study, HES), Hebei province of North China, was conducted [5]. All participants (aged 6–17 years) along with at least one of their parents recruited in HES were included in HOMS between March 2010 and June 2010. Adopted children or children who had moved outside the county at least 6 months prior to this study were excluded. Finally, 878 (70.2 %) of 1238 were recruited [6]. The study followed the tenets of the Declaration of Helsinki, and it was approved by the Ethics Committee of the Handan Eye Hospital. Written, informed-consent was obtained from the children's parents/guardians. In the current study, 836 students who had completed the eye exercises of acupoints questionnaire, the standard CISS questionnaire, and had a cycloplegic refraction were included. Of these, 121 (14.5 %) performed the eye exercises of acupoints in school.

Activity questionnaire
The activity questionnaire used in the Sydney Myopia Study was translated into Chinese with minor modifications [8, 9]. This questionnaire included components such as duration of near and far work, living environment, eating habits, and general health. These activities were grouped into near work and outdoor activities. Details of the activity questionnaire were reported elsewhere [9, 10].

Eye exercises of acupoints questionnaire
The eye exercises of acupoints were performed twice a day (morning and afternoon), each time for 5 continuous minutes in each school day. The participants were also asked to complete an acupoints eye exercise questionnaire. It consisted of 11 items related to motivation, frequency, and attitude towards the eye exercises of acupoints. Details of the eye exercises of acupoints were reported elsewhere [1] (Additional file 1).

Convergence insufficiency symptom survey (CISS)
The CISS consists of 15 items with 5 response categories for each item [11]. It is scored as never (0), infrequently (1), sometimes (2), fairly often (3), and always (4). It covered reading and other near work activities. The total score is obtained as a sum of scores for all 15 items (range from 0 to 60) (Additional file 2).

Refractive error
All students received a cycloplegic autorefraction (*KR8800, Topcon, Tokyo, Japan*), whereas the parents received non-cycloplegic autorefraction due to their age and related reduced accommodation. Cycloplegic autorefraction was performed 20 min after instilling 3 drops of cyclopentolate 1 % (Cyclogyl, Alcon; Fort Worth, TX, USA). Three readings of refractive error were obtained and averaged for further analysis for each eye in all participants.

Data analysis
Due to the high correlation of the cycloplegic refractive error (spherical equivalent, SE = Spherical refraction + ½ cylindrical refraction) between the right and left eyes (Pearson correlation coefficient 0.96, $p < 0.001$), only the SE of the right eye of each student was used in the analysis. Myopia was defined as SE ≤ -0.50D [1, 7]. Parental refractive error was defined as the average of the non-cycloplegic SE of each eye of the father and mother combined.

Both univariate and multiple (after adjusting for putative risk factors for myopia, e.g., children's age, gender, average parental refractive error, time spent on near work and outdoor activity) odds ratio (OR) and the 95 % confidence interval (CI) for myopia for different items of the eye exercises of acupoints question were calculated using generalized linear models (GLMs). Univariate and multiple (adjusting for the same confounding factors) regression analyses were performed for the CISS score with the different items of the eye exercises of acupoints using GLMs.

Results

A total of 836 students (437 males, 52.3 %) with a completed acupoints eye exercise questionnaire, completed convergence insufficiency symptom survey questionnaire (CISS), and a cycloplegic refraction were included in the current analysis. Of these, 121 (14.5 %) students (64 males, 52.9 %) performed the eye exercises of acupoints in school (Table 1). Students who performed the eye exercise in school were older (11.8 ± 2.3 years vs. 10.3 ± 2.4 years, $p < 0.001$), more myopic (-0.40 ± 1.62 D vs. 0.06 ± 1.31 D, $p = 0.004$), and had a higher CISS score (14.3 ± 6.4 vs. 10.7 ± 6.8, $p < 0.001$) compared to those who did not.

Table 2 summarizes the distribution of students' responses against each item of the eye exercises of acupoints questionnaire. It also presents the student's SE, and the univariate and multiple OR for myopia, for each item of the eye exercises questionnaire. Although students who performed the eye exercises in school were more myopic compared to those who did not (-0.40 ± 1.62 D vs. 0.06 ± 1.31 D, $p = 0.004$), performing the eye exercises in school did not reveal a significant effect for myopia per se (multiple OR, 95 % CI: 1.97, 1.19–3.26). Those who performed the eye exercises seriously demonstrated a borderline protective effect for myopia (univariate OR, 95 % CI: 0.46, 0.20–1.05), that is, less myopia. However, this protective effect became *significant* after adjusting for the student's age, gender, average parental refractive error, and time spent on near work and outdoor activity (OR, 95 % CI: 0.12, 0.03–0.49). Moreover, in comparison to students who never performed the eye exercises, those who performed them seriously less than 3 times per week (univariate OR,

95 % CI: 0.41, 0.18–0.93), and every time per week (univariate OR, 95 % CI: 0.28, 0.09–0.87), had less chance of being a myope. Furthermore, after adjusting for the same confounders, students who performed the eye exercises of acupoints seriously each time per week had less chance of being a myope (OR, 95 % CI: 0.17, 0.03–0.99). No other significant effects were observed.

When regression analysis was performed using the children's SE as the dependent variable and items from the eye exercises of acupoints questionnaire as the independent variable, similar results were found. The more often students performed the eye exercises of acupoints per week, the less myopic SE the students had (univariate $\beta = 0.40$, $p = 0.047$). After adjusting for the students' age, gender, average parental refractive error, and time spent on near work and outdoor activity, those with a serious attitude for performing them (multiple $\beta = 0.73$, $p = 0.043$), and with a higher frequency of performing them seriously, still remained borderline significant (multiple $\beta = 0.44$, $p = 0.050$).

Table 3 presents the CISS score, as well as the univariate and multiple β coefficients of the CISS score, for each item of the eye exercises questionnaire. Students who performed the eye exercises of acupoints in school had a higher CISS score (14.3 ± 6.4 vs. 10.7 ± 6.8, $p < 0.001$) compared to those who did not, and this trend remained significant after adjusting for the student's age, gender, average parental refractive error, and time spent on near work and outdoor activity (multiple $\beta = 1.95$, $p = 0.005$). However, no other items related to the eye exercises of acupoints, including a seriousness of attitude of performing them (multiple $\beta = -1.58$, $p = 0.23$), and acupoints acquaintance (multiple $\beta = 0.90$, $p = 0.67$), were found to have an effect on the CISS score; that is, there was no significant effect on relieving the near vision symptoms, in these students. Similar results were found when the student's refractive error was further adjusted.

Discussion

The rural students who performed the eye exercises of acupoints in school were more myopic, and furthermore they had a higher CISS score as compared to those who did not. There could be two possible reasons for this outcome. First, students with a more myopic refractive error might be more determined, or under greater psychological pressure, to perform the eye exercises of acupoints, to stabilize their myopia and to prevent visual symptoms. Second, students who performed these eye exercises in school had a more intense near work load than those who did not (5.43 ± 2.01 vs. 4.66 ± 1.53 h per day, $p < 0.001$).

There were several interesting and important findings in this study, which differed from our Chinese urban study [1]. First, although the eye exercises of acupoints were compulsory in all Chinese school children, only

Table 1 Demographic characteristics of children who performed eye exercises and those who did not performed eye exercises of acupoints in the Handan Offspring Myopia Study

	Children performed eye exercises (n = 121)	Children did not perform eye exercises (n = 715)
Age, years	11.8 ± 2.3	10.3 ± 2.4
Gender, male/female	64/57	373/342
Height, cm	146.3 ± 12.5	138.5 ± 13.5
Weight, kg	39.2 ± 10.4	33.4 ± 10.2
Cycloplegic SE, diopter	−0.40 ± 1.62	0.06 ± 1.31
Myopia, number (%)	50 (41.3)	148 (20.7)
Paternal average SE, diopter	−0.46 ± 0.69	−0.54 ± 0.77
CISS score	14.3 ± 6.4	10.7 ± 6.8

SE spherical equivalent, *CISS* convergence insufficiency symptom survey

Table 2 Children's spherical equivalent (SE) and odds ratio (OR) for myopia for each item of the eye exercises of acupoints questionnaire

	Number (%)	SE (mean ± SD)	Univariate OR (95 % CI)	Multiple OR (95 % CI)[a]
Performed the eye exercises (in school)				
No	715 (85.5)	0.06 ± 1.31		
Yes	121 (14.5)	−0.40 ± 1.62[b]	2.70 (1.80, 4.04)	1.97 (1.19, 3.26)
Times per day (in school)				
< 2	101 (83.5)	−0.45 ± 1.67		
≥ 2	20 (16.5)	−0.14 ± 1.35	1.20 (0.46, 3.15)	0.78 (0.22, 2.76)
Serious or not				
No/ moderate	83 (68.6)	−0.52 ± 1.80		
Yes	38 (31.4)	−0.13 ± 1.12	0.46 (0.20, 1.05)	0.12 (0.03, 0.49)
Serious times per week				
None	53 (43.8)	−0.77 ± 1.81		
< 3	48 (39.7)	−0.12 ± 1.56	0.41 (0.18, 0.93)	0.50 (0.18, 1.41)
Every time	20 (16.5)	−0.09 ± 0.97	0.28 (0.09, 0.87)	0.17 (0.03, 0.99)
Eye exercises were taught by				
Atlas/ classmate	47 (38.8)	−0.65 ± 1.59		
Teacher/doctor/health counselor	74 (61.2)	−0.25 ± 1.64	0.66 (0.32, 1.40)	0.53 (0.20, 1.44)
Speed				
Faster/slower than the broadcast & at will	88 (72.7)	−0.29 ± 1.52		
Following the broadcast	33 (27.3)	−0.68 ± 1.88	1.26 (0.56, 2.83)	1.63 (0.52, 5.13)
Acupoints acquaintance				
No/moderate	106 (87.6)	−0.40 ± 1.67		
Yes	15 (12.4)	−0.37 ± 1.25	0.94 (0.31, 2.83)	1.09 (0.21, 5.78)
Perform additional eye exercises (outside school)				
No	95 (78.5)	−0.39 ± 1.66		
Yes	26 (21.5)	−0.43 ± 1.53	1.57 (0.66, 3.75)	1.36 (0.39, 4.67)

SE spherical equivalent, SD standard deviation, OR odds ratio, CI confidence interval; the first group was the reference group
Multiple OR [a]adjusted for children's age, gender, average parental refractive error, times spent on near work and outdoor
[b]significantly different compared to the first group

approximately 15 % of the rural students actually performed them in school, much less than the 96.6 % among the urban students [1]. Second, there was no association with the CISS score, e.g., ocular-based vision symptoms, and any item of the acupoints eye exercises questionnaire. Third, and most importantly, the more frequently the students performed the eye exercises seriously, the less myopic refractive error they had, which suggested a protective effect for myopia, even after adjusting for possible confounders.

Several Chinese studies have reported on the eye exercises of acupoints and juvenile myopia. One epidemiological study ($n = 612$) reported that the prevalence of myopia was lower in grade 2–6 primary school children who performed the eye exercises regularly, as compared to children who performed them infrequently (29.53 % vs. 38.52 %) [12]. Another study demonstrated that these eye exercises were protective for juvenile myopia [13]. It has

also been reported that having a "serious attitude" towards performing the eye exercises improved visual acuity in grades 1–2 primary school children [14]. However, the underlying mechanism of these eye exercise to reduce myopia remains unclear. One study indicated that they could increase the peak systolic velocity (PSV) in the central retinal and ophthalmic arteries, and thus reduce their resistance index (RI), as observed by color Doppler imaging [15]. In addition, simple cessation of near work to perform the eye exercises provides a short rest period that itself may reduce the visual symptoms [16].

In our previous urban study (BMPS), less myopic refractive error was observed in students who performed the eye exercises of acupoints seriously. However, the protective effect of these eye exercises for myopia was not significant after adjusting for the students' age, gender, parental refractive error, and time spent doing near work and outdoor activity. More importantly, students

Table 3 Children's convergence insufficiency symptom survey scores(CISS) and β coefficientsforeach item of the eye exercises of acupoints questionnaire

	CISS score (mean ± SD)	Univariate β coefficient (p value)	Model 1[a]	Model 2[b]
Performed the eye exercises (in school)				
No	10.7 ± 6.8			
Yes	14.3 ± 6.4[c]	3.63 (<0.001)	1.95 (0.005)	1.88 (0.006)
Times per day (in school)				
< 2	14.1 ± 6.4			
≥ 2	15.4 ± 6.0	1.31 (0.40)	2.30 (0.13)	2.19 (0.15)
Serious or not				
No/moderate	14.6 ± 6.4			
Yes	13.7 ± 6.4	−0.94 (0.45)	−1.58 (0.23)	−1.88 (0.16)
Serious times per week				
None	13.9 ± 6.1			
< 3	15.2 ± 6.3			
Every time	13.1 ± 7.3	−0.06 (0.94)	0.25 (0.76)	0.12 (0.89)
Eye exercises were taught by				
Atlas/classmate	15.7 ± 5.4			
Teacher/doctor/health counselor	13.6 ± 6.8	−2.12 (0.08)	−0.84 (0.49)	−1.00 (0.42)
Speed				
Faster/slower than the broadcast & at will	13.7 ± 6.2			
Following the broadcast	15.9 ± 6.7	2.25 (0.08)	1.43 (0.31)	1.65 (0.25)
Acupoints acquaintance				
No/moderate	14.2 ± 6.2			
Yes	15.3 ± 6.0	1.17 (0.51)	0.90 (0.67)	0.89 (0.67)
Perform additional eye exercises (outside school)				
No	14.1 ± 6.7			
Yes	15.1 ± 5.2	0.98 (0.49)	1.96 (0.18)	1.95 (0.19)

CISS convergence insufficiency symptom survey, *SD* standard deviation
Model 1 [a]adjusted for children's age, gender, average parental refractive error, times spent on near work and outdoor
Model 2 [b]adjusted for Model 1 + children's refractive error
[c]significantly different compared to the first group

who performed the eye exercises seriously, followed the instructions when performing the eye exercises, and were acquainted with the eye exercises, tended to have a lower CISS score, i.e., were less symptomatic when performing near work activities, even after adjusting for the same confounders [1].

Convergence insufficiency is associated with visual symptoms at near, including general eyestrain, blurred vision, diplopia, difficulty concentrating, and reduced comprehension after short periods of reading or performing or other near activities [11, 17, 18]. Studies have demonstrated that the CISS questionnaire is a valid instrument for quantifying near visual symptoms in 9 to 18 year-old children and teenagers [11, 19]. In the present study, unlike the previous urban sample, [1] no association between seriousness of attitude of performing eye exercises of acupoints (multiple β = -1.58, p = 0.23), or acupoints acquaintance (multiple β = 0.90, p = 0.67), and near vision symptoms was found. Due to the correlation between accommodation, vergence, and refractive error, [20] a further multiple regression model with the refractive error adjusted was performed, which yielded similar results.

Consistent with previous studies on the eye exercises of acupoints published in the Chinese literature, [12–14] but different from our previous studies on urban students, [1] rural students in the present study who performed the eye exercises seriously tended to have less change in their myopia. This could be due to a dose-effect of the eye exercises of acupoints for myopia. In the current study, the rural students who performed the eye exercises in school had less myopic refractive error as compared to the urban students (-0.40D vs. -1.70D). Moreover, as compared to urban students, the rural students are exposed to relatively low risk factors for myopia, such as spending less time on near work and more time on outdoor activities, having a more open and spacious living environment, and having fewer myopic parents [21–24]. Lastly, urban student's myopia and related near oculomotor imbalance may be more "embedded" in those with intensive near work demands, and thus less susceptible to any remediation/intervention [25]. Thus, the effect of these daily eye exercises on prevention of myopia for 10 min each day may manifest an effect in the rural, but not in the urban, school students. Also, and again different from the urban students, the eye exercises were not associated with relieving ocular-based visual symptoms.

There were some possible limitations to the present study. First, the two subgroups of students, i.e., those participants versus non-participants in performing the eye exercises at school, were somewhat heterogeneous. The students who performed the eye exercises of acupoints in school were older, more myopic, and had a higher CISS score as compared to those who did not. Second, there was only a relatively small sample of students who actually performed the eye exercises in school. This may have reduced the power to uncover additional associations, e.g., with the CISS score. Third, there may be recall bias, since the questionnaires were used for collecting the information for eye exercises of acupoints, as well as other information (e.g., activities). Fourth, cross-sectional data cannot provide direct evidence on the association between the eye exercises and myopia development. Moreover, the results of this study would be stronger with either a control or additional comparative group. Hence, a randomized controlled trial with a larger sample size, and perhaps different "doses" of acupoints eye exercise schedules, is warranted to understand better the possible effect of eye exercises of acupoints on myopia and related near vision symptomatology.

Conclusions

This cross-sectional study found that the traditional eye exercises of acupoints had a modest protective effect on myopia among these Chinese rural students aged 6–17 years. However, no association between the eye exercises and near vision symptoms was revealed.

Acknowledgments
The authors thank Dr. Xiao Dong Yang (Nanjing Tongren Hospital), Dr. Qian Jia (Handan Eye Hospital), and Hong Jia Zhou (research assistant of The Eye Hospital of Wenzhou Medical University), for their invaluable assistance in data collection.

Funding
This study is being funded by the Innovation Research Project of the Eye Hospital of Wenzhou Medical University (YNCX201308), the Research Startup Project of Wenzhou Medical University (89213008), the Research Startup Project for doctors of the Eye Hospital of Wenzhou Medical University (KYQD131101), the Handan Science & Technology Research Development Program (1113108019), and the Beijing Science and Technology Novel Star Program (2009B44).

Authors' contributions
YBL designed the study protocol and conducted the study as a supervisor. ZL, BV, GYM and KJC participated in the study design, conducted statistical analysis, and drafted the manuscript. SJF, VJ, WH, TYG and YBL participated in the study design, and revised the manuscript. All authors read and approved the final manuscript.

Competing interests
The authors declare that they have no competing interests.

Author details
[1]The Eye Hospital, School of Ophthalmology and Optometry, Wenzhou Medical University, No. 270 West College Road, Wenzhou, Zhejiang 325027, China. [2]College of Optometry, Mid Western University, Glendale, AZ, USA. [3]Handan Eye Hospital, Handan, Hebei, China. [4]School of Environmental Science &Public Health, Wenzhou Medical University, Wenzhou, Zhejiang, China. [5]Department of Ophthalmology and Visual Sciences, The Chinese University of Hong Kong, Hong Kong, China. [6]Department of Biological and Vision Sciences, SUNY College of Optometry, New York, NY, USA.

References
1.   Lin Z, Vasudevan B, Jhanji V, Gao TY, Wang NL, Wang Q, Wang J, Ciuffreda KJ, Liang YB. Eye exercises of acupoints: their impact on refractive error and visual symptoms in Chinese urban children. BMC Complement Altern Med. 2013;13(1):306.
2.   Zhao J, Mao J, Luo R, Li F, Munoz SR, Ellwein LB. The progression of refractive error in school-age children: Shunyi district, China. Am J Ophthalmol. 2002;134(5):735–43.
3.   Lin LL, Shih YF, Hsiao CK, Chen CJ. Prevalence of myopia in Taiwanese schoolchildren: 1983 to 2000. Ann Acad Med Singapore. 2004;33(1):27–33.
4.   He M, Zheng Y, Xiang F. Prevalence of myopia in urban and rural children in mainland China. Optom Vis Sci. 2009;86(1):40–4.
5.   Liang YB, Friedman DS, Wong TY, Wang FH, Duan XR, Yang XH, Zhou Q, Tao Q, Zhan SY, Sun LP, et al. Rationale, design, methodology, and baseline data of a population-based study in rural China: the Handan Eye Study. Ophthalmic Epidemiol. 2009;16(2):115–27.
6.   Gao TY, Zhang P, Li L, Lin Z, Jhanji V, Peng Y, Li ZW, Sun LP, Han W, Wang NL, et al. Rationale, design, and demographic characteristics of the handan offspring myopia study. Ophthalmic Epidemiol. 2014;21(2):124–32.
7.   Lin Z, Vasudevan B, Liang YB, Zhang YC, Qiao LY, Rong SS, Li SZ, Wang NL, Ciuffreda KJ. Baseline characteristics of nearwork-induced transient myopia. Optom Vis Sci. 2012;89(12):1725–33.
8.   Ojaimi E, Rose KA, Smith W, Morgan IG, Martin FJ, Mitchell P. Methods for a population-based study of myopia and other eye conditions in school children: the Sydney Myopia Study. Ophthalmic Epidemiol. 2005;12(1):59–69.
9.   Lin Z, Vasudevan B, Jhanji V, Mao GY, Gao TY, Wang FH, Rong SS, Ciuffreda KJ, Liang YB. Near work, outdoor activity, and their association with refractive error. Optom Vis Sci. 2014;91(4):376–82.
10. Lin Z, Vasudevan B, Ciuffreda KJ, Wang NL, Zhang YC, Rong SS, Qiao LY, Pang CC, Liang YB. Nearwork-induced transient myopia and parental refractive error. Optom Vis Sci. 2013;90(5):507–16.
11. Borsting EJ, Rouse MW, Mitchell GL, Scheiman M, Cotter SA, Cooper J, Kulp MT, London R. Validity and reliability of the revised convergence insufficiency symptom survey in children aged 9 to 18 years. Optom Vis Sci. 2003;80(12):832–8.
12. Ping Z, Wang K, Chunhua Z, Bin Z. The epidemiological investigation of myopia in junior students. Prac J Med Pharm. 2004;21(6):543–5.
13. Changjun L, Wang J, Guo H, Jianzhou W. A survey on prevalence of myopia and its influential factors in middle school students. Mod Prev Med. 2010;37(16):3047–51.
14. Donglin Z, Hui T. Study on the effect of attitude towards the eye exercises on vision. Chin J School Doctor. 2006;20(5):501–3.

15. Jianming L. Observation of ocular haemodynamic change pre and post doing the eye exercises using color Doppler flood image. Chin J Ultrasound Diagn. 2004;5(6):446–7.
16. Ong E, Ciuffreda KJ. Accommodation, Nearwork, and Myopia. Santa Ana: Optometric Extension Program Foundation Press; 1997.
17. Borsting E, Rouse MW, Deland PN, Hovett S, Kimura D, Park M, Stephens B. Association of symptoms and convergence and accommodative insufficiency in school-age children. Optometry. 2003;74(1):25–34.
18. Shin HS, Park SC, Maples WC. Effectiveness of vision therapy for convergence dysfunctions and long-term stability after vision therapy. Ophthalmic Physiol Opt. 2011;31(2):180–9.
19. Rouse M, Borsting E, Mitchell GL, Cotter SA, Kulp M, Scheiman M, Barnhardt C, Bade A, Yamada T. Validity of the convergence insufficiency symptom survey: a confirmatory study. Optom Vis Sci. 2009;86(4):357–63.
20. Allen PM, O'Leary DJ. Accommodation functions: co-dependency and relationship to refractive error. Vision Res. 2006;46(4):491–505.
21. Ip JM, Rose KA, Morgan IG, Burlutsky G, Mitchell P. Myopia and the urban environment: findings in a sample of 12-year-old Australian school children. Invest Ophthalmol Vis Sci. 2008;49(9):3858–63.
22. Pan CW, Ramamurthy D, Saw SM. Worldwide prevalence and risk factors for myopia. Ophthalmic Physiol Opt. 2012;32(1):3–16.
23. Liang YB, Lin Z, Vasudevan B, Jhanji V, Young A, Gao TY, Rong SS, Wang NL, Ciuffreda KJ. Generational difference of refractive error in the baseline study of the Beijing Myopia Progression Study. Br J Ophthalmol. 2013;97(6):765–9.
24. Lin Z, Gao TY, Vasudevan B, Jhanji V, Ciuffreda KJ, Zhang P, Li L, Mao GY, Wang NL, Liang YB. Generational difference of refractive error and risk factors in the handan offspring myopia study. Invest Ophthalmol Vis Sci. 2014;55(9):5711–7.
25. Manas L. Visual analysis. 3rd ed. Chicago: Professional press; 1965. p. 303.

4

The quantity and quality of complementary and alternative medicine clinical practice guidelines on herbal medicines, acupuncture and spinal manipulation

Jeremy Y. Ng, Laurel Liang and Anna R. Gagliardi*

Abstract

Background: Complementary and alternative medicine (CAM) use is often not disclosed by patients, and can be unfamiliar to health care professionals. This may lead to underuse of beneficial CAM therapies, and overuse of other CAM therapies with little proven benefit or known contraindications. No prior research has thoroughly evaluated the credibility of knowledge-based resources. The purpose of this research was to assess the quantity and quality of CAM guidelines.

Methods: A systematic review was conducted to identify CAM guidelines. MEDLINE, EMBASE and CINAHL were searched in January 2016 from 2003 to 2015. The National Guideline Clearinghouse, National Center for Complementary and Integrative Health web site, and two CAM journals were also searched. Eligible guidelines published in English language by non-profit agencies on herbal medicine, acupuncture, or spinal manipulation for adults with any condition were assessed with the Appraisal of Guidelines, Research and Evaluation II (AGREE II) instrument.

Results: From 3,126 unique search results, 17 guidelines (two herbal medicine, three acupuncture, four spinal manipulation, eight mixed CAM therapies) published in 2003 or later and relevant to several clinical conditions were eligible. Scaled domain percentages from highest to lowest were clarity of presentation (85.3 %), scope and purpose (83.3 %), rigour of development (61.2 %), editorial independence (60.1 %), stakeholder involvement (52.0 %) and applicability (20.7 %). Quality varied within and across guidelines. None of the 17 guidelines were recommended by both appraisers; 14 were recommended as Yes or Yes with modifications.

Conclusions: Guidelines that scored well could be used by patients and health care professionals as the basis for discussion about the use of these CAM therapies. In future updates, guidelines that achieved variable or lower scores could be improved according to specifications in the AGREE II instrument, and with insight from a large number of resources that are available to support guideline development and implementation. Future research should identify CAM therapies other than those reviewed here for which guidelines are available. Research is also needed on the safety and effectiveness of CAM therapies.

Keywords: Complementary and alternative medicine, Integrative medicine, Systematic review, AGREE II, Clinical practice guideline

* Correspondence: anna.gagliardi@uhnresearch.ca
Toronto General Hospital Research Institute, University Health Network,
Toronto, Ontario, Canada

Background

It is currently estimated that more than 70 % of North Americans have tried at least one form of complementary and alternative medicine (CAM), [1–3] collectively spending billions of dollars annually on these therapies [4, 5]. CAM has been defined as "a group of diverse medical and health care interventions, practices, products or disciplines that are not generally considered part of conventional medicine" [6]. The National Center for Complementary and Integrative Health (NCCIH) further defines a non-mainstream practice used *together with* conventional medicine as "complementary", a non-mainstream practice used *in place of* conventional medicine as "alternative", and the coordinated delivery or use of conventional and complementary approaches as "integrative" [6]. This study henceforth refers to therapies that fall into all of these categories as CAM.

The past several decades have seen a sharp increase in research on CAM given the strong patient-driven market [7]. Examples of well-studied CAM therapies that show potential benefit include chiropractic spinal manipulation for low back pain and headaches [8–12], and acupuncture for different types of pain [13–18]. Recognizing such benefits, academic institutions are increasingly incorporating CAM into medical education, research and practice [11]. However, a variety of factors appear to influence whether and how CAM is used. Patients may not discuss their use of CAM with health care professionals out of fear of being judged or not seeing this as important to disclose, potentially leading to contraindications with other treatment [19–22]. Many health care professionals were not exposed to CAM in their medical training [23], are unfamiliar with CAM therapies, and find it challenging to discuss use or disuse of CAM with their patients [24, 25]. This is exacerbated by the fact that CAM is comprised of many different and unrelated types of therapies and schools of thought about their use [26]; and the reliability of evidence about safety and effectiveness varies between CAM therapies [27–29]. Given all of these factors, concerns have been raised about legal and ethical issues pertaining to the recommendations that health care professionals offer their patients about using or not using CAM therapies [24, 30]. Hence, patients and health care professionals may benefit from credible, knowledge-based resources upon which to base discussions and decisions about use of CAM.

Health care professionals often rely on evidence-informed clinical practice guidelines to understand whether use of a given therapy is recommended, and as a basis for informed and shared decision-making with patients about associated risks and benefits [31]. Research on a variety of clinical topics has identified that overuse, underuse or misuse of therapies may be associated with guidelines that are of poor quality [32], and

the quality of guidelines has been proven to vary considerably [33]. Few studies have examined CAM guidelines. Content analysis of 10 guidelines on cardiovascular disease and type II diabetes revealed that CAM-relevant information was brief, in some cases unclear, inconclusive and lacking in direction for health care professionals [34]. Analysis of 65 National Institute for Health and Clinical Excellence guidelines available in 2009 found that, among 17 guidelines that mentioned CAM, it was not clinically relevant to most; in 14 of 48 guidelines that did not mention CAM, available evidence on the safety and effectiveness of relevant CAM therapies had not been included [35]. Therefore, no research has thoroughly evaluated the credibility of CAM guidelines. An understanding of the nature of CAM guidelines available to support informed and shared decision-making among patients and providers would help to identify whether such resources are absent and thus needed, or how they could be improved, thereby guiding future guideline development and associated research. The purpose of this study was to assess the quantity and quality of CAM guidelines.

Methods

Approach

A systematic review was conducted to identify CAM guidelines using standard methods [36] and Preferred Reporting Items for Systematic Reviews and Meta-Analyses (PRISMA) criteria [37]. A protocol was not registered. Eligible guidelines were assessed with the widely used and validated Appraisal of Guidelines, Research and Evaluation II (AGREE II) instrument [38]. AGREE II is a tool that assesses the methodological rigour and transparency in which a guideline is developed, and is the international "gold standard" for the assessment of guidelines. Detailed information is available on the AGREE web site [www.agreetrust.org]. It consists of 23 items grouped in six domains: scope and purpose, stakeholder involvement, rigor of development, clarity and presentation, applicability, and editorial independence.

Eligibility criteria

Eligibility criteria for CAM guidelines were based on the Population, Intervention, Comparison and Outcomes framework. Eligible *populations* were adults aged 19 years and older with any diseases or conditions. With respect to *interventions*, guidelines were more likely to have been published on CAM interventions for which evidence has accumulated. We referred to a bibliometric and content analysis of CAM trials in the Cochrane Library by Wieland et al. [39] which found that the CAM therapies most commonly evaluated in trials included herbal supplements (non-vitamin, non-mineral dietary supplements or Chinese herbal medicine), acupuncture, and chiropractic or osteopathic manipulation [39]. For this study, guidelines were eligible if they specifically focused on any of these CAM therapies (category 1 – CAM-specific), or were general CAM guidelines that included at least one recommendation (for or against) at least of these CAM therapies (category 2 – CAM-general). We excluded general guidelines, which includes many hundreds and perhaps thousands, as it would have been challenging to search for and screen them for potential mention of CAM. *Comparisons* pertained to the assessed quality of CAM guidelines. *Outcomes* were AGREE II scores which reflect guideline content and format. The following conditions were also applied to define eligible guidelines: developed by non-profit organizations including academic institutions, government agencies, disease-specific foundations, or professional associations or societies; published in 2003 or later, which corresponds to the publication of AGREE II which provides developers with criteria for developing high-quality guidelines; English language; and either publicly available or could be ordered through our library system. Publications in the form of consensus statements, protocols, abstracts, conference proceedings, letters or editorials; based on primary studies that evaluated CAM therapies; or focused on CAM curriculum, education, training, research, professional certification or performance were not eligible.

Searching and screening

MEDLINE, EMBASE and CINAHL were searched on January 28, 2016 from 2003 to 2015 inclusive. The search strategy (Additional file 1) included Medical Subject Headings and keywords that reflect terms commonly used in the literature to refer to CAM [7]. We also searched the National Guideline Clearinghouse, a publicly available repository of guidelines [http://www.guideline.gov/] using keyword searches restricted based on the eligibility criteria including "acupressure", "acupuncture", "Chinese medicine", "chiropractic", "chiropractor", "herbal medicine", "herbal supplement", "herbal therapy", "osteopath", "phytotherapy", "plant extract" and "spinal manipulation". Next, we searched the NCCIH web site which contained a single list of CAM guidelines [https://nccih.nih.gov/health/providers/clinicalpractice.htm]; and the tables of contents of two CAM journals with the highest impact factors: *BMC Complementary and Alternative Medicine* [https://bmccomplementalternmed.biomedcentral.com/] and the *Journal of Complementary and Alternative Medicine* [http://www.liebertpub.com/overview/journal-of-alternative-and-complementary-medicine-the/26/] from January 2011 and December 2015. All three authors independently screened the titles and abstracts recovered from MEDLINE to standardize screening by discussing and resolving selection differences. Following

this, JYN and LL screened titles and abstracts from all other sources. JYN and ARG screened full-text items to confirm eligibility.

Data extraction and analysis

The following data were extracted from each guideline and summarized: date of publication, country of first author; type of organization that published the guideline (academic institutions, government agencies, disease-specific foundations, or professional associations or societies); topic category 1 (CAM-specific) or category 2 (CAM-general); and guideline topic including type of CAM therapy and disease or condition. Most data were available in the guideline; to assess applicability, the web site of each developer was browsed and searched for any associated knowledge-based resources in support of implementation.

Guideline quality assessment

The extraction and analysis of data from eligible guidelines followed standardized methods for applying the AGREE II instrument [38]. To do this we used the instructional manual provided by AGREE for this purpose. This is a 60-page document that first describes the AGREE instrument, provides instructions on how to apply the instrument then, for each domain, provides detailed guidance on where to look in the guideline for relevant content to judge that domain and how to rate each item in that domain. First a pilot test of the AGREE II instrument was conducted with two guidelines during which all three authors independently assessed both guidelines with the AGREE II instrument. Discrepancies were discussed and resolved. JYN and LL then independently assessed all eligible guidelines for 23 items across six domains using a seven-point Likert scale from strongly disagree (1) to strongly agree (7) that the item is met; rated the overall quality of each guideline (1 to 7); and used that information to recommend for or against use of each guideline. ARG resolved differences. Average appraisal scores were calculated by taking the average rating for all 23 items of a single appraiser of a single guideline, followed by taking the average of this value for both appraisers. Average overall assessments were calculated as the average of both appraisers' "overall guideline assessment" scores for each guideline. Scaled domain percentages were generated for inter-domain comparison, and were calculated by adding both appraisers' ratings of items within each domain, and scaling by maximum and minimum possible domain scores, before converting this into a percentage. Average appraisal scores, average overall assessments and scaled domain percentages for each guideline was tabulated for comparison.

Results

Search results (Fig. 1)

Searches retrieved 3,350 items, 3,126 were unique, and 3,095 titles and abstracts were eliminated, leaving 31 full-text guidelines that were considered. Of those, 14 were not eligible, primarily because they were not focused on CAM (7), they could not be retrieved (3), or did not meet other eligibility criteria (4), leaving 17 guidelines eligible for review.

Guideline characteristics (Table 1)

Eligible guidelines were published in 2003 or later in Canada, the United States, United Kingdom, China, and Australia [40–56]. The guidelines were funded and/or developed by professional associations or societies (13), academic (3), and an international agency (1). Nine guidelines were CAM-specific (2 herbal medicine, three acupuncture, four spinal manipulation) and 8 were CAM-general. Clinical topics included anorexia nervosa, breast cancer, cancer (general) diabetes, headache, herpes zoster, low back pain, lung cancer, major depressive disorder, migraine, multiple sclerosis, neck pain, and Parkinson's disease.

Average appraisal scores, average overall assessments and recommendations regarding use of guidelines

Average appraisal scores, average overall assessments, and recommendation regarding use for each guideline are shown in Additional file 2. The average appraisal scores for each of the 17 guidelines ranged from 3.3 to 5.5 on the seven-point Likert scale (where seven equals strongly agree that the item is met); 14 guidelines

achieved or exceeded an average appraisal score of 4.0, and seven guidelines achieved or exceeded an average appraisal score of 5.0. Average overall assessments for the 17 guidelines ranged between 3.0 (lowest) and 5.5 (highest), including 14 guidelines equalling or exceeding a score of 4.0, and 7 guidelines equalling or exceeding a score of 5.0.

Overall recommendations (Table 2)

None of the 17 guidelines were recommended by both appraisers. Appraisers agreed in their overall recommendation for 13 of 17 guidelines including 2 No [52, 55], and 11 Yes with modifications [40–43, 47–49, 51, 53, 54, 56]. Of the remaining four guidelines, three were rated by the two appraisers as No and Yes with modifications [44, 45, 50], while 1 guideline was rated at Yes and Yes with modifications [46].

Scaled domain percentage quality assessment (Table 3)

With regards to scaled domain percentages, scope and purpose scores were 52.8 to 100.0 %, stakeholder involvement scores were 11.1 to 86.1 %, rigor-of-development scores were 14.6 to 92.7 %, clarity-of-presentation scores ranged from 69.4 to 97.2 %, applicability scores were 0.00 to 60.42 %, and editorial independence scores ranged from 0.0 to 95.8 %.

Scope and purpose

The overall objectives and health questions were generally well-defined in all but one guideline [45]. Authors provided the goal of the guideline, the types of CAM they sought to assess, and the disease or condition that

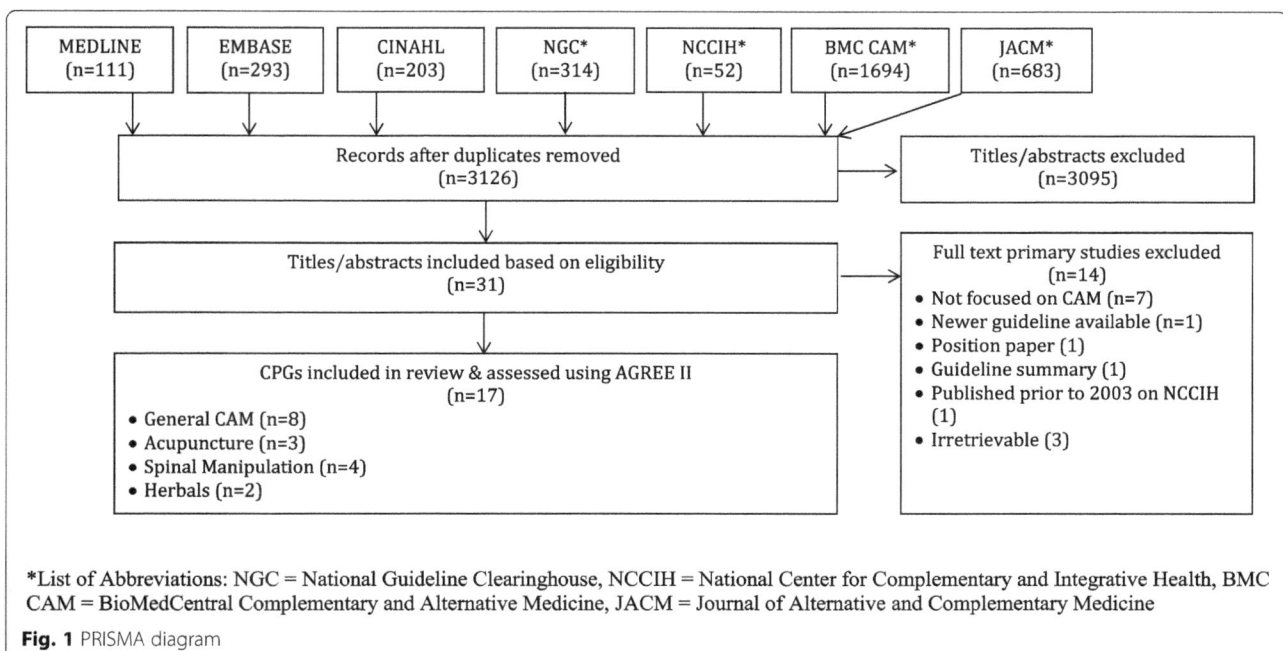

Fig. 1 PRISMA diagram

Table 1 Characteristics of eligible guidelines

Guideline	Country (First Author)	Developer	CAM category	Guideline topic
Fogarty 2015 [40]	Australia	Unclear	Acupuncture	Acupuncture for Anorexia Nervosa
Bryans 2014 [41]	Canada	Canadian Chiropractic Association	Spinal manipulation	Chiropractic Treatment for Neck Pain
Greenlee 2014 [42]	United States	Society for Integrative Oncology	General CAM	Integrative Therapies as Supportive Care in Breast Cancer Patients
Yadav 2014 [43]	United States	American Academy of Neurology	General CAM	Complementary and Alternative Medicine in Multiple Sclerosis
Deng 2013 [44]	United States	American College of Chest Physicians	General CAM	Complementary Therapies and Integrative Medicine in Lung Cancer
Liu 2013 [45]	China	Unclear; Sponsored by World Health Organization	Acupuncture	Acupuncture for Herpes Zoster
Nahas 2013 [46]	Canada	Canadian Diabetes Association	Herbals	Natural Health Products for Diabetes
Holland 2012 [47]	United States	American Academy of Neurology	General CAM	NSAIDs and Complementary Treatments for Episodic Migraine Prevention
Bryans 2011 [48]	Canada	Canadian Chiropractic Association	Spinal manipulation	Chiropractic Treatment of Headache
Seffinger 2010 [49]	United States	American Osteopathic Association	Spinal manipulation	Osteopathic Manipulative Treatment for Low Back Pain
Deng 2009 [50]	United States	Society for Integrative Oncology	General CAM	Complementary Therapies and Botanicals for Integrative Oncology
Ravindran 2009 [51]	Canada	Canadian Psychiatric Association, Canadian Network for Mood and Anxiety Treatments	General CAM	Complementary and Alternative Medicine for the Management of Major Depressive Disorder
Filshie 2006 [52]	United Kingdom	Unclear	Acupuncture	Providing Acupuncture for Cancer Patients
Suchowersky 2006 [53]	Canada	American Academy of Neurology	General CAM	Neuroprotective Strategies and Alternative Therapies for Parkinson Disease
Anderson-Peacock 2005 [54]	Canada	Canadian Chiropractic Association, Canadian Federation of Chiropractic Regulatory Boards	Spinal manipulation	Chiropractic Treatment for Neck Pain
Werneke 2005 [55]	United Kingdom	Unclear	General CAM	Complementary Therapies for Cancer
Mechanick 2003 [56]	United States	American Association of Clinical Endocrinologists	Herbals	Clinical Use of Dietary Supplements and Nutraceuticals

was the target of CAM therapy or therapies. The population to whom the guideline was meant to apply was sometimes less detailed. For example, two guidelines referred to the intended population as "patients" [46, 48].

Stakeholder involvement

Most guidelines thoroughly in detailed the characteristics of the members of the guideline development group, typically including degrees held by, and institutional affiliation of each member, in addition to some of the following: subject discipline, geographical location, and description of member's role in the group [41–44, 46–49, 53–56]. Some guidelines detailed the views and preferences of the target population [44, 46, 53, 56] while most did not [40–43, 45, 47–52, 54, 55]. Target users of the guideline were typically inconsistently defined. Some guidelines offered clear descriptions, for example, type of practitioner, specialty [40, 46, 49, 50, 52, 53, 56], while

other guidelines offered few details about target users [43, 45, 47, 50, 54, 55].

Rigor of development

Systematic methods were almost always used to search for evidence and the criteria for selecting the evidence were almost always clearly described [40–44, 46–51, 53, 54, 56], with the exception of a few guidelines [45, 52, 55]. The strengths and limitations of the body of evidence were clearly described in all guidelines except for one [45]. The methods for formulating the recommendations varied; while some guidelines provided a fair amount of detail on how consensus was reached [40, 42, 46, 48, 49, 53, 54, 56], other guidelines provided minimal information if not none at all [40, 41, 45, 47, 51, 55]. All authors considered some health benefits, side effects, and/or risks in formulating their recommendations, with the exception of one [52]. Nearly all guidelines provided an explicit link between their recommendations and the supporting

Table 2 Overall recommendations for use of appraised guidelines

Guideline	Appraiser 1	Appraiser 2
Fogarty 2015 [40]	Yes with Modifications	Yes with Modifications
Bryans 2014 [41]	Yes with Modifications	Yes with Modifications
Greenlee 2014 [42]	Yes with Modifications	Yes with Modifications
Yadav 2014 [43]	Yes with Modifications	Yes with Modifications
Deng 2013 [44]	No	Yes with Modifications
Liu 2013 [45]	No	Yes with Modifications
Nahas 2013 [46]	Yes with Modifications	Yes
Holland 2012 [47]	Yes with Modifications	Yes with Modifications
Bryans 2011 [48]	Yes with Modifications	Yes with Modifications
Seffinger 2010 [49]	Yes with Modifications	Yes with Modifications
Deng 2009 [50]	No	Yes with Modifications
Ravindran 2009 [51]	Yes with Modifications	Yes with Modifications
Filshie 2006 [52]	No	No
Suchowersky 2006 [53]	Yes with Modifications	Yes with Modifications
Anderson-Peacock 2005 [54]	Yes with Modifications	Yes with Modifications
Werneke 2005 [55]	No	No
Mechanick 2003 [56]	Yes with Modifications	Yes with Modifications

evidence with the exception of two guidelines in which this was inconsistent [49, 52]. While some guidelines explicitly stated that they were externally reviewed by experts prior to publication [41, 46, 54, 56], many did not [42–44, 47, 48, 52, 55]. Some guidelines failed to mention the purpose and intent for, or the methods employed for the external review [40, 45, 49–51, 53]. Most guidelines did not include a procedure for updating the guideline [42, 44, 45, 47, 48, 50–56] and, among those that did, one guideline provided a detailed methodology [46].

Clarity of presentation
Generally, all guidelines offered specific and unambiguous recommendations. However, many typically lacked one or more of the following details: identification of the intent/purpose, relevant population, or caveats. All 17 guidelines scored highly in presenting different options for the management of the condition or health issue, thus

contributing to this high scaled domain percentage [40–56]. Key recommendations were also generally very easily identifiable.

Applicability
One guideline discussed facilitators and barriers to implementation of the recommendations [49]. Three guidelines included advice and/or tools to support implementation of the recommendations [49, 54, 56]. No guidelines addressed the resource implications of implementing the recommendations. Two guidelines provided monitoring and auditing criteria, while 14 guidelines contained little to no such information.

Editorial independence
Guidelines varied in reporting of the funding source or competing interests of the members of the guideline development panel. Several guidelines that declared a funding source did not state whether funding source influenced the content of the guideline [41, 42, 48, 53, 54, 56].

No guidelines explicitly stated that no funding supported their development. Guidelines also varied in reporting of competing interests. Several guidelines did not address competing interests [45, 51, 52, 55, 56]. While remaining guidelines did so, two did not specify how potential competing interests were identified or considered, or how they may have influenced the guideline development process or issuing of recommendations [50, 53].

Discussion
To identify credible, knowledge-based resources upon which patients and health care professionals can base discussions and decisions about use of CAM, the purpose of this research was to assess the quantity and quality of CAM guidelines. This study identified 17 guidelines (nine specific CAM therapy, eight mixed CAM therapies) published in 2003 or later that were relevant to a variety of conditions and diseases. Quality as assessed by the 23-item AGREE II instrument varied widely across guidelines overall and by domain; two guidelines scored 5.0 or higher in both average appraisal score and average overall assessment [46, 49], and three guidelines scored 3.5 or lower in both of these metrics [45, 52, 55] (1 = strongly disagree; 7 = strongly agree that criteria are met).

To our knowledge, no previous studies have assessed the quantity and quality of guidelines on CAM therapies. Thus, we believe that this is the first study to assess the credibility and nature of CAM guidelines. The findings are similar to those of guidelines on other clinical topics. In this study of CAM guidelines, the scaled domain percentages from highest to lowest were clarity of presentation (85.3 %), scope and purpose

Table 3 Scaled domain percentages for appraisers of each guideline

Guideline	Domain score (%)					
	Scope and purpose	Stakeholder involvement	Rigour of development	Clarity of presentation	Applicability	Editorial Independence
Fogarty 2015 [40]	94.4	47.2	65.6	75.0	94.4	47.2
Bryans 2014 [41]	88.9	47.2	75.0	80.6	88.9	47.2
Greenlee 2014 [42]	100.0	72.2	80.2	97.2	100.0	72.2
Yadav 2014 [43]	97.2	47.2	77.1	77.8	97.2	47.2
Deng 2013 [44]	83.3	58.3	60.4	91.7	83.3	58.3
Liu 2013 [45]	52.8	11.1	32.3	88.9	52.8	11.1
Nahas 2013 [46]	75.0	86.1	92.7	91.7	75.0	86.1
Holland 2012 [47]	88.9	30.6	57.3	86.1	88.9	30.6
Bryans 2011 [48]	69.4	41.7	74.0	80.6	69.4	41.7
Seffinger 2010 [49]	97.2	66.7	69.8	91.7	97.2	66.7
Deng 2009 [50]	58.3	69.4	51.0	97.2	58.3	69.4
Ravindran 2009 [51]	94.4	30.6	60.4	88.9	94.4	30.6
Filshie 2006 [52]	83.3	38.9	14.6	72.2	83.3	38.9
Suchowersky 2006 [53]	94.4	72.2	66.7	80.6	94.4	72.2
Anderson-Peacock 2005 [54]	97.2	47.2	77.1	77.8	97.2	47.2
Werneke 2005 [55]	69.4	50.0	27.1	69.4	69.4	50.0
Mechanick 2003 [56]	77.8	72.2	71.9	94.4	77.8	72.2

(83.3 %), rigour of development (61.2 %), editorial independence (60.1 %), stakeholder involvement (52.0 %) and applicability (20.7 %). In a previous study we found that, among 137 guidelines on a wide variety of clinical topics published from 2008 to 2013, the scaled domain percentages were ordered in similar fashion from highest (clarity of presentation 76.3 %) to lowest (applicability 43.6 %) [33]. Previous studies that examined a total of 654 guidelines published from 1980 to 2007 [57, 58], and 1,046 guidelines produced between 2005 and 2013 by 130 Australian guideline developers [59] also reported similar findings. Therefore the variable and sub-optimal quality of guidelines is not a unique phenomenon.

Notable strengths of this study included the use of a comprehensive systematic review to identify eligible CAM guidelines and the use of the validated AGREE II instrument by which to assess their quality, which is the internationally-accepted gold standard for appraising guidelines [38]. The interpretation of these findings may be limited by the fact that guidelines were independently assessed by two appraisers instead of four as recommended by the AGREE II instrument to optimize reliability. To mitigate this and standardize scoring, ARG, JYN and LL conducted an initial pilot-test during which they independently appraised the same two guidelines, then discussed the results and achieved consensus on how to apply the AGREE II instrument. Following appraisal of the 17 guidelines, ARG met with JYN and LL to discuss and resolve any uncertainties without unduly modifying legitimate discrepancies. This review does not address all CAM therapies; three therapies were chosen (herbal medicine, acupuncture, chiropractic or osteopathic manipulation) because they were identified as having the largest evidence base, and were therefore considered more likely to be the subject of guidelines [39]. We may not have identified all guidelines that included these three types of CAM therapy because, to establish a feasible scope, we did not search for guidelines on specific clinical topics and then peruse them for CAM-related content, and we did not search all CAM journals or the Guidelines International Network guideline library. We included CAM topics for which there was likely to be available evidence such as guidelines. Many patients use CAM lacking supporting evidence, therefore, it may be useful to examine guidelines on a broader range of CAM topics to evaluate the basis for recommending those therapies.

By describing the quantity and quality of CAM guidelines, this study revealed that few CAM guidelines are available to support informed and shared decision-making among patients and health care professionals. This likely reflects the lack of research on CAM therapies. Others have identified numerous factors that challenge CAM research including negative attitudes about CAM therapies [60–65] and a lack of targeted funding [66–69]. However, this is expected to change given that CAM therapies continue to be used by more than 40 % of the population in some regions of the world

[70, 71]; and patients continue to use CAM despite documented risks associated with some CAM therapies [22, 70–75]. As research emerges, so too will guidelines that focus on CAM therapies [10].

This study also revealed that the quality of CAM guidelines varied across domains within individual guidelines, and across different guidelines. This finding is relevant to those who will produce CAM guidelines in the future, and to developers of existing CAM guidelines that, when updated, could be improved. Apart from the AGREE II instrument, numerous principles, frameworks, criteria and checklists are available to help guideline developers, including CAM guideline developers, to generate the highest-quality products [76–81].

Conclusions

This study identified 17 guidelines published since 2003 on CAM therapies including herbal medicines, acupuncture, and chiropractic or osteopathic manipulation. Appraisal of these guidelines with the AGREE II instrument revealed that quality varied within and across guidelines. Some of these guidelines that achieved higher AGREE II scores and favourable overall recommendations could be used by patients and health care professionals as the basis for discussion about the use of these CAM therapies. In future updates, guidelines that achieved variable or lower scaled domain percentage and overall recommendations could be improved according to specifications in the AGREE II instrument, and with insight from a large number of resources that are available to support guideline development and implementation [75–80]. However, the fact that few CAM guidelines are available to support informed and shared decision-making between patients and health care professionals may continue to foster underuse of beneficial CAM therapies, and overuse or contraindicated use of other CAM for which there is no proven benefit or potential associated risks. This finding justifies the need for greater research on the safety and effectiveness of CAM therapies. Future research should also identify CAM therapies other than those reviewed here which are supported by sufficient evidence to serve as the basis for guideline development.

Additional files

Additional file 1: MEDLINE Search Strategy for CAM guidelines executed Jan 28, 2016.

Additional file 2: Average appraisal scores and average overall assessments of each guideline.

Abbreviations

AGREE II: Appraisal of guidelines for research & evaluation II; BMC CAM: BioMedCentral complementary and alternative medicine; CAM: Complementary and alternative medicine; JACM: Journal of complementary and alternative medicine; NCCIH: National Center for Complementary and Integrative Health; NGC: National Guideline Clearinghouse; PICO: Patients, intervention, comparison and outcomes; PRISMA: Preferred reporting items for systematic reviews and meta-analyses

Acknowledgements

Not applicable.

Funding

Not applicable.

Authors' contributions

JYN: made contributions to the design of the study, collected and analysed data, drafted the manuscript, and gave final approval of the version to be published. LL: contributed to study design and planning, assisted with the collection and analysis of data, and gave final approval of the version to be published. ARG: made substantial contributions to the design of the study, the collection of data as well as interpretation and analysis of the data, revised the manuscript critically, and gave final approval of the version to be published.

Competing interests

The authors declare that they have no competing interests.

References

1. Public Health Agency of Canada. Complementary and alternative health. http://www.phac-aspc.gc.ca/chn-rcs/cah-acps-eng.php. (2008). Accessed 28 Jan 2016.
2. Barnes PM, Powell-Griner E, McFann K, Nahin RL. Complementary and alternative medicine use among adults: United States, 2002. Semin Integr Med. 2004;2(2):54–71.
3. Eisenberg DM, Davis RB, Ettner SL, Appel S, Wilkey S, Van Rompay M, Kessler RC. Trends in alternative medicine use in the United States, 1990-1997: Results of a follow-up national survey. JAMA. 1998;280(18):1569–75.
4. Nahin RL, Barnes PM, Stussman BJ, Bloom B. Costs of complementary and alternative medicine (CAM) and frequency of visits to CAM practitioners: US 2007. Hyattsville: Diane Publishing; 2010.
5. Esmail N. Complementary and alternative medicine in Canada: trends in use and public attitudes, 1997-2006. Vancouver: Fraser Institute; 2007.
6. National Institutes of Health, National Centre for Complementary and Integrative Health (NCCIH). Complementary, alternative, or integrative health: What's in a name? https://nccih.nih.gov/health/integrative-health (2016). Accessed 28 Jan 2016.
7. Ng JY, Boon HS, Thompson AK, Whitehead CR. Making sense of "alternative", "complementary", "unconventional" and "integrative" medicine: exploring the terms and meanings through a textual analysis. BMC Complement Altern Med. 2016;16(134):1.
8. Chaibi A, Tuchin PJ, Russell MB. Manual therapies for migraine: a systematic review. J Headache Pain. 2011;12(2):127–33.
9. Walker BF, French SD, Grant W, Green S. A Cochrane review of combined chiropractic interventions for low-back pain. Spine J. 2011;36(3):230–42.
10. Bronfort G, Haas M, Evans R, Leininger B, Triano J. Effectiveness of manual therapies: the UK evidence report. Chiropr Man Therap. 2010;18(1):3.
11. Bronfort G, Assendelft WJ, Evans R, Haas M, Bouter L. Efficacy of spinal manipulation for chronic headache: a systematic review. J Manipulative Physiol Ther. 2001;24(7):457–66.
12. Cherkin DC, Mootz RD. Chiropractic in the United States: training, practice, and research. Rockville: AHCPR Publication; 1997.

13. Liu L, Skinner M, McDonough S, Mabire L, Baxter GD. Acupuncture for low back pain: an overview of systematic reviews. Evid Based Complement Alternat Med. 2015;2015:328196.

14. Manyanga T, Froese M, Zarychanski R, Abou-Setta A, Friesen C, Tennenhouse M, Shay BL. Pain management with acupuncture in osteoarthritis: a systematic review and meta-analysis. BMC Complement Altern Med. 2014;14(1):312.

15. Vickers AJ, Cronin AM, Maschino AC, Lewith G, MacPherson H, Foster NE, Sherman KJ, Witt CM, Linde K. Acupuncture for chronic pain: individual patient data meta-analysis. Arch Intern Med. 2012;172(19):1444–53.

16. Cherkin DC, Sherman KJ, Avins AL, Erro JH, Ichikawa L, Barlow WE, Delaney K, Hawkes R, Hamilton L, Pressman A, Khalsa PS. A randomized trial comparing acupuncture, simulated acupuncture, and usual care for chronic low back pain. Arch Intern Med. 2009;169(9):858–66.

17. Yuan J, Purepong N, Kerr DP, Park J, Bradbury I, McDonough S. Effectiveness of acupuncture for low back pain: a systematic review. Spine J. 2008;33(23):E887–900.

18. Witt CM, Jena S, Brinkhaus B, Liecker B, Wegscheider K, Willich SN. Acupuncture for patients with chronic neck pain. Pain. 2006;125(1):98–106.

19. Ventola CL. Current issues regarding complementary and alternative medicine (CAM) in the United States: Part 1: The widespread use of CAM and the need for better-informed health care professionals to provide patient counseling. Pharmacol Ther. 2010;35(8):461.

20. Barraco D, Valencia G, Riba AL, Nareddy S, Draus CB, Schwartz SM. Complementary and alternative medicine (CAM) use patterns and disclosure to physicians in acute coronary syndromes patients. Complement Ther Med. 2005;13(1):34–40.

21. Coulter ID, Willis EM. The rise and rise of complementary and alternative medicine: a sociological perspective. Med J Aust. 2004;180(11):587.

22. Tsai HH, Lin HW, Simon Pickard A, Tsai HY, Mahady GB. Evaluation of documented drug interactions and contraindications associated with herbs and dietary supplements: A systematic literature review. Int J Clin Pract. 2012;66(11):1056–78.

23. Cowen VS, Cyr V. Complementary and alternative medicine in US medical schools. Adv Med Educ Pract. 2015;6:113–7.

24. Adams KE, Cohen MH, Eisenberg D, Jonsen AR. Ethical considerations of complementary and alternative medical therapies in conventional medical settings. Ann Intern Med. 2002;137(8):660–4.

25. Wilkinson S, Gomella LG, Smith JA, Brawer MK, Dawson NA, Wajsman Z, Dai L, Chodak GW. Attitudes and use of complementary medicine in men with prostate cancer. J Urol. 2002;168(6):2505–9.

26. Fisher P, Ward A. Complementary medicine in Europe. BMJ. 1994;309(6947):107.

27. Pearson NJ, Chesney MA. The CAM education program of the national center for complementary and alternative medicine: an overview. Acad Med. 2007;82(10):921–6.

28. Kroll DJ. ASHP statement on the use of dietary supplements. Am J Health Syst Pharm. 2004;61(16):1707–11.

29. Halcón LL, Chlan LL, Kreitzer MJ, Leonard BJ. Complementary therapies and healing practices: faculty/student beliefs and attitudes and the implications for nursing education. J Prof Nurs. 2003;19(6):387–97.

30. Weir M. Legal issues for medical doctors in the provision of complementary and alternative medicine. Med Law. 2007;26(4):817–28.

31. Shekelle P, Woolf S, Grimshaw JM, Schunemann H, Eccles MP. Developing clinical practice guidelines: reviewing, reporting, and publishing guidelines; updating guidelines; and the emerging issues of enhancing guideline implementability and accounting for comorbid conditions in guideline development. Implement Sci. 2012;7:62.

32. Mickan S, Burls A, Glasziou P. Patterns of "leakage" in the utilization of clinical guidelines: a systematic review. Postgrad Med J. 2011;87(1032):670–9.

33. Gagliardi AR, Brouwers MC. Do guidelines offer implementation advice to target users? A systematic review of guideline applicability. BMJ Open. 2015;5(2):e007047.

34. Team V, Canaway R, Manderson L. Integration of complementary and alternative medicine information and advice in chronic disease management guidelines. Aust J Prim Health. 2011;17(2):142–9.

35. Ernst E. Assessments of complementary and alternative medicine: the clinical guidelines from NICE. Int J Clin Pract. 2010;64(10):1350–8.

36. Higgins JPT, Green S, editors. Cochrane Handbook for Systematic Reviews of Interventions Version 5.1.0. London: The Cochrane Collaboration; 2011.

37. Moher D, Liberati A, Tetzlaff J, Altman DG. Preferred reporting items for systematic reviews and meta-analyses: the PRISMA statement. Ann Intern Med. 2009;151(4):264–9.

38. Brouwers MC, Kho ME, Browman GP, Burgers JS, Cluzeau F, Feder G, Fervers B, Graham ID, Grimshaw J, Hanna SE, Littlejohns P. AGREE II: advancing guideline development, reporting and evaluation in health care. Can Med Assoc J. 2010;182(18):E839–42.

39. Wieland LS, Manheimer E, Sampson M, Barnabas JP, Bouter LM, Cho K, Lee MS, Li X, Liu J, Moher D, Okabe T. Bibliometric and content analysis of the Cochrane complementary medicine field specialized register of controlled trials. Syst Rev. 2013;2:51.

40. Fogarty S, Ramjan LM. Practice guidelines for acupuncturists using acupuncture as an adjunctive treatment for anorexia nervosa. Complement Ther Med. 2015;23(1):14–22.

41. Greenlee H, Balneaves LG, Carlson LE, Cohen M, Deng G, Hershman D, Mumber M, Perlmutter J, Seely D, Sen A, Zick SM. Clinical practice guidelines on the use of integrative therapies as supportive care in patients treated for breast cancer. J Natl Cancer Inst Monogr. 2014;50(2014):346–58.

42. Bryans R, Decina P, Descarreaux M, Duranleau M, Marcoux H, Potter B, Ruegg RP, Shaw L, Watkin R, White E. Evidence-based guidelines for the chiropractic treatment of adults with neck pain. J Manipulative Physiol Ther. 2014;37(1):42–63.

43. Yadav V, Bever C, Bowen J, Bowling A, Weinstock-Guttman B, Cameron M, Bourdette D, Gronseth GS, Narayanaswami P. Summary of evidence-based guideline: complementary and alternative medicine in multiple sclerosis. J Neurol. 2014;82(12):1083–92.

44. Deng G, Rausch SM, Jones LW, Gulati A, Kumar NB, Greenlee H, Pietanza MC, Cassileth BR. Complementary therapies and integrative medicine in lung cancer: diagnosis and management of lung cancer: American College of Chest Physicians evidence-based clinical practice guidelines. Chest. 2013;143 Suppl 5:e420S–36.

45. Liu ZS, Peng WN, Liu BY, Wang J, Wang Y, Mao M, Deng YH, Yu JN, Liaw Y, Mu Y, Luo Y. Clinical practice guideline of acupuncture for herpes zoster. Chin J Integr Med. 2013;19(1):58–67.

46. Nahas R, Goguen J. Natural health products. Can J Diabetes. 2013;37 Suppl 1:S97–9.

47. Holland S, Silberstein SD, Freitag F, Dodick DW, Argoff C, Ashman E. Evidence-based guideline update: NSAIDs and other complementary treatments for episodic migraine prevention in adults Report of the Quality Standards Subcommittee of the American Academy of Neurology and the American Headache Society. Neurology. 2012;78(17):1346–53.

48. Bryans R, Descarreaux M, Duranleau M, Marcoux H, Potter B, Ruegg R, Shaw L, Watkin R, White E. Evidence-based guidelines for the chiropractic treatment of adults with headache. J Manipulative Physiol Ther. 2011;34(5):274–89.

49. Seffinger MA, Buser BR, Licciardone JC. American Osteopathic Association guidelines for osteopathic manipulative treatment (OMT) for patients with low back pain. Clinical guideline subcommittee on low back pain. J Am Osteopath Assoc. 2010;110(11):653–66.

50. Ravindran AV, Lam RW, Filteau MJ, Lespérance F, Kennedy SH, Parikh SV, Patten SB. Canadian Network for Mood and Anxiety Treatments (CANMAT) Clinical guidelines for the management of major depressive disorder in adults.: V. Complementary and alternative medicine treatments. J Affect Disord. 2009;117 Suppl 1:S54–64.

51. Deng GE, Frenkel M, Cohen L, Cassileth BR, Abrams DI, Capodice JL, Courneya KS, Dryden T, Hanser S, Kumar N, Labriola D. Evidence-based clinical practice guidelines for integrative oncology: complementary therapies and botanicals. J Soc Integr Oncol. 2009;7(3):85.

52. Filshie J, Hester J. Guidelines for providing acupuncture treatment for cancer patients–a peer-reviewed sample policy document. Acupunct Med. 2006;24(4):172–82.

53. Suchowersky O, Gronseth G, Perlmutter J, Reich S, Zesiewicz T, Weiner WJ. Practice Parameter: Neuroprotective strategies and alternative therapies for Parkinson disease (an evidence-based review) Report of the quality standards subcommittee of the American Academy of Neurology. J Neurol. 2006;66(7):976–82.

54. Anderson-Peacock E, Blouin JS, Bryans R, Danis N. Chiropractic clinical practice guideline: evidence-based treatment of adult neck pain not due to whiplash. J Can Chiropr Assoc. 2005;49(3):158.

55. Werneke U. A guide to using complementary alternative medicines in cancer. Drugs. 2005;101(5):1403–11.

56. Mechanick JI, Brett EM, Chausmer AB, Dickey RA, Wallach S, Bergman DA, Garber JR, Hamilton CR, Handelsman Y, Holdy KE, Kukora JS. American Association of Clinical Endocrinologists medical guidelines for the clinical use of dietary supplements and nutraceuticals. Endocr Pract. 2003;9(5):417–70.

57. Alonso-Coello P, Irfan A, Solà I, Gich I, Delgado-Noguera M, Rigau D, Tort S, Bonfill X, Burgers J, Schunemann H. The quality of clinical practice guidelines over the last two decades: a systematic review of guideline appraisal studies. Qual Saf Health Care. 2010;19(6):1–7.

58. Knai C, Brusamento S, Legido-Quigley H, Saliba V, Panteli D, Turk E, Car J, McKee M, Busse R. Systematic review of the methodological quality of clinical guideline development for the management of chronic disease in Europe. Health Policy. 2012;107(2):157–67.

59. National Health and Medical Research Council (NHMRC). Annual report on Australian clinical practice guidelines. Canberra: National Health and Medical Research Council; 2014.

60. Weisleder P. Unethical prescriptions: alternative therapies for children with cerebral palsy. Clin Pediatr. 2010;49(1):7–11.

61. Singh S, Ernst E. Trick or treatment: the undeniable facts about alternative medicine. New York: WW Norton & Company; 2008.

62. Chatfield K, Partington H, Duckworth J. The place of the university in the provision of CAM education. Aust J Homeopathic Med. 2012;24(1):16–20.

63. Colquhoun D. Science degrees without the science. Nature. 2007;446(7134):373–4.

64. Offit PA. Studying complementary and alternative therapies. JAMA. 2012;307(17):1803–4.

65. Colquhoun D. Should NICE evaluate complementary and alternative medicines. BMJ. 2007;334:506–7.

66. Fischer FH, Lewith G, Witt CM, Linde K, von Ammon K, Cardini F, Falkenberg T, Fønnebø V, Johannessen H, Reiter B, Uehleke B. High prevalence but limited evidence in complementary and alternative medicine: guidelines for future research. BMC Complement Altern Med. 2014;14(1):1.

67. Ernst E, Cohen MH, Stone J. Ethical problems arising in evidence based complementary and alternative medicine. J Med Ethics. 2004;30(2):156–9.

68. Ernst E. Obstacles to research in complementary and alternative medicine. Med J Aust. 2003;179(6):279–80.

69. Nissen N, Manderson L. Researching alternative and complementary therapies: mapping the field. Med Anthropol. 2013;32(1):1–7.

70. Clarke TC, Black LI, Stussman BJ, Barnes PM, Nahin RL. Trends in the use of complementary health approaches among adults: United States, 2002–2012. Natl Health Stat Report. 2015;10(79):1–16.

71. Harris PE, Cooper KL, Relton C, Thomas KJ. Prevalence of complementary and alternative medicine (CAM) use by the general population: a systematic review and update. Int J Clin Pract. 2012;66(10):924–39.

72. Werneke U, Earl J, Seydel C, Horn O, Crichton P, Fannon D. Potential health risks of complementary alternative medicines in cancer patients. Br J Cancer. 2004;90(2):408–13.

73. Ernst E. Harmless herbs? A review of the recent literature. Am J Med. 1998;104(2):170–8.

74. Patel DN, Low WL, Tan LL, Tan MM, Zhang Q, Low MY, Chan CL, Koh HL. Adverse events associated with the use of complementary medicine and health supplements: An analysis of reports in the Singapore Pharmacovigilance database from 1998 to 2009. Clin Toxicol. 2012;50(6):481–9.

75. Angell M, Kassirer JP. Alternative medicine-the risks of untested and unregulated remedies. N Engl J Med. 1998;339(12):839–40.

76. Schünemann HJ, Oxman AD, Brozek J, Glasziou P, Bossuyt P, Chang S, Muti P, Jaeschke R, Guyatt GH. GRADE: assessing the quality of evidence for diagnostic recommendations. Evid Based Med. 2008;13(6):162–3.

77. Shiffman RN, Dixon J, Brandt C, Essaihi A, Hsiao A, Michel G, O'Connell R. The GuideLine Implementability Appraisal (GLIA): development of an instrument to identify obstacles to guideline implementation. BMC Med Inform Decis Mak. 2005;5(1):23.

78. Schünemann HJ, Wiercioch W, Etxeandia I, Falavigna M, Santesso N, Mustafa R, Ventresca M, Brignardello-Petersen R, Laisaar KT, Kowalski S, Baldeh T. Guidelines 2.0: systematic development of a comprehensive checklist for a successful guideline enterprise. Can Med Assoc J. 2014;186(3):E123–42.

79. Gagliardi AR, Brouwers MC, Bhattacharyya O. A framework of the desirable features of guideline implementation tools (GItools): Delphi survey and assessment of GItools. Implement Sci. 2014;9:98.

80. Gagliardi AR, Brouwers MC, Bhattacharyya OK. The development of guideline implementation tools: a qualitative study. CMAJ Open. 2015;3(1):e127–33.

81. Gagliardi AR, Marshall C, Huckson S, James R, Moore V. Developing a checklist for guideline implementation planning: A review and synthesis of guideline development and implementation advice. Implement Sci. 2015;10:19.

5

Acupuncture with different acupoint combinations for chemotherapy-induced nausea and vomiting

Lili Gao[1,2†], Bo Chen[1,2†], Qiwen Zhang[1,2], Tianyi Zhao[1,2], Bo Li[1,2], Tao Sha[1], Jinxin Zou[1,2], Yongming Guo[1,2], Xingfang Pan[1,2*] and Yi Guo[1,2*]

Abstract

Background: Acupuncture is beneficial for controlling chemotherapy-induced nausea and vomiting (CINV). However, the effect of different acupoint combinations on controlling CINV remains unknown. This study aims to compare the effects of distal-proximal point association and local distribution point association on controlling CINV.

Methods/design: The study is a single-center, randomized controlled trial. A total of 240 participants will be randomly divided into four groups. The control group will receive standard antiemetic only, whereas three acupuncture groups will receive four electro-acupuncture treatments once a day with the standard antiemetic. Acupuncture group I and II will receive distal-proximal point association ("Neiguan (PC6) and Zhongwan (CV12)", and "Zusanli (ST36) and CV12", respectively); Acupuncture group III will receive local distribution point association ("Shangwan (CV13) and CV12"). The primary outcome measures are the frequency and distress of nausea and vomiting. The secondary outcome measures are the grade of constipation and diarrhea, electrogastrogram, quality of life, etc. Assessment is scheduled from the day before chemotherapy to the fifth day of chemotherapy. Follow-ups are performed from the sixth day to the twenty-first day of chemotherapy.

Discussion: Results of this trial will help in evaluating the efficacy and safety of electro-acupuncture with different acupoint combinations in the management of CINV.

Trial registration: ClinicalTrials.gov identifier: NCT02478047.

Keywords: Acupuncture, Chemotherapy-induced nausea and vomiting, Acupoint combination, Randomized controlled trial

Background

Chemotherapy-induced nausea and vomiting (CINV) are common side-effects of many antineoplastic regimens and can occur for several days after treatment [1]. CINV significantly impacts the patient' quality of life and nutritional status, and may lead to dose reduction or treatment discontinuation, subsequently increasing the risk of disease progression [2]. Although effective guidelines for CINV prevention exist for both moderately and highly emetogenic chemotherapies, adherence to these guidelines is not widely practiced because of their expensive costs and side-effects, such as headaches, dizziness, constipation, and insomnia [1].

Acupuncture treatment is one of the most sought-after therapeutic modalities in complementary and alternative medicine [3]. It is a safe medical procedure with minimal side effects. Evidence for the therapeutic effects of acupuncture on CINV exists [4]. Electroacupuncture for CINV management has been recommended by the American Society of Clinical Oncology [5]. Based on Traditional Chinese Medicine (TCM), the combination

---
* Correspondence: panxingfang@163.com; guoyi_168@163.com
†Equal contributors
[1]College of Acupuncture and Massage, Tianjin University of Traditional Chinese Medicine, No. 312, Anshan West Road, Nankai District, Tianjin 300193, China
Full list of author information is available at the end of the article

of acupoints can strengthen the essential and comprehensive therapeutic effects of acupuncture [6]. However, no consensus currently exists on the optimal acupoint combination for controlling CINV. For example, Gottschling S [7] found that stimulating PC6 (Neiguan), CV12 (Zhongwan), ST36 (Zusanli) and LI4 (Hegu) may effectively prevent CINV; Shen J [8] concluded that electro-acupuncture on PC6 (Neiguan) and ST36 (Zusanli) is more effective in controlling emesis than antiemetic pharmacotherapy alone. Therefore, we propose a randomized, controlled trial to determine the optimal combination of acupoints for CINV management.

In this trial, we aim to determine whether different acupoint combinations similarly manage CINV. We also aim to determine whether distal-proximal point association or local distribution point association more efficiently manages CINV.

Methods/design
Objectives
This study aims to: (1) assess the clinical efficacy and safety of distal-proximal point association and local distribution point association by electro-acupuncture for CINV management; (2) assess the patients' quality of life, anxiety, and depression, as well as other side effects of chemotherapy, such as diarrhea and constipation.

Hypothesis
According to the theory of TCM, the combination of acupoints can achieve a synergistic effect. In addition, distal-proximal point association and local distribution point association are the classic methods for combinating acupoints. We hypothesize that distal-proximal point association will achieve better therapeutic effect by reducing toxicity and enhance efficacy in CINV management.

Design
This is a four-armed parallel randomized controlled trial (RCT). 240 participants will be randomly assigned to four groups (a control group and three acupuncture groups) through central randomization in a 1:1:1:1 ratio. The flow chart is shown in Fig. 1.

Recruitment
All participants will be recruited from the Tianjin Medical University Cancer Institute and Hospital, and the clinical trial information will be posted on notice boards of the hospital. Our trial started on June 2015, and the first participant was recruited on 26 June 2015. For eligible participants who meet all required criteria, it will be requested to sign the written informed consent before randomization, meanwhile they will be given enough time to decide whether they willing to join this study.

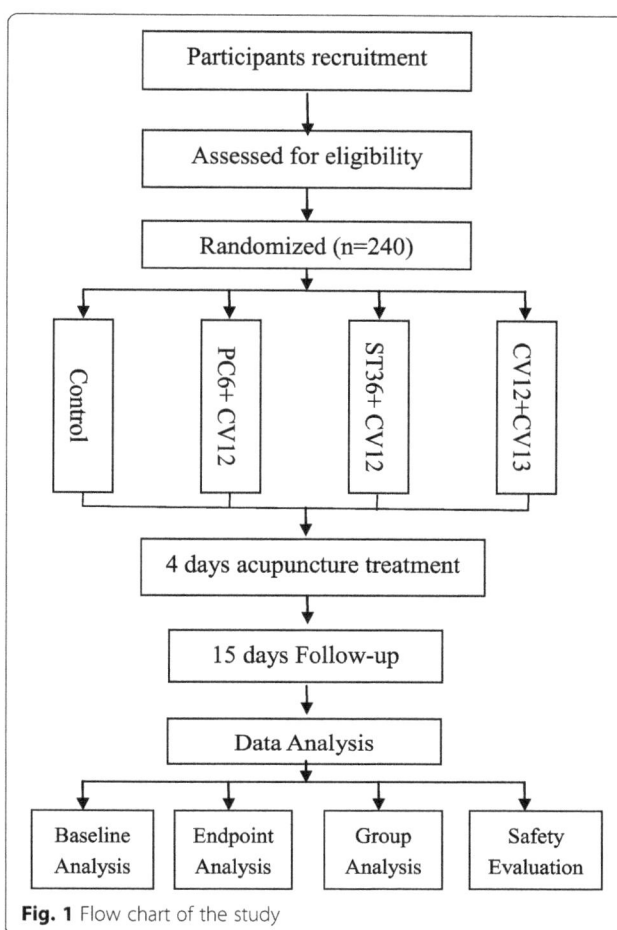

Fig. 1 Flow chart of the study

Inclusion and exclusion criteria
Inclusion criteria
Participants who meet all of the following criteria will be considered for enrollment. The inclusion criteria are as follows: (1) Diagnosed with cancer and need chemotherapy. (2) The score of Karnofsky (KPS) ≥ 70. (3) Between 18 and 80 years old (either sex). (4) Receiving chemotherapy as outpatients or inpatients. (5) Receiving chemotherapy for one or multiple cycles, but the patient will be taken into the study only once. (6) Patients receiving chemotherapy containing cis-platinum (cis-platinum $\geq$ 75 mg/m^2) or antharcycline-combined chemotherapy (doxorubicin ≥ 40 mg/m^2 or epirubicin ≥ 60 mg/m^2). (7) Life expectancy ≥ 6 months. (8) Willing to participate in the study and be randomly allocated into one of the four study groups.

Exclusion criteria
Participants who meet any of the following will be excluded: (1) Receiving radiotherapy concurrently with chemotherapy. (2) Gastrointestinal tumors. (3) Liver disease with serious complications, or with serious abnormal hepatorenal function (glutamic oxalacetic transaminase

(AST), glutamic-pyruvic transaminase (ALT), or total bilirubin (TBIL) three times higher than normal, blood urea nitrogen (BUN) or urine creatinine (Cr) two times higher than normal). (4) Presence of cardiac pacemaker. (5) Active skin infection. (6) Nausea and/or vomiting resulting from opioids or metabolic imbalances, such as electrolyte disturbances. (7) Unable to provide self-care or communicate, or have mental illness. (8) Nausea and/or vomiting resulting from mechanical risk factors, such as, intestinal obstructions. (9) Brain metastases or intracranial hypertension. (10) Pregnant or lactating.

Randomization
After signing an informed consent and evaluating the inclusion and exclusion criteria, participants will be randomly assigned to one of four groups by center randomization. The central randomized system will be used and performed by the Clinical Evaluation Center at China Academy of Chinese Medical Science in Beijing. A random number and group assignment will be immediately obtained through the website at http://118.144.35.11/crivrs/index.htm. Then the practitioner will assign the participant to that intervention and the evaluator will perform a baseline evaluation.

Blinding
The evaluator and the statistician are blinded to the intervention a participant accepts. Acupuncturists and patients are not blinded to the treatments they deliver because of the nature of the intervention.

Intervention
There are four arms in this randomized controlled trial. The control group is supplied with standard antiemetic alone, and the other three arms consist of antiemetic drug and acupuncture.

Control groups
Participants in the control group received standard antiemetic alone. Standard antiemetic for all groups is based on the American Society of Clinical Oncology Clinical Practice Guideline [9]. 5-hydroxytryptamine-3 (5-HT3) antagonist (Ramosetron, Tropisetron) and dexamethasone will be administered before the chemotherapy treatment.

Acupuncture groups
Three acupuncture groups will receive electro-acupuncture with different acupoint combinations: Acupuncture group I and II will receive distal-proximal point association, and Acupuncture group III will receive local distribution point association. The acupuncturists are the members who hold a Chinese medicine practitioner license from the Ministry of Health of the People's Republic of China.

Acupuncture group I: acupoints "PC6+ CV12" plus antiemetic drug
Participants in Acupuncture group I will receive electro-acupuncture at the Neiguan (PC6) point and Zhongwan (CV12) point. The location of Neiguan (PC6) is on the anterior aspect of the forearm, between the tendons of the palmaris longus and the flexor carpi radialis, 2 B-cun proximal to the palmar wrist crease [10]. The location of Zhongwan (CV12) is on the upper abdomen, 4 B-cun superior to the center of the umbilicus, on the anterior median line [10].

Acupuncture group II: acupoints "ST36+ CV12" plus antiemetic drug
Participants in Acupuncture group II will receive electroacupunture at Zusanli (ST36) and Zhongwan (CV12) points. The location of Zusanli (ST36) is on anterior aspect of the leg, on the line connecting ST35 with ST41, 3 B-cun inferior to ST35 [10]. The location of Zhongwan (CV12) has been introduced above.

Acupuncture group III: acupoints "CV12+ CV13" plus antiemetic drug
Participants in Acupuncture group III will receive electroacupuncture at Zhongwan (CV12) point and Shangwan (CV13) points. The location of Shangwan (CV13) is on the upper abdomen, 5 B-cun superior to the center of the umbilicus, on the anterior median line [10]. The location of Zhongwan (CV12) has been introduced above.

Disposable, stainless steel acupuncture needles will be used in this trial. The acupuncturists will first insert needles into the acupoints, then the needles will be manipulated until"de qi"sensation is achieved. Next, the needle will be connected to an electroacupuncture apparatus. The positive pole is linked to the needle, and the reference pole is secured approximately one cm in the proximity of the acupoint with a plaster. The electro-acupuncture treatment will use a frequency of 2/10 Hz, and the intensity of stimulation will be adjusted according to the patient's tolerance. The electric current will be set at less than 10 mA. The procedure will last for 30 min. Treatment is scheduled to occur 30–60 min before chemotherapy infusion and will last for 4 days. Detailed information on acupuncture treatment is summarized based on the revised STRICTA recommendations [11] in Table 1.

Participant timeline
Enrollment will be conducted the day before chemotherapy (day 0). The electro -acupuncture intervention will be given once daily from day 1 to day 4. The schedule of enrollment, interventions, and assessments is shown in Table 2.

Table 1 Acupuncture treatment details based on the STRICTA checklist [11]

Item	Detail
1.Acupuncture rationale	1a) Style of acupuncture
	- electro-acupuncture
	1b) Reasoning for treatment provided, based on historical context, literature sources, and/or consensus methods, with references where appropriate
	- electro-acupuncture treatment based on the theory of TCM, literature sources, and clinical experience in acupuncture and CINV, such as references [16] and [17].
	1c) Extent to which treatment was varied
	- The treatment was not varied.
2. Details of needling	2a) Number of needle insertions per subject per session (mean and range where relevant)
	- From 2 to 3.
	2b) Names (or location if no standard name) of points used (uni/bilateral)
	- Four points used: ST36 (bilateral); PC6 (bilateral) ;CV12(unilateral); CV13 (unilateral).
	2c) Depth of insertion, based on a specified unit of measurement, or on a particular tissue level
	- PC6: 0.5 body-inches; ST36: 1-1.5 body-inches; CV12 and CV13: 1-1.5 body-inches.
	2d) Response sought (e.g., de qi or muscle twitch response)
	- 'De qi' sensation will be achieved by lifting and thrusting combined with twirling and rotating the needles.
	2e) Needle stimulation (e.g., manual, electrical)
	- Electrical stimulation: the frequency is 2/10 Hz, and the intensity of stimulation is adjusted according to the patient's tolerance (maximum of 10 mA).
	2f) Needle retention time
	- Thirty minutes
	2g) Needle type (diameter, length, and manufacturer or material)
	- A disposable stainless steel acupuncture needle, 0.25mm × 40 mm (Huatuo, Suzhou Medical Co. Ltd., Jiangsu, China).
3.Treatment regimen	3a) Number of treatment sessions
	- Four treatment sessions in acupuncture groups.
	3b) Frequency and duration of treatment sessions
	- Once daily for 4 days, 30 minutes for each session.
4. Other components of treatment	4a) Details of other interventions administered to the acupuncture group (e.g., moxibustion, cupping, herbs, exercises, lifestyle advice)
	- No other interventions.
	4b) Setting and context of treatment, including instructions to practitioners, and information and explanations to patients
	- University hospitals. - Participants will be informed about acupuncture treatment in the study as follows: "In this study, eletroacupuncture for CINV will be used based on traditional Chinese medicine."
5.Practitioner background	5) Description of participating acupuncturists (qualification or professional affiliation, years in acupuncture practice, other relevant experience)
	- The participating acupuncturists have all majored in acupuncture, have an acupuncture degree, and are qualified doctors of Tradition Chinese Medicine. All have at least 3 years of experience, and will have been trained in the standard operating procedure of electro-acupuncture on CINV. Thus, they are able to provide identical acupuncture treatment in accordance with a pre-defined protocol.
6. Control or comparator interventions	6a) Rationale for the control or comparator in the context of the research question, with sources that justify this choice
	- The control group is supplied with standard antiemetic alone, so as to provide patients with conventional treatment for CINV.
	6b) Precise description of the control or comparator. If sham acupuncture or any other type of acupuncture-like control is used, provide details as for items 1 to 3 above.
	- Participants in the control group will not receive acupuncture treatment.

Table 2 The schedule of enrollment, interventions, and assessments

Time points	Enrolment -t1	Allocation t0	Post-allocation t1	t2	t3	t4	t5	t6-t20	Close-out t21
Enrollment									
Eligibility screen	√								
Informed consent	√								
Allocation		√							
Interventions									
Control group									
Experimental group I			√	√	√	√			
Experimental group II			√	√	√	√			
Experimental group III			√	√	√	√			
Assessments									
Baseline variables	√	√							
The frequency of nausea and vomiting		√	√	√	√	√	√	√	√
The grading of nausea and vomiting		√	√	√	√	√	√	√	√
Rhodes Index of nausea, vomiting and retching		√	√	√	√	√	√	√	√
The grading of constipation and diarrhea		√						√	√
eletrogastrogram		√						√	√
quality of life		√						√	√
anxiety and depression		√						√	√
Other adverse effect during the chemotherapy								√	√
The adverse effects of acupuncture			√	√	√	√			

t0, the day before chemotherapy; t1-t5, the first day to the fifth day of chemotherapy; t6-t21, the sixth day to the 21st day of chemotherapy

Outcome measures

The observation period will cover the day before chemotherapy (day 0) to the fifth day of chemotherapy (day 5). Follow-ups will be conducted from the sixth day (day 6) to the twenty first day (day 21) of chemotherapy. Participants will be asked to keep CINV diaries from the sixth day (day 6) to the twentieth day of chemotherapy (day 20).

Primary outcome measures

The primary outcome measures are as follows:

(1) Frequency of nausea and vomiting: total nausea and vomiting episodes per person over the 6-day study period will be recorded. The frequency of nausea and vomiting is the most valuable measurement for evaluation.
(2) Grading of nausea and vomiting: nausea and vomiting will be graded by Common Terminology Criteria for Adverse Events Version 4.0 [12].
(3) Rhodes Index of Nausea, Vomiting and Retching: nausea, vomiting and retching will be measured as separate entities by Rhodes Index of Nausea, Vomiting and Retching, which have 8 items with 5-point Likert scales. The frequency and distress of all entities are measured, as well as the duration of nausea and the amount of vomitius. [13]

Secondary outcome measures

Secondary outcome measures include the following:

(1) Grading of constipation and diarrhea: constipation and diarrhea will be evaluated by Common Terminology Criteria for Adverse Events Version 4.0 [12].
(2) Electrogastrogram: gastrointestinal motility will be monitored by electrogastrogram.
(3) Assessment of quality of life: the Functional Assessment of Cancer Therapy- General (FACT-G) [14] will be applied to assess four domains of patient quality of life, including physical, social/family, emotional, and functional well-being.
(4) Assessment of anxiety and depression: the Hospital Anxiety and Depression Scale [15] will be used to assess anxiety with seven items and depression with another seven items.
(5) Other adverse effects, including appetite, will be assessed by Common Terminology Criteria for Adverse Events Version 4.0 [12].

Sample size calculation

A sample size calculation was performed based on the result of a trial by Shen J [8] and the results of a pilot study. To detect a significant difference between any two groups with a power of 90 % and type I error of 5 %, the calculated number of patients is 192. Considering a 20 % drop-out rate, the total sample size needs 240 patients and 60 patients in each group.

Statistical analysis

Statistical analysis will also be performed by the Clinical Evaluation Center at China Academy of Chinese Medical Science. The statistician is blinded from the allocation of groups. The Kruskal-Wallis test will be employed in the analysis of skewed distribution data. Chi-square analysis will be used for categorical variables, and Analysis of variance (ANOVA) for numerical variables. Repeated measures analysis will be used in the different time point assessment. A P value less than 0.05 is regarded as statistically significant.

Data management

To promote data quality, the data will be collected by well-trained assessor and the double entry of the data will be implemented by clinical research coordinators.

Safety

Participants will also be monitored for any adverse events, including swelling, pain, bruise at the sites of needle insertion, or discomfort, palpitation, dizziness, etcetera after acupuncture treatment. Adverse effects will be recorded in the case report forms (CRF).

Quality control

All researchers will be required to undergo special training classes to guarantee the quality of the study. The training classes will introduce researchers to the trial's details. For example, researchers will be trained to use the central randomized system, to fully understand the inclusion and exclusion criteria, and to fill in the CRFs. Additionally, clinical monitors will also check the trial processes and CRFs. Patient drop-outs and their reasons will be fully recorded.

Ethics and dissemination

Medical Ethics Committees at Tianjin University of Traditional Chinese Medicine has approved this protocol (approval number is TJUTCM-EC20140006 and). Patients' data will be stored securely and the results of the present study will be published in a peer-reviewed journal.

Discussion

This study protocol expands current literature regarding the efficacy of acupuncture on CINV. Previous reviews showed that acupoint stimulation has a certain effect on CINV. However, the effects of different acupoint combinations are inconsistent. We designed our trial to compare the effects of distal-proximal point association and local distribution point association.

More than 300 acupuncture points are located on the body and each point has its own therapeutic indication. The correct selection and combination of acupoints are the keys to the curative effects of acupuncture [6]. Before developing the trial protocol, we screened a range of published articles and ancient books. Our literature search showed that PC6, ST36, and CV12 are the most commonly used acupoints for managing CINV [16, 17]. We selected PC6 and ST36 as the distal acupoints, and CV12 as the local acupoint. Based on the theory of Chinese acupuncture, distal-proximal acupoint association and local distribution point association are the two classic methods for combining acupoints. Distal-proximal acupoint association is also the most commonly used method in clinical applications. In this trial, there are three different acupuncture groups: "PC6 and CV12" and "ST36 and CV12" are the two disal-proximal acupoint association groups, and "CV12 and CV13" is the local distribution point association group. Therefore, we expect that distal-proximal point association ("PC6 and CV12" or "ST36 and CV12") will have better effect than local distribution point association ("CV12 and CV13"). Furthermore, we can screen the most effective acupoint combination for clinical application from these three groups.

Although the manipulators and participants cannot be blinded to the group allocation in this study, all outcome measures will be administered and collected by a blinded estimator, and statisticians blinded to group assignment will perform data analysis. With respect to clinical quality control, the manipulators, estimators and statisticians will work independently to reduce the adverse impacts of artificial factors on data. A third party has been invited to manage data independently and to design a central randomization system for minimizing bias and enhancing clinical research quality.

In conclusion, the results of this trial are expected to assess the clinical efficacy and safety of distal-proximal point association and the local distribution point association by electro-acupuncture in the management of CINV.

Trial status

The first participant was recruited on 26 June 2015. This study is currently recruiting participants.

Abbreviations

ALT: Glutamic-pyruvic transaminase; ANOVA: Analysis of Variance; AST: Glutamic oxalacetic transaminase; BUN: Blood urea nitrogen; CINV: Chemotherapy- induced nausea and vomiting; Cr: Urine creatinine; CRF: Case Report Form; CV12: The acupoint of Zhongwan; CV13: The acupoint of Shangwan; FACT-G: The Functional Assessment of Cancer Therapy - General; KPS: The scoring of Karnofsky; LI4: The acupoint of Hegu; PC6: The acupoint of Neiguan; RCT: Randomized Controlled trial; ST36: The acupoint of Zusanli; STRICTA: Standards for Reporting Interventions in Clinical Trials of Acupuncture; TBIL: Total bilirubin; TCM: Traditional Chinese Medicine

Acknowledgments

We acknowledge Tianjin Medical University Cancer Institute and Hospital. We also appreciate the help and efforts for all research staffs participating in this trial.

Funding

This research was supported by National Basic Research Program of China under Grant No. 2014CB543201, and the National Natural Science Foundation of China (NSFC) No. 81330088. The funding source had no role in the design of this study and will not have any role during its execution, analyses, interpretation of the data, or decision to submit results.

Authors' contributions

GL carried out the evaluation, participated in the conception and design of the trial and drafted the manuscript. BC participated in the conception and design of the trial and helped to draft the manuscript. QZ participated in the patient recruitment. TZ participated in the statistical analysis. BL carried out the acupuncture practice. TS participated in drafting and proofreading the manuscript. JZ is in charge of random allocation. YG monitored the trial and Case Report Forms. XP participated in the design of the study and performed the statistical analysis. YG conceived of the study, and participated in its design and coordination and helped to draft the manuscript. YG and XFP are the correspondence authors. All authors read and approved the final manuscript.

Competing interests

The authors declare that they have no competing interests.

Author details

[1]College of Acupuncture and Massage, Tianjin University of Traditional Chinese Medicine, No. 312, Anshan West Road, Nankai District, Tianjin 300193, China. [2]Acupuncture Research Center, Tianjin University of Traditional Chinese Medicine, No. 312, Anshan West Road, Nankai District, Tianjin 300193, China.

References

1. Schwartzberg LS, Modiano MR, Rapoport BL, Chasen MR, Gridelli C, Urban L, et al. Safety and efficacy of rolapitant for prevention of chemotherapy-induced nausea and vomiting after administration of moderately emetogenic chemotherapy or anthracycline and cyclophosphamide regimens in patients with cancer: a randomised, active-controlled, double-blind, phase 3 trial. Lancet Oncol. 2015;16(9):1071–8.
2. Bloechl-Daum B, Deuson RR, Mavros P, Hansen M, Herrstedt J. Delayed nausea and vomiting continue to reduce patients' quality of life after highly and moderately emetogenic chemotherapy despite antiemetic treatment. J Clin Oncol. 2006;24(27):4472–8.
3. Han G, Ko SJ, Park JW, Kim J, Yeo I, Lee H, et al. Acupuncture for functional dyspepsia: study protocol for a two-center, randomized controlled trial. Trials. 2014;15:89.
4. Wu X, Chung VC, Hui EP, Ziea ET, Ng BF, Ho RS, et al. Effectiveness of acupuncture and related therapies for palliative care of cancer: overview of systematic reviews. Sci Rep. 2015;5:16776.
5. Naeim A, Dy SM, Lorenz KA, Sanati H, Walling A, Asch SM. Evidence-based recommendations for cancer nausea and vomiting. J Clin Oncol. 2008;26(23):3903–10.
6. Zhao JS. Chinese acupuncture and moxibustion. 1st ed. Shanghai: Publishing house of Shanghai University of Traditional Chinese Medicine; 2002.
7. Gottschling S, Reindl TK, Meyer S, Berrang J, Henze G, Graeber S, et al. Acupuncture to alleviate chemotherapy-induced nausea and vomiting in pediatric oncology-a randomized multicenter crossover pilot trial. Klin Padiatr. 2008;220(6):365–70.
8. Shen J, Wenger N, Glaspy J, Hays RD, Albert PS, Choi C, et al. Electroacupuncture for control of myeloablative chemotherapy-induced emesis: A randomized controlled trial. JAMA. 2000;284(21):2755–61.
9. Basch E, Prestrud AA, Hesketh PJ, Kris MG, Feyer PC, Somerfield MR, et al. Antiemetics: American Society of Clinical Oncology clinical practice guideline update. J Clin Oncol. 2011;29(31):4189–98.
10. World Health Organization, WHO standard acupuncture point locations in the Western Pacific Region. Manila: World Health Organization Regional Office for the Western Pacific; 2008.
11. MacPherson H, Altman DG, Hammerschlag R, Li YP, Wu TX, White A, et al. Revised STandards for Reporting Interventions in Clinical Trials of Acupuncture (STRICTA): extending the CONSORT statement. PLoS Med. 2010;7(6):e1000261.
12. US Department of Health and Human Services, Common terminology criteria for adverse events (CTCAE) version 4.0. Bethesda: National Institutes of Health, National Cancer Institute; 2009.
13. Rhodes VA, McDaniel RW. The index of nausea, vomiting, and retching: a new format of the index of nausea and vomiting. Oncol Nurs Forum. 1999;26(5):889–94.
14. Fairclough DL, Cella DF. Functional Assessment of Cancer Therapy (FACT-G): non-response to individual questions. Qual Life Res. 1996;5(3):321–9.
15. Snaith RP. The hospital anxiety and depression scale. Health Qual Life Outcomes. 2003;1:29.
16. An Q, Chen B, Guo Y, Pan XF, Guo YM. A preliminary discussion on rules of clinical acupoint selection of acupuncture for the treatment of chemotherapy-induced nausea and vomiting. World J Acupunct Moxibustion. 2015;25(2):39–44. 66.
17. Bao T. Use of acupuncture in the control of chemotherapy-induced nausea and vomiting. J Natl Compr Canc Netw. 2009;7(5):606–12.

6

Safe needling depths of upper back acupoints in children

Yi-Chun Ma[1,2], Ching-Tien Peng[3], Yu-Chuen Huang[4,5], Hung-Yi Lin[3] and Jaung-Geng Lin[4,6]*

Abstract

Background: Acupuncture is applied for treating numerous conditions in children, but few studies have examined the safe needling depth of acupoints in the pediatric population. In this study, we investigated the depths to which acupuncture needles can be inserted safely in the upper back acupoints of children and the variations in safe depth according to sex, age, weight, and body mass index (BMI).

Methods: We retrospectively studied computed tomography (CT) images of patients aged 4 to 18 years who underwent chest CT at China Medical University Hospital between December 2004 and May 2013. The safe depths of 23 upper back acupoints in the Governor Vessel (GV), Bladder Meridian (BL), Small Intestine Meridian (SI), Gallbladder Meridian (GB) and Spleen Meridian (SP) were measured directly from the CT images. The relationships between the safe depths of these acupoints and sex, age, body weight, and BMI were analyzed.

Results: The results indicated significant differences in safe needling depth between boys and girls in most upper back acupoints, except at BL42, BL44, BL45, BL46, GB21 and SP21. Safe depths differed significantly depending on age ($p < 0.001$), weight ($p \leq 0.01$), and BMI ($p < 0.05$). Multiple regression analysis revealed that weight was the most crucial factor in determining the safe depth.

Conclusions: Sex, age, weight, and BMI are relevant factors in determining the safe needling depths of upper back acupoints in children. Physicians should pay attention to wide variations in needle depth when performing acupuncture.

Keywords: Acupuncture, Safe depth, Children, Upper back

Background

Acupuncture is a traditional Chinese medical practice that has been used to treat numerous diseases in China for thousands of years. The practice has gained popularity in Western countries and become one of the most popular forms of complementary and alternative therapy. Acupuncture has been applied to treat several conditions in children, including pain, nocturnal enuresis, postoperative nausea and vomiting, allergic rhinitis, laryngospasm, and neurological disorders [1, 2]. Thus, the safety of acupuncture is critical and should be considered carefully regarding pediatric patients.

Acupuncture may cause serious adverse events including subarachnoid hemorrhages, pneumothorax, cardiac ruptures, nerve impairment, intestinal obstruction, hemoptysis, reversible comas, and infection [3]. Pneumothorax is the most frequent organ injury caused by acupuncture [4]. Acupoints over upper back used to be applied for cough, dyspnea, backache and shoulder pain. Hence, studying the safe depths of acupoints over upper back is critical to prevent serious and common complications, such as pneumothorax from acupuncture.

The depths of acupuncture needling recorded in ancient references have variations and there was no difference between different body sizes. Besides, no references were specific for children. In clinical practice, the depths of needling were usually performed according to practitioners' experiences and patients' responses. However, children usually cannot response properly to the needling stimulation. There were risks for serious complications such as pneumothorax or organ damage. Therefore, we want to establish data of the safe needling depth, considering the factors of sex, age, weight and BMI in children.

* Correspondence: jglin@mail.cmu.edu.tw
[4]School of Chinese Medicine, College of Chinese Medicine, China Medical University, Taichung, Taiwan, ROC
[6]China Medical University, No.91, Xueshi Rd., North Dist., Taichung City 40402, Taiwan, ROC
Full list of author information is available at the end of the article

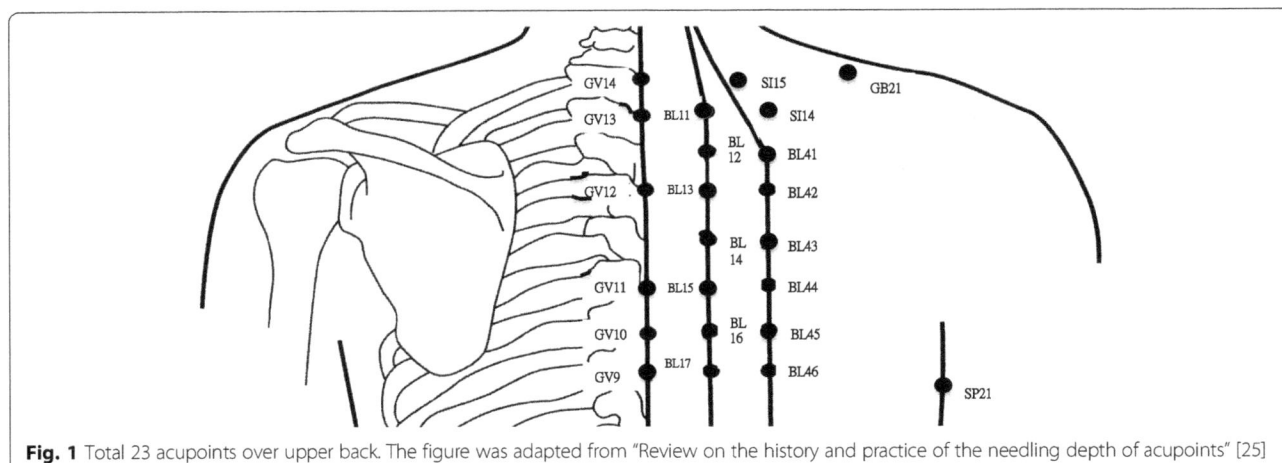

Fig. 1 Total 23 acupoints over upper back. The figure was adapted from "Review on the history and practice of the needling depth of acupoints" [25]

In children, the physical development process may cause changes in lean muscle mass and fat volume [5]. Particularly during puberty, the sexual dimorphism of body composition and the wide time range of pubertal onset cause wide variations in fat volume, muscle mass, and their distribution [6]. Such variations may be highly complex and may influence safe needling depth. Such difficulties are not encountered when treating adults.

Most previous studies on safe needling depth have involved small sample sizes and adult groups [7, 8]. One study measured the safe depths of back loci in adults, finding differences depending on body size but not sex

[9]. Few studies have evaluated safe needling depth in children. Only two studies measuring the safe depths and therapeutic depths of abdomen acupoints have included pediatric populations [10, 11]. In this study, we included large sample sizes of children and measured the safe depths of upper back acupoints by analyzing

Table 1 General characteristics of patients

Characteristics	Subjects numbers
Gender	
Male	205
Female	114
Age (years old)	
4–6	79
7–9	45
10–12	30
13–15	56
16–18	109
Weight	
<3rd percentile	32
3–<85th percentile	215
85–<97th percentile	42
≥97th percentile	29
BMI	
Underweight	52
Healthy weight	186
Overweight	18
Obesity	30

Table 2 Safe depths of 23 upper back acupoints of sexes

Acupoints	Boys Mean ± S.D.	Girls Mean ± S.D.	P value
GV9	27.78 ± 8.88	24.87 ± 7.83	0.003[a]
GV10	28.54 ± 8.47	26.02 ± 7.67	0.009[a]
GV11	28.17 ± 8.21	25.88 ± 7.04	0.009[a]
GV12	30.45 ± 9.90	28.03 ± 8.24	0.028[a]
GV13	33.61 ± 10.07	30.59 ± 9.11	0.008[a]
GV14	33.81 ± 10.57	30.70 ± 10.68	0.012[a]
BL11	33.39 ± 10.48	28.95 ± 8.67	<0.001[a]
BL12	35.61 ± 9.61	32.33 ± 8.09	0.001[a]
BL13	28.54 ± 7.08	26.41 ± 5.38	0.003[a]
BL14	24.92 ± 7.95	22.69 ± 6.63	0.008[a]
BL15	25.48 ± 6.57	23.93 ± 5.41	0.024[a]
BL16	24.15 ± 7.19	21.89 ± 6.24	0.004[a]
BL17	25.37 ± 6.87	23.62 ± 6.20	0.021[a]
BL41	30.86 ± 9.20	28.21 ± 7.89	0. 010[a]
BL42	28.02 ± 8.69	26.48 ± 7.25	0.110
BL43	24.68 ± 7.54	22.95 ± 6.75	0.043[a]
BL44	20.31 ± 7.79	19.19 ± 7.01	0.202
BL45	18.45 ± 7.07	17.62 ± 6.50	0.300
BL46	18.16 ± 6.63	16.96 ± 6.12	0.111
SI14	36.82 ± 12.23	32.51 ± 10.81	0.002[a]
SI15	38.75 ± 12.10	34.74 ± 10.47	0.003[a]
GB21	28.01 ± 9.37	26.61 ± 8.81	0.192
SP21	19.48 ± 4.39	18.84 ± 4.56	0.216

Unit of mean ± SD: mm
[a]Statistically significant

computed tomography (CT) scans. We also evaluated the variations in safe depth according to sex, age, weight, and body mass index (BMI).

Methods

Study population

All patients aged 4 to 18 years who underwent chest CT between December 2004 and May 2013 at China Medical University Hospital (CMUH) were identified. These patients underwent CT scans for evaluating an acute chest or upper back condition such as acute accidental injuries, pneumothorax, pneumonia, and cardiac diseases. Patients with back trauma or chronic oncological diseases were excluded because of the possible effect on the thickness of subcutaneous tissues and muscles in the back. Thus, we included 4 to 18 years patients who underwent chest CT between December 2004 and May 2013 at CMUH without back trauma or chronic oncological diseases.

The age, sex, height and body weight of each patient were obtained from chart records. BMI was measured according to weight (kg)/height^2 (m^2). Patients were divided into five groups according to age in years: 4–6, 7–9, 10–12, 13–15, and 16–18 on the basis of previous references [10, 11]. Patients were also divided into four weight groups according to growth charts for Taiwanese children and adolescents [12]: below the third percentile, from the third percentile up to the 85th percentile, from the 85th percentile up to the 97th percentile, and at or above the 97th percentile. Patients were divided into four BMI groups according to the same charts: underweight, defined as below the fifth percentile; healthy weight, defined as from the fifth percentile up to the 85th percentile; overweight, defined as from the 85th percentile up to the 95th percentile; and obese, defined as at or above the 95th percentile [12, 13]. The data were anonymized and this study was approved by the Research Ethics Committee of CMUH.

Measurement of safe depths at upper back acupoints

Acupoints were located according to a classic Chinese acupuncture technique called Tong Shen Cun (cun).

Table 3 Safe depths of 23 upper back acupoints of age groups

Points	4–6 y/o (n = 79) Mean ± S.D.	7–9 y/o (n = 45) Mean ± S.D.	10–12 y/o (n = 30) Mean ± S.D.	13–15 y/o (n = 56) Mean ± S.D.	16–18 y/o (n = 109) Mean ± S.D.	P value
GV9	19.31 ± 2.84	23.32 ± 6.17	27.20 ± 7.54	29.83 ± 8.04	31.83 ± 8.55	<0.001[a]
GV10	20.70 ± 3.62	23.64 ± 4.93	28.86 ± 6.12	29.88 ± 7.74	32.84 ± 8.31	<0.001[a]
GV11	22.14 ± 4.80	22.96 ± 4.52	27.70 ± 6.19	29.56 ± 7.56	31.71 ± 8.29	<0.001[a]
GV12	22.26 ± 4.54	25.93 ± 5.59	30.75 ± 7.58	32.40 ± 8.73	34.63 ± 10.16	<0.001[a]
GV13	23.02 ± 5.59	29.18 ± 7.70	35.75 ± 8.25	35.78 ± 7.99	38.26 ± 8.65	<0.001[a]
GV14	23.26 ± 4.95	26.57 ± 8.05	33.20 ± 9.48	37.83 ± 8.79	39.29 ± 9.54	<0.001[a]
BL11	24.93 ± 5.44	28.71 ± 8.00	31.29 ± 7.86	36.07 ± 10.53	36.01 ± 10.63	<0.001[a]
BL12	28.54 ± 8.50	32.57 ± 8.48	34.43 ± 8.24	37.74 ± 8.56	37.78 ± 8.33	<0.001[a]
BL13	24.82 ± 2.74	25.01 ± 3.00	26.53 ± 4.55	29.17 ± 7.57	30.68 ± 8.04	<0.001[a]
BL14	18.90 ± 2.66	21.35 ± 4.32	24.67 ± 6.53	26.42 ± 8.14	27.71 ± 8.48	<0.001[a]
BL15	20.94 ± 3.46	23.42 ± 4.57	24.45 ± 5.36	26.72 ± 6.45	27.65 ± 6.78	<0.001[a]
BL16	18.23 ± 2.76	21.12 ± 5.04	23.96 ± 5.37	25.32 ± 7.26	26.79 ± 7.50	<0.001[a]
BL17	19.14 ± 2.85	22.56 ± 4.03	25.60 ± 5.33	26.98 ± 6.76	28.33 ± 6.89	<0.001[a]
BL41	24.77 ± 3.51	25.32 ± 5.99	27.74 ± 6.44	33.75 ± 8.96	34.17 ± 9.95	<0.001[a]
BL42	21.97 ± 3.88	24.86 ± 5.50	28.20 ± 7.28	29.49 ± 8.15	31.30 ± 9.28	<0.001[a]
BL43	19.41 ± 3.74	21.92 ± 4.32	24.29 ± 6.19	25.60 ± 7.95	27.46 ± 8.14	<0.001[a]
BL44	15.21 ± 5.67	18.72 ± 5.42	19.68 ± 5.99	21.65 ± 7.61	22.99 ± 8.04	<0.001[a]
BL45	13.14 ± 3.39	15.84 ± 4.47	19.43 ± 6.47	20.26 ± 6.46	21.32 ± 7.53	<0.001[a]
BL46	12.74 ± 2.35	15.24 ± 3.58	19.34 ± 6.04	19.53 ± 6.45	21.01 ± 7.00	<0.001[a]
SI14	26.30 ± 6.29	30.88 ± 9.25	34.18 ± 10.28	40.32 ± 11.41	41.31 ± 11.91	<0.001[a]
SI15	26.92 ± 4.94	31.77 ± 7.65	39.52 ± 9.72	43.85 ± 12.10	43.17 ± 10.54	<0.001[a]
GB21	20.84 ± 3.25	23.70 ± 4.99	30.16 ± 9.14	28.94 ± 8.97	32.45 ± 10.06	<0.001[a]
SP21	16.97 ± 2.89	16.88 ± 2.18	19.89 ± 3.25	19.99 ± 4.44	21.34 ± 5.17	<0.001[a]

Unit of mean ± SD: mm
[a]Statistically significant

The back transverse Tong Shen Cun is one-sixth of the shortest distance between the two scapulae. The back vertical Tong Shen Cun is located using vertebral spinous processes. The safe depths of acupoints in the Governor Vessel (GV) are defined as the distance from the skin surface of the acupoint to the epidural layer. The safe depths of other acupoints in the upper back are defined as the distance from the skin surface of acupoints to the pleura.

Twenty-three back acupoints located in the GV, Bladder Meridian (BL), Small Intestine Meridian (SI), Gallbladder Meridian (GB) and Spleen Meridian (SP) were measured. Patients diagnosed with pneumothorax were measured on the healthy side of their backs. GV14, GV13, GV12, GV11, GV10, and GV9 were located at the central points between the spinous processes of C7 and T1, T1 and T2, T3 and T4, T5 and T6, T6 and T7, and T7 and T8, respectively. The BL was 1.5 and 3 cun lateral to the GV. For example, BL13 and BL42 were 1.5 and 3 cun lateral to the GV12. SI15 was 2 cun lateral to GV14 and SI14 was 3 cun lateral to GV13. GB21 was located at the midpoint of the line between the C7 and the lateral end of acromion. Sp21 was located at intersection of the sixth intercostal space and the midaxillary line (Fig. 1).

The CT machines used at CMUH were the Optima Speed CT Scanner (GE Healthcare, General Electric, USA), Optima CT660 (GE Healthcare) and Light Speed 16 CT Scanner (GE Healthcare). All CT images were captured in the transverse plane and body positions of all the participants were supine. The section thickness between each image was 5 mm. Safe depths were measured by examining the CT images on a Picture Archiving and Communication System (PACS) monitor (Realsync, Taiwan).

Statistical analysis

The safe depths of acupoints among different age, weight, and BMI groups were analyzed using a one-way analysis of variance. Student's t tests were used to compare the safe depths of acupoints between boys and girls. Multiple regression models were used to analyze

Table 4 Safe depths of 23 upper back acupoints in different weight groups

Points	<3rd (n = 32)	3–<85th (n = 215)	85–<97th (n = 42)	≥97th (n = 29)	P value
	Mean ± S.D.	Mean ± S.D.	Mean ± S.D.	Mean ± S.D.	
GV9	23.95 ± 5.74	26.00 ± 7.55	29.07 ± 9.61	32.00 ± 13.69	<0.001[a]
GV10	25.88 ± 5.85	26.45 ± 7.16	30.51 ± 8.18	34.18 ± 13.32	<0.001[a]
GV11	24.98 ± 5.10	26.41 ± 6.55	29.28 ± 8.97	34.25 ± 12.74	<0.001[a]
GV12	27.58 ± 6.53	28.12 ± 6.65	32.47 ± 9.81	38.48 ± 19.01	<0.001[a]
GV13	30.21 ± 8.23	31.25 ± 8.44	35.47 ± 9.16	40.42 ± 16.13	<0.001[a]
GV14	31.31 ± 9.68	31.66 ± 9.36	34.88 ± 12.04	38.63 ± 16.11	0.004[a]
BL11	29.99 ± 9.18	30.87 ± 8.57	33.96 ± 10.81	37.51 ± 16.68	0.003[a]
BL12	33.08 ± 9.92	33.58 ± 8.33	36.21 ± 8.89	39.23 ± 12.94	0.007[a]
BL13	26.25 ± 4.70	26.96 ± 4.99	29.26 ± 6.82	33.51 ± 12.84	<0.001[a]
BL14	21.86 ± 5.44	23.45 ± 6.48	25.99 ± 8.42	28.99 ± 12.37	<0.001[a]
BL15	22.86 ± 4.42	24.13 ± 5.20	27.28 ± 6.72	29.73 ± 10.12	<0.001[a]
BL16	21.36 ± 5.25	22.50 ± 5.90	25.42 ± 7.59	28.89 ± 10.86	<0.001[a]
BL17	22.23 ± 4.57	24.13 ± 6.07	26.70 ± 6.78	29.35 ± 9.86	<0.001[a]
BL41	26.45 ± 5.32	29.14 ± 7.03	31.83 ± 10.67	36.77 ± 15.45	<0.001[a]
BL42	24.59 ± 5.71	26.38 ± 6.55	29.53 ± 6.86	35.74 ± 15.50	<0.001[a]
BL43	22.17 ± 4.95	23.00 ± 5.34	26.11 ± 8.25	30.98 ± 13.86	<0.001[a]
BL44	17.10 ± 4.24	19.06 ± 6.13	22.28 ± 8.10	25.90 ± 13.45	<0.001[a]
BL45	15.01 ± 4.16	17.28 ± 5.57	20.52 ± 7.03	24.72 ± 11.74	<0.001[a]
BL46	15.41 ± 4.58	16.80 ± 4.87	20.12 ± 6.69	23.66 ± 12.14	<0.001[a]
SI14	31.64 ± 9.57	33.98 ± 9.68	37.57 ± 12.13	45.52 ± 20.78	<0.001[a]
SI15	35.12 ± 10.03	36.39 ± 10.09	38.22 ± 12.86	45.15 ± 18.52	0.001[a]
GB21	25.40 ± 9.45	26.32 ± 7.88	31.09 ± 9.68	33.27 ± 13.27	<0.001[a]
SP21	17.97 ± 4.26	18.83 ± 4.12	20.26 ± 4.15	22.46 ± 5.89	<0.001[a]

Unit of mean ± SD: mm
[a]Statistically significant

whether sex, age, weight, or BMI are relevant factors in determining the safe depths of acupoints. Statistical analyses were performed using the SPSS software package, Version 18.0 (SPSS Inc., Chicago, IL), and $p < 0.05$ was considered significant.

Results

A total of 319 patients (205 boys and 114 girls) aged 4 to 18 years were included in this study. The general characteristics of the patients are shown in Table 1.

The mean and standard deviation of the safe depths of boys and girls at 23 back acupoints are listed in Table 2. The shallowest and greatest depths of both sexes were at BL46 and SI15, respectively. Among the upper back acupoints, the deepest safe depth was 2.13 times in boys and 2.05 times in girls than the shallowest one. The safe depths of most back acupoints differed significantly between boys and girls, except BL42, BL44, BL45, BL46,

GB21 and SP21. All 23 acupoints in boys were deeper than in girls.

Safe depths significantly differed among age groups ($p < 0.001$; Table 3). Almost all safe depths significantly correlated with an increase in age. The safe depth was greater in those who are older.

Safe depths significantly differed between weight groups ($p < 0.01$; Table 4) and significantly increased with weight at all 23 acupoints. Safe depths among those weighing above the 97th percentile were between 1.19 (BL12) and 1.65 (BL45) times deeper than among those weighing below the third percentile.

Safe depths also significantly varied between BMI groups ($p < 0.05$; Table 5). An increase in BMI was significantly correlated with increased safe depth. Safe depths in the obese group were between 1.18 (BL12) and 1.47 (BL44) times deeper than in the underweight group.

Table 5 Safe depth of 23 upper back acupoints of BMI groups

Points	Underweight[a] (n = 52) Mean ± S.D.	Healthy weight[b] (n = 186) Mean ± S.D.	Overweight[c] (n = 18) Mean ± S.D.	Obesity[d] (n = 30) Mean ± S.D.	P value
GV9	24.40 ± 5.94	26.21 ± 7.73	29.42 ± 10.63	30.92 ± 12.99	0.003[e]
GV10	25.27 ± 5.47	26.75 ± 7.21	30.51 ± 8.62	33.58 ± 12.14	<0.001[e]
GV11	25.23 ± 5.02	26.38 ± 6.94	30.47 ± 8.26	33.40 ± 11.82	<0.001[e]
GV12	26.91 ± 5.80	28.54 ± 6.89	32.23 ± 9.25	36.78 ± 17.38	<0.001[e]
GV13	30.62 ± 7.26	31.61 ± 8.36	34.86 ± 9.39	38.70 ± 14.71	<0.001[e]
GV14	30.26 ± 9.19	31.84 ± 9.39	33.86 ± 13.01	38.80 ± 14.75	0.002[e]
BL11	30.25 ± 8.39	30.90 ± 8.96	33.94 ± 11.20	37.66 ± 15.18	0.003[e]
BL12	32.78 ± 9.13	33.86 ± 8.52	33.92 ± 8.54	38.57 ± 11.70	0.037[e]
BL13	26.09 ± 4.78	27.06 ± 4.89	28.94 ± 7.44	33.22 ± 12.10	<0.001[e]
BL14	22.72 ± 5.91	23.33 ± 6.60	26.68 ± 8.13	29.00 ± 11.85	<0.001[e]
BL15	22.62 ± 3.81	24.57 ± 5.35	26.70 ± 6.67	29.78 ± 9.61	<0.001[e]
BL16	21.98 ± 5.31	22.37 ± 6.17	26.30 ± 6.86	28.62 ± 10.07	<0.001[e]
BL17	23.21 ± 4.98	24.20 ± 6.00	26.35 ± 6.94	29.03 ± 9.72	<0.001[e]
BL41	27.33 ± 5.67	29.16 ± 7.41	32.41 ± 10.18	35.88 ± 14.86	<0.001[e]
BL42	25.42 ± 6.23	26.60 ± 6.51	30.06 ± 6.90	32.92 ± 13.70	<0.001[e]
BL43	21.98 ± 4.87	22.90 ± 5.56	27.11 ± 6.64	30.25 ± 13.17	<0.001[e]
BL44	17.59 ± 4.86	18.99 ± 6.29	23.29 ± 7.90	25.85 ± 12.07	<0.001[e]
BL45	15.98 ± 4.77	17.42 ± 5.63	21.73 ± 6.97	22.89 ± 11.49	<0.001[e]
BL46	16.15 ± 4.54	16.94 ± 5.00	19.67 ± 6.69	22.71 ± 11.53	<0.001[e]
SI14	32.40 ± 9.29	33.88 ± 9.94	39.87 ± 12.20	42.61 ± 18.58	<0.001[e]
SI15	35.25 ± 9.01	36.41 ± 10.49	39.54 ± 11.60	45.26 ± 18.02	<0.001[e]
GB21	26.43 ± 8.52	26.67 ± 8.11	31.23 ± 11.01	31.41 ± 12.84	0.012[e]
SP21	19.36 ± 4.86	18.76 ± 4.03	20.40 ± 4.55	20.68 ± 5.50	0.086

Unit of mean ± SD: mm
[a]Underweight: patients with BMI below the fifth percentile
[b]Healthy weight: patients with BMI from the 5th percentile up to the 85th percentile
[c]Overweight: patients with BMI from the 85th percentile up to the 95th percentile
[d]Obese: patients with BMI at or above the 95th percentile
[e]Statistically significant

We performed multiple regression models to analyze whether age, sex, weight, and BMI are relevant factors in determining the safe depths of acupoints. The results revealed that weight was significantly correlated with safe depth at all 23 acupoints. (Table 6) Thus, weight was the most crucial factor in determining the safe depths of upper back acupoints.

Discussion

Performing acupuncture on back acupoints has been demonstrated to be an effective alternative therapy for local myofascial pain [14, 15], asthma, allergic rhinitis [16], and tuberculosis consumptive diseases [17]. As the popularity of acupuncture increases, the importance of determining the safe depths of acupoints also increases, particularly the safe depths in the upper back. Acupuncture on the upper back may cause pleural and lung injuries [18, 19]. In pediatric groups, safe needling depths vary largely because of rapid changes in body size and shape. This study is the first to estimate the variations in the safe depths of upper back acupoints according to sex, age, weight, and BMI in children aged 4 to 18 years. We observed boys had deeper safe depth than girls. The safe depths were greater among older groups, heavier weight groups, and higher BMI groups.

The safe depths of all upper back acupoints in boys were deeper than in girls, and all such differences were significant, except at BL42, BL44, BL45, BL46, GB21 and SP21. Girls tend to accumulate more total body and subcutaneous fat, which is deposited mainly in the gynoid region and thigh during and after puberty. However, among boys, more fat is deposited in the upper segment of the body, both subcutaneously and intraabdominally, and more total lean and muscle mass is developed in this period [5, 20]. The greater amount of muscle mass and trunk fat among boys could explain this difference between the sexes, which has not been observed in studies on pediatric abdomen acupoints [10] or adult back acupoints [9].

Table 6 Multiple regression analysis for safe depths of 23 upper back acupoints

Points	Variables in multiple regression model			
	Age	Weight	BMI	Sex (male vs female)
	β (95 % CI)	β (95 % CI)	β (95 % CI)	β (95 % CI)
	P value	P value	P value	P value
GV9	−0.06 (−0.38–0.26) 0.716	0.33 (0.22–0.43) <0.001*	0.08 (−0.16–0.32) 0.527	−0.60 (−2.15–0.95) 0.446
GV10	−0.01 (−0.31–0.28) 0.927	0.28 (0.18–0.38) <0.001*	0.23 (0.01–0.45) 0.038*	−0.85 (−2.27–0.57) 0.241
GV11	−0.25 (−0.55–0.05) 0.100	0.31 (0.22–0.41) <0.001*	0.19 (−0.04–0.41) 0.098	−1.05 (−2.49–0.39) 0.152
GV12	−0.14 (−0.48–0.20) 0.412	0.34 (0.23–0.45) <0.001*	0.21 (−0.04–0.47) 0.101	−1.41 (−3.06–0.24) 0.093
GV13	0.27 (−0.07–0.60) 0.114	0.27 (0.16–0.38) <0.001*	0.27 (0.02–0.52) 0.035*	−0.82 (−2.45–0.81) 0.324
GV14	0.46 (0.05–0.86) 0.027*	0.26 (0.13–0.39) <0.001*	0.17 (−0.13–0.48) 0.261	−0.61 (−2.58–1.36) 0.544
BL11	−0.07 (−0.50–0.37) 0.757	0.29 (0.15–0.44) <0.001*	0.10 (−0.22–0.43) 0.531	1.34 (−0.78–3.46) 0.213
BL12	0.18 (−0.24–0.60) 0.395	0.19 (0.06–0.33) 0.005*	0.02(−0.30–0.33) 0.927	1.06 (−0.97–3.09) 0.304
BL13	−0.51 (−0.78–−0.24) <0.001*	0.31 (0.22–0.40) <0.001*	0.04 (−0.16–0.24) 0.700	−0.52 (−1.83–0.80) 0.442
BL14	−0.32 (−0.62–−0.01) 0.044*	0.32 (0.22–0.42) <0.001*	0.037 (−0.19–0.27) 0.755	−0.82 (−2.31–0.68) 0.284
BL15	−0.33 (−0.58–−0.09) 0.008*	0.25 (0.17–0.33) <0.001*	0.20 (0.01–0.38) 0.035*	−0.77 (−1.96–0.42) 0.201
BL16	−0.16 (−0.44–0.12) 0.253	0.24 (0.15–0.33) <0.001*	0.20 (−0.01–0.40) 0.065	−0.142 (−1.48–1.20) 0.835
BL17	−0.22 (−0.47–0.03) 0.078	0.29 (0.21–0.37) <0.001*	0.05 (−0.14–0.23) 0.609	−1.16 (−2.36–0.04) 0.057
BL41	−0.51 (−0.86–−0.16) 0.005*	0.43 (0.31–0.54) <0.001*	−0.08 (−0.35–0.19) 0.553	−1.14 (−2.86–0.57) 0.191
BL42	−0.32 (−0.64–−0.01) 0.046*	0.33 (0.23–0.44) <0.001*	0.06 (−0.17–0.30) 0.598	−1.69 (−3.23–−0.14) 0.032*
BL43	−0.32 (−0.62–−0.02) 0.036*	0.28 (0.19–0.38) <0.001*	0.13 (−0.09–0.36) 0.242	−0.97 (−2.42–0.47) 0.186
BL44	−0.36 (−0.68–−0.04) 0.026*	0.29 (0.18–0.39) <0.001*	0.138 (−0.10–0.38) 0.256	−1.62 (−3.17–−0.07) 0.040*
BL45	−0.40 (−0.67–−0.14) 0.003*	0.34 (0.25–0.42) <0.001*	0.00 (−0.20–0.20) 1.000	−2.25 (−3.53–−0.98) 0.001*
BL46	−0.31 (−0.55–−0.07) 0.012*	0.31 (0.23–0.38) <0.001*	−0.01 (−0.19–0.18) 0.938	−1.66 (−2.84–−0.47) 0.006*
SI14	−0.10 (−0.56–0.36) 0.674	0.41 (0.26–0.56) <0.001*	0.13 (−0.22–0.47) 0.473	0.03 (−2.21–2.27) 0.978
SI15	0.20 (−0.26–0.66) 0.383	0.34 (0.20–0.49) <0.001*	0.18 (−0.16–0.53) 0.300	−0.22 (−2.45–2.00) 0.846
GB21	−0.26 (−0.64–0.13) 0.189	0.39 (0.26–0.51) <0.001*	−0.17 (−0.46–0.12) 0.249	−2.12 (−3.99–−0.25) 0.026*
SP21	−0.04 (−0.24–0.16) 0.695	0.14 (0.08–0.21) <0.001*	−0.07 (−0.22–0.09) 0.389	−0.57 (−1.55–0.41) 0.254

*Statistically significant β regression coefficient, CI confidence interval

Safe depth significantly differed among age groups and was significantly correlated with an increase in age for nearly all acupoints. Age influences safe depths because muscle mass and subcutaneous adipose tissue increase with age [5] among children. However, age need not be considered when determining the safe depths in adults.

Safe depths significantly differed between weight groups and significantly increased with weight at all 23 acupoints. Thicker fat or muscle tissue layers in heavier children may explain this observation, which is compatible with the results of an adult study in which the safe depths of back acupoints were related to body size [9]. At BL42, BL44, BL45, and BL46, the safe depths of patients weighing above the 97th percentile were approximately 1.5–1.6 times the safe depths of those weighing below the third percentile. Clinicians should be aware of these weight-related differences and the risk of pneumothorax when performing acupuncture in this area of the body.

The BMI characterizes the relative proportion of child's weight and height percentile for age and sex. The BMI is the optimal clinical standard for diagnosing obesity in children and adolescents [21, 22]. We found that increasing BMI was significantly correlated with increased safe depths. At BL43, BL44, BL45, and BL46, the safe depths in the obesity group were approximately 1.4–1.5 times deeper than those in the underweight group. This result was similar to that in the weight group.

Multiple regression analysis revealed that weight was the most critical factor in determining the safe depths of upper back acupoints. Previous studies have observed that BMI percentile changes may not accurately reflect changes in adiposity in children, particularly among male adolescents and children with lower BMIs [23]. The BMI is limited in its usefulness in predicting adiposity by its inability to distinguish fat mass from lean body mass in pediatric populations. We used growth charts for Taiwanese children and adolescents [12, 13] for decreasing ethnic differences, but BMI was also influenced by age, sex and pubertal status [24]. This might explain why BMI was less crucial than weight in influencing safe depths in this study.

This study has three noteworthy strengths. First, the study included larger pediatric sample sizes. Second, we studied factors such as sex, age, weight, and BMI that influence safe depth. Finally, the study determined safe depths by examining in vivo CT images, a more accurate method than recording measurements from cadavers. Depths from cadavers are unreliable because the tissues dries and contracts after freezing, anticorrosive positioning, and dyeing processes.

This study has limitations. First, the study used a retrospective design. Second, the examined children were patients, not healthy children. However, to increase validity, patients with diseases that might have affected

the thickness of the subcutaneous tissues or muscles in their backs were excluded. Third, the sample size of the overweight group was small. Finally, this study was conducted in a single medical center, limiting its population generalizability.

Conclusions

This study determined that the safe depths of most upper back acupoints significantly differ between the sexes. Safe depths significantly differed among age groups and significantly increased with weight and BMI. Acupuncturists should consider wide variations in safe needling depth in the upper backs of children to balance treatment effects and complications.

Competing interests
The authors declare that they have no competing interests.

Authors' contributions
YCM designed the study and drafted the initial manuscript. JGL helped the study's conception, and reviewed and revised the manuscript. CTP helped to conduct the literature review and supervised the field activities, quality assurance and control. YCH designed the study's analytic strategy and conducted the data analysis. HYL helped to measure the depth of acupoints. All authors read and approved the final manuscript.

Author details
[1]Graduate Institute of Chinese Medicine, College of Chinese Medicine, China Medical University, Taichung, Taiwan, ROC. [2]Department of Pediatrics, Tai-An Hospital, Taichung, Taiwan. [3]Children's Hospital of China Medical University, Taichung, Taiwan, ROC. [4]School of Chinese Medicine, College of Chinese Medicine, China Medical University, Taichung, Taiwan, ROC. [5]Department of Medical Research, China Medical University Hospital, Taichung, Taiwan, ROC. [6]China Medical University, No.91, Xueshi Rd., North Dist., Taichung City 40402, Taiwan, ROC.

References
1. Libonate J, Evans S, Tsao JC. Efficacy of acupuncture for health conditions in children: a review. Sci World J. 2008;8:670–82.
2. Jindal V, Ge A, Mansky PJ. Safety and efficacy of acupuncture in children: a review of the evidence. J Pediatr Hematol Oncol. 2008;30(6):431–42.
3. Adams D, Cheng F, Jou H, Aung S, Yasui Y, Vohra S. The safety of pediatric acupuncture: a systematic review. Pediatrics. 2011;128(6):e1575–87.
4. He W, Zhao X, Li Y, Xi Q, Guo Y. Adverse events following acupuncture: a systematic review of the Chinese literature for the years 1956–2010. J Altern Complement Med. 2012;18(10):892–901.
5. Staiano AE, Katzmarzyk PT. Ethnic and sex differences in body fat and visceral and subcutaneous adiposity in children and adolescents. Int J Obes. 2012;36(10):1261–9.
6. Loomba-Albrecht LA, Styne DM. Effect of puberty on body composition. Curr Opin Endocrinol Diabetes Obes. 2009;16(1):10–5.
7. Lin JG, Chou PC, Chu HY. An exploration of the needling depth in acupuncture: the safe needling depth and the needling depth of clinical efficacy. Evid Based Complement Alternat Med. 2013;2013:740508.
8. Chou PC, Chu HY, Lin JG. Safe needling depth of acupuncture points. J Altern Complement Med. 2011;17(3):199–206.
9. Lin JG, She CY, Huang WS. [Detecting the safety depth on human back loci by computer tomographic scanning]. Zhong Xi Yi Jie He Za Zhi. 1991;11(1):10–3.

10. Chen HN, Lin JG, Yang AD, Chang SK. Safe depth of abdominal acupoints in pediatric patients. Complement Ther Med. 2008;16(6):331–5.

11. Chen HN, Lin JG, Ying LC, Huang CT, Lin CH. The therapeutic depth of abdominal acupuncture points approaches the safe depth in overweight and in older children. J Altern Complement Med. 2009;15(9):1033–7.

12. Chen W, Chang MH. New growth charts for Taiwanese children and adolescents based on World Health Organization standards and health-related physical fitness. Pediatr Neonatol. 2010;51(2):69–79.

13. Body mass index of children and adolescents. Health Promotion Administration, Ministry of Health and Welfare. 2013. http://www.hpa.gov.tw/BHPNet/Web/HealthTopic/TopicArticle.aspx?id=201308300012&parentid=201109290001.

14. Kung YY, Chen FP, Chaung HL, Chou CT, Tsai YY, Hwang SJ. Evaluation of acupuncture effect to chronic myofascial pain syndrome in the cervical and upper back regions by the concept of Meridians. Acupunct Electrother Res. 2001;26(3):195–202.

15. Chen L. [A new thinking of acupuncture and moxibustion treatment of shoulder pain after hemiplegia]. Zhongguo Zhen Jiu. 2006;26(9):669–71.

16. Zhou RL, Zhang JC. [An analysis of combined desensitizing acupoints therapy in 419 cases of allergic rhinitis accompanying asthma]. Zhongguo Zhong Xi Yi Jie He Za Zhi. 1997;17(10):587–9.

17. Guo YJ, Gu J, Liu LG. [Analysis on characteristics of ancient acupuncture and moxibustion treatment of tuberculosis consumptive diseases]. Zhongguo Zhen Jiu. 2005;25(2):135–7.

18. Tagami R, Moriya T, Kinoshita K, Tanjoh K. Bilateral tension pneumothorax related to acupuncture. Acupunct Med. 2013;31(2):242–4.

19. Inayama M, Shinohara T, Hino H, Yoshida M, Ogushi F. Chylothorax caused by acupuncture. Intern Med. 2011;50(20):2375–7.

20. Slyper AH. Childhood obesity, adipose tissue distribution, and the pediatric practitioner. Pediatrics. 1998;102(1):e4.

21. Force USPST. Screening and interventions for overweight in children and adolescents: recommendation statement. Pediatrics. 2005;116(1):205–9.

22. Reilly JJ. Assessment of obesity in children and adolescents: synthesis of recent systematic reviews and clinical guidelines. J Hum Nutr Diet. 2010;23(3):205–11.

23. Demerath EW, Schubert CM, Maynard LM, Sun SS, Chumlea WC, Pickoff A, et al. Do changes in body mass index percentile reflect changes in body composition in children? Data from the Fels Longitudinal Study. Pediatrics. 2006;117(3):e487–95.

24. Weber DR, Moore RH, Leonard MB, Zemel BS. Fat and lean BMI reference curves in children and adolescents and their utility in identifying excess adiposity compared with BMI and percentage body fat. Am J Clin Nutr. 2013;98(1):49–56.

25. Lin JG. Review on the history and practice of the needling depth of acupoints. 1st ed. Beitou: National Research Institute of Chinese Medicine; 2012.

7

Acupuncture for acute moderate thalamic hemorrhage

Chengwei Wang[1], Chao You[2], Lu Ma[2], Mengyue Liu[1], Meng Tian[2] and Ning Li[1*]

Abstract

Background: Thalamic hemorrhage (TH) is a neurological insult with a high rate of morbidity and mortality. Moderate TH (10–30 ml) accounts for more than half of all TH. Treatment remains controversial. The role of acupuncture in patients with moderate TH is not clear.

Methods: We will conduct a single-center, randomized, parallel group, and assessor-blinded clinical trial. A total of 488 patients with moderate TH will be randomly assigned to one of eight groups: 10–15 cc left sided TH study group ($N = 61$) and a corresponding control group ($N = 61$), 10–15 cc right sided TH study group ($N = 61$) and a corresponding control group, 15–30 cc left sided TH study group ($N = 61$) and a corresponding control group ($N = 61$), and 15–30 cc right sided TH study group ($N = 61$) and a corresponding control group. Study groups will receive acupuncture in addition to standard treatment, while control groups will receive standard treatment alone. The primary outcome will be change in National Institutes of Health Stroke Scale scores at 30 and 90 days after TH. The secondary outcomes will be death or major disability, defined as a score of 3 to 6 on the modified Rankin scale (in which a score of 0 indicates no symptoms, a score of 5 indicates severe disability, and a score of 6 indicates death) at 90-days, need for surgery at 30-days, Glasgow Outcome Scale (GOS) score at 90-days following TH onset, and the results of several additional group specific tests. The rate of adverse events will then be compared between the groups.

Discussion: This study will attempt to answer the question of whether or not acupuncture can improve neurologic outcome following moderate TH.

Trial registration: Chinese clinical trial registry (ChiCTR-IOR-16008362)

Keywords: Acupuncture, Intracranial hemorrhage, Moderate thalamic hemorrhage, RCT

Background

Spontaneous intracerebral hemorrhage (ICH), non-iatrogenic ICH without trauma, is the second most common and the most devastating form of all strokes with the poorest prognosis [1, 2]. Approximately 15% of all cases of spontaneous ICH occur in the thalamus [3–5]. The thalamus is a deep brain structure and is an important center for the transmission of neural signals [3, 6]. Due to its anatomical location and the vital functions that it performs, the decision of conservative or surgical management for TH remains controversial [2, 7, 8]. Management is influenced mainly by the clinical experience of the treating surgeon and the volume of the hematoma [9]. Patients with minor TH, especially volumes less than 10 cc, usually obtain favorable outcomes when treated with conservative measures. However, patients with major TH, greater than 30 cc, have mortality rates of more than 80%, no matter what treatment is selected [10]. Moderate TH (10–30 mL) constitutes more than half of all cases of TH, and these patients have a mortality rate of more than 30% [11]. As moderate TH is the most common form of TH, its prognosis carries the greatest weight in calculating the prognosis of all forms of TH. In patients with moderate TH, conservative

* Correspondence: zhenjiuhuaxi@163.com
[1]Department of Integrated Traditional and Western Medicine, West China Hospital, Sichuan University, Chengdu, China
Full list of author information is available at the end of the article

treatment alone versus surgical treatment is naturally a difficult decision to make. Because surgical treatment is invasive, adjacent structures may be damaged and neural pathways may be disrupted during surgical evacuation of a hematoma, thereby aggravating the degree of neurologic deficits or creating new ones. Meanwhile, conservative treatment alone does not offer the involved thalamic tissue the same type of relief that evacuation offers and is therefore felt to be a limited strategy in improving neurologic function. The limitations of both therapeutic strategies provide considerable room for better approaches or combinations of approaches.

Two recognized mechanisms of brain injury from ICH have been established [12, 13]. Primary injury happens at the time of initial hemorrhage when direct damage to brain tissue occurs either secondary to the hematoma itself or to its mass effect on surrounding brain tissue. Secondary injury happens at some time following initial hemorrhage and includes neuronal death from either the inflammatory response to the hematoma, the release of toxic materials and other cytokines, the breakdown of the brain blood barrier, apoptosis, or the development of edema. While the pathophysiology of ICH provides many potential approaches for its treatment, enlargement of the hematoma and the development of surrounding edema have been identified as major contributors to the high morbidity and mortality of ICH and have thus been the major focus of potential treatment strategies [14–17].

Acupuncture, one of the major branches of Traditional Chinese Medicine (TCM), has long been used to treat acute stroke, including hemorrhagic stroke, in China as well as in many other East Asian countries. Acupuncture's utility in the treatment of non-hemorrhagic stroke, which is now documented by the WHO (World Health Organization, 2002), has been widely researched [18]. In recent years, a number of studies using modern technologies have shown that acupuncture may have neuroprotective effects following hemorrhagic stroke as well [19–22]. One preclinical systematic review of 19 animal studies showed that GV20 (Baihui) based acupuncture can improve neurologic outcome by regulating the inflammatory response to a hematoma, inhibiting neuronal apoptosis, reducing cerebral edema, maintaining ATP supply, promoting nerve regeneration, maintaining neuronal membrane integrity, and promoting hematoma resorption [23]. In another animal study, acupuncture at the DU20 acupoint was reported to have a neuroprotective effect on cerebral hemorrhage by inhibiting Notch-Hes signaling in rat basal ganglia [24]. It has also been reported that electro-acupuncture treatment at the Zusanli (ST36) acupoint may accelerate ICH-induced angiogenesis via the up-regulation of the HIF-1α protein and therefore may enhance recovery following hemorrhagic cerebral injury [25]. A separate study confirmed that treatment at the

ST36 acupoint may aid recovery following central nervous system intracerebral hemorrhage in rats [26]. Although animal studies have led to progress in determining how acupuncture exerts its benefits in the treatment of acute hemorrhagic stroke, the determination of its clinical value remains incompletely assessed [27–30].

To our knowledge, no organized study has reported on the effects of acupuncture in patients with acute moderate TH. Specifically, no prior study has examined whether or not the use of acupuncture combined with conventional treatments improves the prognosis of moderate TH patients compared to conventional treatments alone.

Methods/Design

Aims

We hypothesize that the addition of acupuncture to conventional treatments will improve neurological prognosis in TH patients. To test this hypothesis, we will compare study and control groups created based on the size and side of the TH. The study groups will receive acupuncture in addition to standard treatments, while the control groups will receive standard treatments alone.

Study design

This study will be a single-center, randomized, placebo-controlled, parallel group, and patient-assessor-blinded clinical trial. After completing informed consent, 488 eligible patients will be recruited and randomized to one of eight groups: 10–15 cc left sided TH study group ($N = 61$) and a corresponding control group ($N = 61$), 10–15 cc right sided TH study group ($N = 61$) and a corresponding control group, 15–30 cc left sided TH study group ($N = 61$) and a corresponding control group ($N = 61$), and 15–30 cc right sided TH study group ($N = 61$) and a corresponding control group. The patients in each of the study groups will receive 36 sessions of Chinese acupuncture in addition to standard treatments for TH, which include anticonvulsant therapy, antihypertensives, osmotic diuretics for the management of intracranial pressure, and invasive treatments as necessary. The patients in each of the control groups will receive standard treatments only. Patients' neurologic status will be assessed at baseline and at the end of treatment as well as at 30 day and 90 day follow-up intervals. CT imaging will be performed on admission and at 90 days follow up. All patients will be required to complete written informed consent prior to enrollment. If patients are unable to complete written informed consent, it will be obtained from their relatives. A flow chart demonstrating an outline of the study is included in Fig. 1.

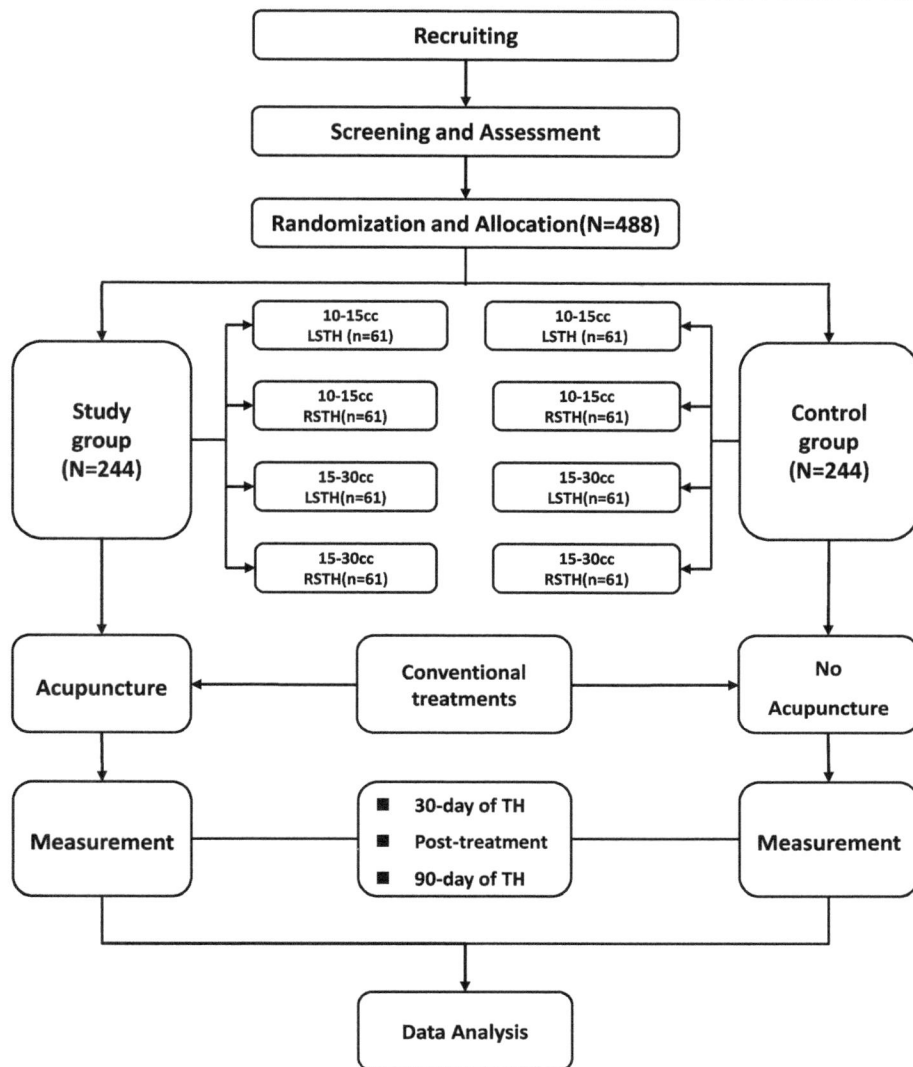

Fig. 1 The flow chart. Patients in acupuncture group will receive 36 sessions acupuncture treatment, 6 days a weeks for 6 weeks, in addition to conventional treatments and patients in control group will receive conventional TH treatments only. LSTH, left-sided thalamic hemorrhage; RSTH, right-sided thalamic hemorrhage

Study setting
This study will be conducted on a neurosurgery unit in Sichuan University's West China (Hua Xi) Hospital in Chengdu, China. With 4300 beds and more than 300 surgical operations per day, the hospital is one of the largest in China. The neurosurgery department is the largest in southwest China, with 181 surgical beds, 100 beds for rehabilitation and/or postoperative recovery, and more than 3800 craniotomies performed per year.

Ethics
This trial will be carried out in accordance with the ethical standards described in the 2013 updated Declaration of Helsinki. The study was approved by the West China Hospital, Sichuan University clinical research and

biomedical ethics committees (ethics reference: 2016-044). Written and signed informed consent will be obtained from all participants prior to their inclusion in the study. This trial has also been registered on www.chictr.org.cn (ChiCTR-IOR-16008362) and will be reported in compliance with the CONSORT statement (www.consort-statement.org) [31] as well as STRICTA (Standards for Reporting Interventions in Clinical Trials of Acupuncture) [32].

Participants
Patients with moderate TH will be recruited from the neurosurgery unit at Huaxi Hospital in China. The diagnosis of TH and the side of the hemorrhage will be determined based on computer tomography. TH volume

will be calculated by the neurosurgeon for all patients. Patients who meet eligibility criteria will be enrolled in the study, and written informed consent will be obtained prior to their enrollment.

Subject enrollment

The nurses responsible for the neurosurgery patients at Huaxi Hospital will be thoroughly educated regarding moderate TH. Patients and/or their legal guardians will be able to contact the project leader at any time should they desire additional information. After obtaining signed informed consent, the project leader will collect certain baseline information (including age, diagnosis, side of hemorrhage (left or right), hematoma volume, medical history, CT report, etc..) and determine whether or not the patient meets the eligibility criteria for the trial or not. Only participants who meet the inclusion criteria and do not possess any of the exclusion criteria will be enrolled. A total of 488 patients with TH who are admitted to the neurosurgical unit of our hospital will be enrolled in the trial.

Randomization and blinding

Randomization of subjects to the study and control groups will be computer-generated, using the Package for Encyclopaedia Medical Statistics 3.1 (PEMS 3.1) software. Stratified block randomization will not be performed. Concealed allocation will be achieved by having an assigned researcher not to have any contact with patients. Group assignments will be placed in opaque sealed envelopes. Subjects with 10–15 cc left TH, 10–15 cc right TH, 15–30 cc left TH, and 15–30 cc right TH will thus be assigned to either an acupuncture plus conventional treatment group or a conventional treatment alone group, in a 1:1 ratio based on the size and side of their hemorrhage. The primary researchers will be blinded to the type of intervention that each patient has received. The acupuncture practitioners will not provide any clues regarding group assignments to either the researchers or to the statistician.

Inclusion criteria

Patients with ICH who meet the following inclusion criteria will be enrolled in the trial:

(1) First ever TH verified by computer tomography (CT)
(2) Moderate TH (10 ~ 30 ml);
(3) Unilateral primary TH;
(4) Hematoma originating and confined to the thalamus;
(5) Age between 18 and 70 years;
(6) Acupuncture treatment can be applied within 72 h after TH;
(7) Voluntarily willing to sign informed consent.
(8) Right handed.

(9) All bleeding has stopped at the time of acupuncture initiation.

Exclusion criteria

Patients meeting any of the following criteria will be excluded from the study:

(1) Traumatic TH;
(2) Bilateral TH;
(3) Hematoma originates in another location and extends to the thalamus or hematoma originates in the thalamus and extends beyond the thalamus;
(4) Other areas of cerebral infarction, cerebral hemorrhage, or tumor on admission CT/MRI;
(5) Unable to determine the location of the origin of the hematoma on admission CT;
(6) Minor TH (<10 ml) or major TH (>30 ml);
(7) Heart, liver, or renal failure;
(8) Refusal to sign written informed consent;
(9) Unable to undergo randomized enrollment.
(10) Left handed.
(11) Continued bleeding at the time of acupuncture administration.

Procedure

Eligible patients will be randomized to either study groups (acupuncture plus conventional treatment) or control groups (conventional treatment alone) based on the size and side of their TH. After successful randomization, neurological assessments will occur at four time points: before treatment sessions begin, 30 days after onset of TH, at the end of treatment (6 weeks), and 90 days after onset of TH.

Intervention

Participants in both groups will receive conventional Western medical treatments as recommended by the guidelines for the management of spontaneous intracerebral hemorrhage including blood pressure management, ICP monitoring, appropriate prophylaxis, and surgical treatment as necessary for life-threatening hemorrhages [2]. In addition to conventional treatment, patients in the study group will receive 36 sessions (once a day, 6 days a week for 6 weeks) of acupuncture.

Acupuncture

Acupuncture treatment will be started within 72 h after TH onset, and applied once a day, 6 days a week for 6 weeks (a total of 36 sessions). The sessions will be performed by an experienced acupuncture doctor with over 10 years of working experience and 7 years of acupuncture training. This doctor will also receive training prior to the start of the trial. The acupuncture protocol was designed by a Sichuan University Huaxi Hospital professor with more than 25 years of practical experience, in accordance with guidelines from published papers and clinical experience. It will follow the Standards for Reporting Interventions in Clinical Trials for Acupuncture 2010 checklist, as shown in Table 1. Acupuncture points are identified by the point location method as described by the World Health Organization (WHO standard) [33].

Both scalp and body acupuncture will be performed in this trial. The parameters for scalp acupuncture will be as follows: two or three needles penetrating through the top midline, the motor region of the affected side, and the sensory region on the side of the lesion. The acupoints on the affected side of the body only and not on the contralateral side will be as follows: LI15 (Jian Yu), LI11 (Qu Chi), SJ5 (Wai Guan), and LI4 (He Gu) in the upper extremity; ST34 (Liang Qiu), ST36 (Zu San Li), GB34 (Yang Ling Quan), SP6 (San Yin Jiao), and LV3 (Tai Chong) in the lower extremity (Table 1). Additional acupoints will be added as follows: RN23 (Lian Quan), bilateral GB20 (Feng Chi), and ST9 (Ren Ying) for dysphagia; ST6 (Jia Che) and ST5 (Di Cang) on the affected side for facial paralysis (Table 2).

Stimulation will be applied to both the scalp and body acupoints until the patient experiences de qi (obtains qi). A patient's experience of de qi may take on multiple unique manifestations at the needle site itself and/or around the site of needle manipulation including soreness, aching, numbness, tingling, and even warmth.

Huatuo brand needles (size 0.25 mm × 40 mm) made by Suzhou Medical Appliances in Suzhou, Jiangsu province, China, will be used to perform the acupuncture treatments. Electrical stimulation of acupuncture needles will be done at low frequency (1–3 Hz) in order to ensure patient comfort.

Control group

Subjects in the control groups will not receive acupuncture treatments. They will receive conventional TH treatments only. Control group participants will then be assessed neurologically at each follow-up visit.

Table 1 Acupoints to be used in the study

Acupoint	Location	Major indication and function
MS 5 (Dingzhonxian)	At the top of the head, along the middle line of the head, connecting DU 20 to DU 21.	Prolapse, sacral and lumbar problems, paralysis, cortical polyuria, gastroptosis, hyperostosis, hypertension
MS 6 (Dingnieqianxiexian)	1 cun anterior from DU 20 to GB 6.	Treats motor function disorders
MS 7 (Dingniehouxiexian)	1 cun posterior to MS6, from DU 20 to GB 7.	Treats sensory function disorders
LI15 (Jian Yu)	On the shoulder girdle, in the depression between the anterior end of the lateral border of the acromion and the greater tubercle of the humerus.	Shoulder pain, paralysis
LI11 (Qu Chi)	On the lateral aspect of the elbow, at the midpoint of the line connecting LU5 with the lateral epicondyle of the humerus.	Upper extremity palsies, relaxes and strengthens tendons
SJ5 (Wai Guan)	On the posterior aspect of the forearm, at the midpoint of the interosseous space between the radius and the ulna, 2 B-cun proximal to the dorsal wrist crease.	Tinnitus, paralysis of the arms, upper extremity pain;
LI4 (He Gu)	On the dorsum of the hand, in the depression radial and proximal to the second metacarpophalangeal joint.	Spasm in the fingers
ST34 (Liang Qiu)	On the anterolateral aspect of the thigh, between the vastus lateralis muscle and the lateral border of the rectus femoris tendon, 2 B-cun superior to the base of the patella.	Gastrospasm, leg muscle atrophy
ST36 (Zu San Li)	On the anterior aspect of the leg, on the line connecting ST35 with ST41, 3 B-cun inferior to ST35.	Constipation or diarrhea, paralysis of the lower limbs
GB34 (Yang Ling Quan)	On the fibular aspect of the leg, in the depression anterior and distal to the head of the fibula.	Inhibited ability to flex and stretch
SP6 (San Yin Jiao)	On the tibial aspect of the leg, posterior to the medial border of the tibia, 3 B-cun superior to the prominence of the medial Malleolus.	Irregular menstruation, paralysis of the lower limbs
LV3 (Tai Chong)	On the dorsum of the foot, between the first and second metatarsal bones, in the depression distal to the junction of the bases of the two bones, over the dorsalis pedis artery.	Hypertension, paralysis

Table 2 Interventions details according to Standards for Reporting Interventions in Clinical Trials of Acupuncture (STRICTA) guidelines

Item	Detail	Detail response
1. Acupuncture rationale (Explanations and examples)	1a) Style of acupuncture (e.g. Traditional Chinese Medicine, Japanese, Korean, Western medical, Five Element, ear acupuncture, etc)	Traditional needle acupuncture
	1b) Reasoning for treatment provided, based on historical context, literature sources, and/or consensus methods, with references where appropriate	Selected traditional acupuncture points in the 12 meridian system and scalp points based on literature review and clinical experience
	1c) Extent to which treatment was varied	No variation
2. Details of needling (Explanations and examples)	2a) Number of needle insertions per subject per session (mean and range where relevant)	13–19 insertions per session
	2b) Names (or location if no standard name) of points used (uni/bilateral)	Scalp points: motor region and sensory region, unilateral on the side of the lesion Acupoints on limbs:LI15 (Jian Yu), LI11 (Qu Chi), SJ5 (Wai Guan), LI4 (He Gu), ST34 (Liang Qiu), ST36 (Zu San Li), GB34 (Yang Ling Quan), SP6 (San Yin Jiao), LV3 (Tai Chong),all unilateral on the affected side Modification: for dysphagia, GB20 (Feng Chi), RN23 (Lian Quan), and ST9 (Ren Ying); for facial paralysis, ST6 (Jia Che) and ST5 (Di Cang), unilateral on the affected side
	2c) Depth of insertion, based on a specified unit of measurement, or on a particular tissue level	Depth of needle insertion is at least 5 to 10 mm
	2d) Response sought (e.g. *de qi* or muscle twitch response)	De-qi sensation felt by practitioner and subject
	2e) Needle stimulation (e.g. manual, electrical)	Manual
	2f) Needle retention time	30 min
	2 g) Needle type (diameter, length, and manufacturer or material)	Needles: 0.25×40 mm, stainless steel (Huatuo brand, made by Suzhou Medical Appliances, China)
3. Treatment regimen (Explanations and examples)	3a) Number of treatment sessions	36 sessions
	3b) Frequency and duration of treatment sessions	6 times per week, interval of 1 day between sessions
4. Other components of treatment (Explanations and examples)	4a) Details of other interventions administered to the acupuncture group (e.g. moxibustion, cupping, herbs, exercises, lifestyle advice)	None
	4b) Setting and context of treatment, including instructions to practitioners, and information and explanations to patients	The same practitioner will treat every subject every session at the patient's bedside
5. Practitioner background (Explanations and examples)	5) Description of participating acupuncturists (qualification or professional affiliation, years in acupuncture practice, other relevant experience)	Licensed Traditional Chinese medicine doctor at Huaxi Hospital of Sichuan University with more than 10 years of acupuncture treatment experience
6. Control or comparator interventions (Explanations and examples)	6a) Rationale for the control or comparator in the context of the research question, with sources that justify this choice	No acupuncture will be performed on the control group
	6b) Precise description of the control or comparator. If sham acupuncture or any other type of acupuncture-like control is used, provide details as for Items 1 to 3 above.	No sham acupuncture will be performed on the control group

Dropout criteria

Participants who meet any of the following criteria will be removed from the study: (1) study group subjects who miss more than three sessions (out of a total of 36) of acupuncture; (2) patients who withdraw their consent; (3) patients who experience severe adverse events making their further inclusion in the trial unsustainable; (4) patients whose neurological condition deteriorates making it difficult for them to continue participating in the trial; (5) patients who experience decompensation related to accompanying and/or additional diseases; or (6) patients whose further participation in the trial is felt to be impossible as determined by the principal investigator.

Outcome measures

Primary outcome measure

The primary outcome measure will be NIHSS score, a measure of neurological status, at the end of treatment, at 30 days after TH, and at 90 days after TH. NIHSS is used to describe neurological deficits in stroke patients, and it strongly predicts the likelihood of a patient's recovery after stroke. The NIHSS is comprised of 11 test items including level of consciousness, gaze, visual field defects, facial palsy, upper extremity motor, lower extremity motor, limb ataxia, sensory ability, language, dysphagia, and neglect. Total score ranges from 0 to 42, with scores above 25 indicating very severe neurological impairment, scores of 5 to 24 indicating moderately severe to severe impairment, and scores below 5 indicating mild impairment.

Secondary outcome measures

Secondary outcome measures are as follows:

1. Poor outcome, defined as death or major disability, is defined as a score of 3 to 6 on the modified Rankin scale at 90 days after onset of TH. Scores on the modified Rankin scale range from 0 to 6, with a score of zero indicating no symptoms; a score of five indicating severe disability, confinement to bed, or incontinence; and a score of six indicating death.
2. The rate of surgery at 30 days is defined as the incidence of neurological deterioration requiring surgical intervention.
3. The Glasgow Outcome Scale (GOS) at 90 days after onset of TH is a measure of long-term outcome and includes five grades: 5, good recovery; 4, moderate disability; 3, severe disability; 2, persistent vegetative state; and 1, death.
4. The Barthel activities of daily living (ADL) index and the Rivermead Mobility Index will be performed on

each patient at the end of treatment, at 30 days after TH, and at 90 days after TH.
5. Patients with left thalamic hemorrhages will also be evaluated with several language tests including the Boston Naming Test, the Boston Diagnostic Aphasia Exam, the Western Aphasia Battery, and the Mount Wilga High Level Language Screening Test at the end of treatment, at 30 days after TH, and at 90 days after TH.
6. Patients with right thalamic hemorrhages will also be evaluated for visual neglect with the Behavioral In-attention Test (BIT) at the end of treatment, at 30 days after TH, and at 90 days after TH.

Safety evaluation

Any adverse events or abnormalities will be recorded on case report forms no matter what intervention is used. The severity of such adverse events will be described as mild, moderate, or severe, and the relation of the events to the intervention will be evaluated as not related, possibly related, or related. If any serious adverse events occur as the result of a certain intervention, that intervention will be stopped immediately and appropriate corrective action will be taken. Any serious adverse events will be reported promptly to the institutional review board, according to the protocol.

Sample size calculation

Using the variable NIHSS score, the primary outcome measure of the study, PS Power and Sample Size software (version 3.0) was used to determine an appropriate sample size for the study. In a previous study, NIHSS scores in each subject group exhibited a normal distribution with a standard deviation of 4.2 points [11]. This assumes a difference of 2.3 points between the groups, as shown in a previous study on moderate TH. A sample size of 488 provides 80% power ($\alpha = 0.05$) to detect a beneficial effect of early acupuncture therapy on the primary outcome, assuming a 10% non-adherence to treatment and a 3% loss to follow-up.

Statistical analysis

The results will be presented as mean score plus or minus standard deviation and as percentages. Categorical data will be analyzed with Fisher's exact test or the Mann-Whitney U test where appropriate. Continuous data will be analyzed with the Student's t test or Pearson's test where appropriate. Multi-ranked data will be analyzed using the Mann-Whitney U test. Differences will be considered statistically significant at $P < 0.05$ (two-tailed). All statistical analyses will be performed using the Statistical Package for the Social Sciences (version 13.0; SPSS; Chicago, Illinois, USA).

Discussion

In this randomized controlled trial, we will observe the effect of acupuncture therapy on patients with acute TH. The findings of this project are expected to provide evidence for the efficacy of acupuncture in improving the prognosis of patients with moderate TH. To minimize bias, stratified block randomization will be used according to sex and age, and the outcomes reviewer will be blinded. Subjects will be treated alone in a treatment room in order to avoid any communication with other subjects.

Generally speaking, no ideal placebo-controlled acupuncture trials have been performed previously [34]. Because recent acupuncture trials have examined so-called sham acupuncture techniques, including: needling of acupuncture points through non-penetrating needles, needling of non-acupuncture points, and needling of acupuncture points that are not indicated for that specific condition, these prior trials have not accurately reflected TCM theory and therefore have not properly assessed it [34]. Further complicating things is that sham acupuncture has been shown to have some efficacy [35]. In China, many patients and their families have had acupuncture at some time in their lives or are at least familiar with the acupuncture process. Therefore, it would be difficult to design a trial assessing the utility of sham acupuncture versus real acupuncture while keeping the patient blinded.

The decision was made to examine patients with left sided TH separately from patients with right sided TH. In the majority of patients, Broca's cortical area and Wernicke's cortical area are located in the left hemisphere. Therefore, patients with left hemisphere stroke (ischemic or hemorrhagic) are at risk for language deficits. Similarly, patients with right sided insults are at risk for symptoms of visual neglect. Both language deficits and visual neglect can have a profound impact on the way a patient responds to treatment and rehabilitation of other neurologic deficits. Therefore, to account for the potentially confounding effects of language deficits and visual neglect respectively, patients were subdivided into right and left TH subgroups.

Along the same lines, not all patients have their language centers located in their left hemisphere. While the majority of left handed patients have their language centers in the left hemisphere, some do have them in the right hemisphere. Therefore, in this study, we have only included right handed patients.

Another potentially confounding factor is the involvement of adjacent brain tissue as a secondary result of the initial thalamic insult. Adjacent brain tissue can necrose either directly via extension of the thalamic bleed or indirectly via mass effect from the thalamic bleed and/or edema related to the thalamic bleed. Areas at specifically high risk include the genu of the internal capsule which lies lateral to the thalamus, the posterior limb of the internal capsule which lies posterolateral to the thalamus, the anterior limb of the internal capsule which lies anterolateral to the thalamus, and the peri-thalamic/peri-ventricular white matter which lies superior to the thalamus. Involvement of the genu of the internal capsule, the posterior limb of the internal capsule, and adjacent white matter could result in paralysis. Involvement of the posterior limb of the internal capsule could also result in sensory loss or impaired comprehension [36]. Finally, involvement of the anterior limb of the internal capsule could result in cognitive issues. Involvement of any of these areas could potentially impact how a patient recovers and/or sway the post-stroke assessment scores in one direction or another depending on how many of the affected patients ended up in the control group or the intervention group. To combat this, we utilized two mechanisms. First, we excluded patients from the study whose TH on admission CT demonstrated extension of the insult beyond the thalamus. However, admission CT often does not disclose the true area affected by the insult. CT performed 90 days later is much more sensitive in demonstrating the insult's true encompassment. We therefore further subdivided the groups by size. While all subjects in the study have moderate thalamic hemorrhage, groups were further subdivided into subjects with 10–15 cc of TH and 15–30 cc of TH. Patients with 10–15 cc of TH are much less likely to experience insults to brain tissue external to the thalamus than patients with 15–30 cc of TH as a result of the smaller size of the initial bleed. We also plan to retrospectively analyze the results of CT scans performed 90 days following the insult to determine what percent of patients in each group experienced extension of their primary insult to tissue beyond the thalamus and how this may have affected the results in that group. After dividing patients by side of hemorrhage and size of hemorrhage four intervention groups were established, and along with the corresponding four control groups, this totaled eight distinct subject groups.

Previous research has demonstrated that patients with hand paresis only following stroke may not only be the most likely to benefit from acupuncture therapy but also the most likely to experience complete resolution of their neurologic symptoms [37]. As a result, it is important, if able, to determine the results of our intervention in patients with hand paresis only. As only patients with moderate thalamic hemorrhage will be enrolled in this trial, it is unlikely that our study will include many, if any, subjects with hand paresis only. However, if there are subjects with hand paresis, the results of our intervention will be analyzed retrospectively following conclusion of the trial.

The primary outcome measure is NIHSS result. While the NIHSS is a fine test, its comprehensiveness is somewhat lacking. In fact, previous studies examining interventions in stroke patients may have failed due to their sole reliance on the NIHSS as an outcome measure [38]. Therefore, additional tests measuring paralysis, language, visual neglect, and stroke outcome were also included in this study.

Under strict quality control, this trial will attempt to answer the question of whether or not acupuncture can improve neurologic outcome following moderate TH.

Trial status

Recruitment commenced in January 2017, and it is anticipated that the trial will be completed by March 2021.

Funding
None.

Authors' contributions
CWW participated in study design and drafted this protocol. CY and NL contributed to the conception of the study. NL was responsible for the standardization of acupuncture therapy. LM will screen the potential subjects. MYL revised the manuscript and will finish acupuncture manipulation. MT will independently assess the effect and the safety of the intervention. All of the authors have read and approved the final version of the manuscript.

Competing interests
The authors declare that they have no competing interests.

Author details
[1]Department of Integrated Traditional and Western Medicine, West China Hospital, Sichuan University, Chengdu, China. [2]Neurosurgery, West China Hospital, Sichuan University, Chengdu, China.

References
1. Lee SH, Park KJ, Kang SH, Jung YG, Park JY, Park DH. Prognostic Factors of Clinical Outcomes in Patients with Spontaneous Thalamic Hemorrhage. Med Sci Monit. 2015;21:2638–46.
2. Hemphill 3rd JC, Greenberg SM, Anderson CS, Becker K, Bendok BR, Cushman M, Fung GL, Goldstein JN, Macdonald RL, Mitchell PH, et al. Guidelines for the Management of Spontaneous Intracerebral Hemorrhage: A Guideline for Healthcare Professionals From the American Heart Association/American Stroke Association. Stroke. 2015;46(7):2032–60.
3. Broderick J, Connolly S, Feldmann E, Hanley D, Kase C, Krieger D, Mayberg M, Morgenstern L, Ogilvy CS, Vespa P, et al. Guidelines for the management of spontaneous intracerebral hemorrhage in adults: 2007 update: a guideline from the American Heart Association/American Stroke Association Stroke Council, High Blood Pressure Research Council, and the Quality of Care and Outcomes in Research Interdisciplinary Working Group. Circulation. 2007;116(16):e391–413.
4. Greenberg M, Arredondo N. Handbook of neurosurgery. 6th ed. New York: Thieme; 2006.
5. van Asch CJ, Luitse MJ, Rinkel GJ, van der Tweel I, Algra A, Klijn CJ. Incidence, case fatality, and functional outcome of intracerebral haemorrhage over time, according to age, sex, and ethnic origin: a systematic review and meta-analysis. Lancet Neurol. 2010;9(2):167–76.
6. Gaab MR. Intracerebral hemorrhage (ICH) and intraventricular hemorrhage (IVH): improvement of bad prognosis by minimally invasive neurosurgery. World Neurosurg. 2011;75(2):206–8.
7. Kanno T, Sano H, Shinomiya Y, Katada K, Nagata J, Hoshino M, Mitsuyama F. Role of surgery in hypertensive intracerebral hematoma: a comparative study of 305 nonsurgical and 154 surgical cases. J Neurosurg. 1984;61(6):1091–9.
8. Nakano T, Ohkuma H. Surgery versus conservative treatment for intracerebral haemorrhage—is there an end to the long controversy? Lancet. 2005;365(9457):361–2.
9. Cho DY, Chen CC, Lee HC, Lee WY, Lin HL. Glasgow Coma Scale and hematoma volume as criteria for treatment of putaminal and thalamic intracerebral hemorrhage. Surg Neurol. 2008;70(6):628–33.
10. Mori S, Sadoshima S, Ibayashi S, Fujishima M, Iino K. Impact of thalamic hematoma on six-month mortality and motor and cognitive functional outcome. Stroke. 1995;26(4):620–6.
11. Chen M, Wang Q, Zhu W, Yin Q, Ma M, Fan X, Li Y, Ni G, Liu C, Liu W, et al. Stereotactic aspiration plus subsequent thrombolysis for moderate thalamic hemorrhage. World Neurosurg. 2012;77(1):122–9.
12. Keep RF, Hua Y, Xi G. Intracerebral haemorrhage: mechanisms of injury and therapeutic targets. Lancet Neurol. 2012;11(8):720–31.
13. Xi G, Keep RF, Hoff JT. Mechanisms of brain injury after intracerebral haemorrhage. Lancet Neurol. 2006;5(1):53–63.
14. Aronowski J, Zhao X. Molecular pathophysiology of cerebral hemorrhage: secondary brain injury. Stroke. 2011;42(6):1781–6.
15. Gebel JM, Jauch EC, Brott TG, Khoury J, Sauerbeck L, Salisbury S, Spilker J, Tomsick TA, Duldner J, Broderick JP. Relative Edema Volume Is a Predictor of Outcome in Patients With Hyperacute Spontaneous Intracerebral Hemorrhage. Stroke. 2002;33(11):2636–41.
16. Qureshi AI, Mendelow AD, Hanley DF. Intracerebral haemorrhage. Lancet. 2009;373(9675):1632–44.
17. Mehdiratta M, Kumar S, Hackney D, Schlaug G, Selim M. Association between serum ferritin level and perihematoma edema volume in patients with spontaneous intracerebral hemorrhage. Stroke. 2008;39(4):1165–70.
18. World Health Organization. Acupuncture: review and analysis of reports on controlled clinical trials. Geneva; 2002.
19. Chen F, Qi Z, Luo Y, Hinchliffe T, Ding G, Xia Y, Ji X. Non-pharmaceutical therapies for stroke: mechanisms and clinical implications. Prog Neurobiol. 2014;115:246–69.
20. He T, Zhu W, Du SQ, Yang JW, Li F, Yang BF, Shi GX, Liu CZ. Neural mechanisms of acupuncture as revealed by fMRI studies. Auton Neurosci. 2015;190:1–9.
21. Chen JC. The effects of acupuncture and traditional Chinese medicines on apoptosis of brain tissue in a rat intracerebral hemorrhage model. Physiol Behav. 2015;151:421–5.
22. Litscher G. Ten years evidence-based high-tech acupuncture—a short review of peripherally measured effects. Evid Based Complement Alternat Med. 2009;6(2):153–8.
23. Li HQ, Li JH, Liu AJ, Ye MY, Zheng GQ. GV20-based acupuncture for animal models of acute intracerebral haemorrhage: a preclinical systematic review and meta-analysis. Acupunct Med. 2014;32(6):495–502.
24. Zou W, Chen QX, Sun XW, Chi QB, Kuang HY, Yu XP, Dai XH. Acupuncture inhibits Notch1 and Hes1 protein expression in the basal ganglia of rats with cerebral hemorrhage. Neural Regen Res. 2015;10(3):457–62.
25. Luo JK, Zhou HJ, Wu J, Tang T, Liang QH. Electroacupuncture at Zusanli (ST36) accelerates intracerebral hemorrhage-induced angiogenesis in rats. Chin J Integr Med. 2013;19(5):367–73.
26. Cho NH, Lee JD, Cheong BS, Choi DY, Chang HK, Lee TH, Shin MC, Shin MS, Lee J, Kim CJ. Acupuncture suppresses intrastriatal hemorrhage-induced apoptotic neuronal cell death in rats. Neurosci Lett. 2004;362(2):141–5.
27. Sun F, Wang J, Wen X. Acupuncture in stroke rehabilitation: Literature retrieval based on international databases. Neural Regen Res. 2012;7(15):1192.
28. Wu HM, Tang JL, Lin XP, Lau J, Leung PC, Woo J, Li Y. Acupuncture for stroke rehabilitation. Cochrane Database Syst Rev. 2006;3.

29. Ernst E, Lee MS. Acupuncture during stroke rehabilitation. Stroke. 2010;41(8): e549.

30. Zhuang L, He J, Zhuang X, Lu L. Quality of reporting on randomized controlled trials of acupuncture for stroke rehabilitation. BMC Complement Altern Med. 2014;14(1):1.

31. Schulz KF, Altman DG, Moher D, Group C. CONSORT 2010 Statement: updated guidelines for reporting parallel group randomised trials. BMC Med. 2010;8:18.

32. MacPherson H, Altman DG, Hammerschlag R, Youping L, Taixiang W, White A, Moher D. Revised standards for reporting interventions in clinical trials of acupuncture (STRICTA): extending the CONSORT statement. J Evid Based Med. 2010;3(3):140–55.

33. Pacific WROftW. WHO standard acupuncture point locations in the Western Pacific Region. Geneva: World Health Organization; 2008.

34. Appleyard I, Lundeberg T, Robinson N. Should systematic reviews assess the risk of bias from sham–placebo acupuncture control procedures? Eur J Integr Med. 2014;6(2):234–43.

35. Moffet HH. Sham acupuncture may be as efficacious as true acupuncture: a systematic review of clinical trials. J Altern Complement Med. 2009;15(3): 213–6.

36. Naeser MA, Palumbo CL. Neuroimaging and language recovery in stroke. J Clin Neurophysiol. 1994;11(1):150–74.

37. Naeser MA, Alexander MP, Stiassny-Eder D, Galler V, Hobbs J, Bachman D. Acupuncture in the treatment of paralysis in chronic and acute stroke patients–improvement correlated with specific CT scan lesion sites. Acupunct Electrother Res. 1994;19(4):227–49.

38. Zivin JA, Sehra R, Shoshoo A, Albers GW, Bornstein NM, Dahlof B, Kasner SE, Howard G, Shuaib A, Streeter J, Richieri SP, Hacke W. NeuroThera efficacy and safety trial-3 (NEST-3). Int J Stroke. 2014;9(7):950–5.

8

Treatment of allergic rhinitis with acupoint herbal plaster: an oligonucleotide chip analysis

Horng-Sheng Shiue[1], Yun-Shien Lee[2], Chi-Neu Tsai[1] and Hen-Hong Chang[3,4*]

Abstract

Background: Allergic rhinitis is regarded as an imbalanced Th1/Th2 cell-mediated response. The present study used microarray analysis to compare gene expression levels between allergic rhinitis patients before and after a series of acupoint herbal plaster applications.

Methods: In this experimental pilot study, volunteers experiencing sneezing, runny nose, and congestion for more than 9 months in the year following initial diagnoses were included after diagnostic confirmation by otolaryngologists to exclude patients with sinusitis and nasal polyps. Patients with persistent allergic rhinitis each received four acupoint herbal plaster treatments applied using the moxibustion technique. Clinical outcomes were evaluated using the Rhinitis Quality of Life Questionnaire (RQLQ). Peripheral blood samples were analyzed using an ImmunoCAP Phadiatop test, and patients were classified as phadiatop (Ph)-positive or -negative. Microarray results were analyzed for genes that were differentially expressed between (1) Ph-positive and -negative patients treated with herbal plaster; and (2) before and after herbal plaster treatment in the Ph-positive patient group. Unsupervised and supervised methods were used for gene-expression data analysis.

Results: Nineteen Ph-positive and four Ph-negative participants with persistent allergic rhinitis were included in the study. RQLQ results indicated that the 19 Ph-positive volunteers experienced improvement in six of seven categories following acupoint herbal plaster treatments, whereas the four Ph-negative participants reported improvement in only two categories. Hierarchical clustering and principle component analysis of the gene expression profiles of Ph-positive and –negative participants indicated the groups exhibited distinct physiological responses to acupoint herbal treatment. Evaluation of gene networks using MetaCore identified that the "Immune response_IL-13 signaling via JAK-STAT" and the "Inflammation_Interferon signaling" were down- and up-regulated, respectively, among Ph-positive subjects.

Conclusions: In this preliminary study, we find that the IL-13 immune response via JAK-STAT signaling and interferon inflammation signaling were down- and upregulated, respectively, in the Ph-positive group. Further studies are required to verify these pathways in Ph-positive patients, and to determine the mechanism of such pathway dysregulation.

Trial registration: ClinicalTrials.gov: NCT02486159. Registered 30 Jun 2015.

Keywords: Allergic rhinitis, Acupoint herbal plaster, Oligonucleotide chip

* Correspondence: tcmchh55@gmail.com
[3]School of Post-Baccalaureate Chinese Medicine, and Research Center for Chinese Medicine and Acupuncture, China Medical University, Taichung, Taiwan
[4]Departments of Chinese Medicine, China Medical University Hospital, Taichung, Taiwan
Full list of author information is available at the end of the article

Background

Many patients with allergic rhinitis have chosen complementary and alternative medicine (CAM), including traditional Chinese medicine (TCM) or acupuncture [1, 2], as they have found CAM to be more attractive and less invasive [1]. The World Health Organization (WHO) published an article examining CAM therapies for allergic rhinitis and asthma [2], which include major contributions from TCM and deserve our continued study to assess therapeutic efficacies and mechanisms. In addition to acupuncture and TCM to treat allergic rhinitis, acupoint herbal plaster applications have recently been used widely in Taiwan [3–5] and mainland China [6, 7] due to the non-invasive and easy to manipulate nature of these treatments. An herbal plaster is applied with a drug applicator using a technique akin to moxibustion, stimulating the skin at specific acupuncture points [3, 4]. Acupoint herbal plaster methods have been recommend for allergic rhinitis beginning in 2009 [8], and practitioners throughout Taiwan and China use similar approaches in the composition of herbal medicine, the herbal medicine application operating process [9] and what acupoints are used [10]. Clinical research regarding the application of acupoint therapy for allergic rhinitis has increased, and evidence-based methods have validated its efficacy and safety [7, 9–11]. However, the majority of these studies are clinical trials; therefore, the efficacy and mechanisms of acupoint herbal plaster treatment need to be validated via mechanistic, molecular methods [2, 9, 12].

We previously studied the effect of herbal plaster treatment for allergic rhinitis [13]. Ours was the first comprehensive clinical outcome assessment of acupoint herbal plaster therapy for allergic rhinitis using the Rhinoconjunctivitis and Rhinitis Quality of Life Questionnaire (RQLQ) [14]. We showed that acupoint herbal plaster for the treatment of allergic rhinitis is safe, effective, and associated with high compliance rates. Here, we aimed to perform a pilot study for acupoint herbal plaster treatment based on our previous microarray experience. Our laboratory has rich microarray experience that combines the Genomic Medicine Research Core Laboratory (GMRCL) [15], clinicians in the Department of Chinese Medicine at Chang Gung Memorial Hospital, and bioinformatics specialists. We performed chip analysis before and after acupuncture treatment in allergic rhinitis patients [16, 17]. We used cDNA microarray and oligonucleotide microarray analyses to investigate the influence of acupuncture on RNA expression profiles using blood samples from patients with allergic rhinitis. We used the RQLQ and statistical analysis to assess clinical outcomes [14]. The results of our microarray analysis were associated with the RQLQ to obtain our final conclusions.

Following exposure to allergens, allergic rhinitis patients exhibit immunoglobulin E (IgE), mast cell, and T helper (Th)2 lymphocyte immune responses related to (1) sensitization and memory, (2) the early phase, and (3) the late phase [18, 19]. The early phase can induce sneezing, nasal itching, runny and congested nasal passages, and other symptoms. The late phase contributes to patient fatigue, malaise, irritability, and other symptoms. Allergic rhinitis is regarded as an imbalanced Th1/Th2 cell-mediated response [20, 21]. Th1 cells primarily secrete IL-2, IFNγ, IL-3, and GM-CSF; whereas Th2 cells secrete IL-3, IL-4, IL-5, IL-10, IL-13, and GM-CSF [22]. Dominant Th2 cytokines can enhance allergen-specific IgE, which plays an important role in allergic inflammation [18, 20]. Studies using DNA microarray have indicated an imbalance in the T-helper cell-mediated immune system in patients with allergic rhinitis [23, 24]. Genes encoding chemokines and their receptors were elevated in this analysis; these genes play important roles in the Th2 response [24, 25].

According to our previous study, peripheral blood samples collected from allergic rhinitis patients before and after acupuncture treatment and analyzed by cDNA microarray analysis indicated an improvement in the counterbalance between pro-inflammatory cytokines derived from Th1 cells and anti-inflammatory cytokines derived from Th2 cells [16]. Nasal allergic reactions in patients with allergic rhinitis were inhibited by Th1 cells and were not promoted by Th2 cells following acupuncture treatment [16]. Although strengthening the Th1 response is regarded as a novel therapeutic target for allergic rhinitis, it has not yet been applied in clinical practice [19, 21]. We have published that acupuncture treatment may be another way to restructure Th1 and Th2 responses in patients with allergic rhinitis [16]. ImmunoCAP Phadiatop is a blood test widely used by ENT specialists in Taiwan to detect serum allergen-specific IgE antibodies [26, 27]. Among normal controls and atopic patients, the frequency of Ph-positive patients was 1 of 47 and 49 of 53, respectively [26]. In our previous study [17], Th1 and Th2 cells were suppressed after acupuncture treatment with group differences between Phadiatop (Ph)-positive and Ph-negative patients regarding gene expression characteristics and physiological responses. Studies have shown that the reduction in allergic inflammation and the restored Th1/Th2 (and Treg/Th2) equilibrium following acupuncture are sustained [17].

In this pilot study, we examined changes in gene expression associated with acupoint herbal plaster for allergic rhinitis. Using microarray, we compared gene expression levels in allergic rhinitis patients before and after a series of acupoint herbal plaster applications. This study applies EBM and supports the use of acupoint herbal therapy to treat allergic rhinitis.

Methods

Acupoint herbal plaster treatment

This pilot study was designed using an intervention model with single group assignment. Allergic rhinitis patients were included after their diagnoses were confirmed, and were treated with four applications of herbal plaster. The clinical portion of this study was conducted at the Department of Acupuncture and Moxibustion, Center for Traditional Chinese Medicine, Chang Gung Memorial Hospital from October 2009 to March 2010. Patients (age, 18–45 y) were eligible who met the following criteria: (1) exhibited sneezing, runny nose, and congestion for more than 9 months of the year [18]; (2) did not take medication in the previous month; and (3) provided written consent to enter a Chang Gung Memorial Hospital Institutional Review Board (IRB)-approved human trial. Patient diagnoses were confirmed by the following clinical and biochemical tests, which were performed by otolaryngologists: (1) physical examination; (2) anterior rhinoscopy; (3) ImmunoCAP Phadiatop (InVitroSight, Phadia AB, Uppsala, Sweden), determination of specified serum IgE antibodies to detect inhalant allergens [26, 27]. Patients were included in the trial after their initial diagnoses were confirmed [18, 28]. Patients with sinusitis or nasal polyps, or those who were unwilling or unable to complete the full course of treatment were excluded from the trial. All included patients were diagnosed with allergic rhinitis that was consistent with persistent allergic rhinitis according to ARIA's new classification system. The ARIA system includes the following rhinitis symptoms and quality of life variables: duration, which includes intermittent or persistent allergic rhinitis; and nasal allergy symptoms, which must occur more than 4 days per week for 4 months per year to qualify as persistent allergic rhinitis [29, 30].

In total, 23 study patients received acupoint herbal plaster applications every 7–10 days over a 4-week period for a total of 4 applications. The herbal plaster consisted of mustard seed, fumarate, asarum, angelica, cinnamon, and ginger at a ratio of 3:3:2:2:0.5:4, respectively. The treatment was prepared by dissolving the ginger in water and adding the powder to form a plaster. Mixtures were formed into cakes of approximately $1.5 \times 1.5 \times 0.5$ cm^3 [13] and were held in position using plastic sheets. The following nine acupoints were selected: Dazhui (GV14), Feishu (BL13, both sides), Gaohuang (BL43, both sides), Shenshu (BL23, both sides), and Pishu (BL20, both sides). Each patching time lasted 1–3 h, depending on the patient's tolerance. When drug cakes were removed, patients typically exhibited local skin redness and experienced slight burning sensations. Subsequent water exposure, including bathing, was avoided for 1–2 h following treatment to prevent skin aggravation. Patient drug tolerance varies, and adhering the cake for too long occasionally led to blisters. Blisters resulting from this treatment were coated with povidone iodine syrup and were protected with sterile gauze bandages.

Outcome evaluation

Clinical symptoms were indexed as follows: (1) assess symptoms before the first acupoint herbal plaster application, (2) determine rhinoconjunctivitis and rhinitis symptoms at the third and fourth acupoint herbal plaster applications. Clinical outcomes were evaluated using the RQLQ, which has been proven to be effective [14, 31] and includes 28 questions in 7 categories. The RQLQ was designed to measure the impact of rhinitis on quality of life. It considers that allergic rhinitis patients often are troubled by nasal symptoms, eye symptoms, sleep problems, emotional problems, social issues, and other symptoms [14, 29].

ImmunoCAP Phadiatop blood test

Prior to treatment at Chang Gung Memorial Hospital, all 23 allergic rhinitis patients were assessed by clinical pathologists using the ImmunoCAP Phadiatop blood test. Patients were evaluated for the presence of IgE antibodies against the following allergens: *Dermatophagoides pteronyssinus*, cat dander, dog dander, the German cockroach, and Moulds. Detection of IgE antibodies exceeding 0.35 kUA/L indicated a positive result.

RNA extraction and microarray

Patient peripheral blood samples were obtained in 5-ml volumes at the following 6 times (T0–T5) during the study: (1) before (T0) and 24 h after the first (T1) acupoint herbal plaster application; (2) before (T2) and 24 h after the third (T3) acupoint herbal plaster application; and (3) before (T4) and 24 h after the fourth (T5) acupoint herbal plaster application.

From each 5-ml blood sample, 2.5-ml aliquots were analyzed by the Clinical Pathology Department of Chang Gung Memorial Hospital for the following: complete blood count/differential count (CBC/DC):total white blood count; differential counts for neutrophils, lymphocytes, monocytes, eosinophils, and basophils; red blood cell count; platelet count; hemoglobin, hematocrit, and erythrocyte indices (mean corpuscular volume, mean corpuscular hemoglobin, mean corpuscular hemoglobin concentration, and red cell distribution width [RDW]). Total serum IgE levels were tracked before the first acupoint herbal plaster application and 24 h after the fourth acupoint herbal plaster application.

The remaining 2.5-ml blood samples were stored at room temperature in PAXgene Blood RNA collection tubes (Qiagen, Valencia, CA, USA), containing an RNA stabilizer. RNA was extracted from blood samples using the PAXgene Blood RNA System (Qiagen), according to the manufacturer's recommendations, and samples were stored at –80 °C. RNA samples then were isolated using an RNeasy MinElute kit (Qiagen), and RNA quality and quantity were analyzed using a Bioanalyzer 2100 (Agilent Technologies, Santa Clara, CA, USA).

Owing to the IRB's limitation that no more than 5-ml peripheral blood could be collected from each study volunteer, we were unable to obtain sufficient RNA quantities to analyze individual participants. Therefore, we applied pre-amplification pooled mRNA samples to a single microarray chip, a method that has been used frequently in microarray analysis [23]. Although pooling could potentially confound signals by mixing cell populations and individuals, it avoids variation within individuals [32]. Because a microarray using pooled RNA only identifies genes that change dramatically, this approach highlights the most differentially expressed signaling pathways between diseased and control individuals [25]. In our study, equal quantities of mRNA were pooled from individuals with similar clinical diagnosis and IgE levels, thereby increasing RNA homogeneity. Each pooled sample corresponded to the blood RNA from 2 to 3 patients. Samples were analyzed using a GeneChip Human Genome U133 Plus2 array (Affymetrix, Santa Clara, CA, USA) containing approximately 54,675 probes. Samples from the 23 patients were divided into 7 pooled groups for each of the 6 blood collection time points and were applied to 42 chips.

Statistical analysis
Changes in RQLQ and IgE were compared to the first time point (T0; before first herbal plaster) via a paired Student's t-test and a Mann Whitney U-test, respectively.

Microarray data analysis
Unsupervised (hierarchical clustering and principal component analysis) and supervised (Student's t-test) methods have traditionally been used to analyze gene-expression data [33]. In this study, data were analyzed by hierarchical clustering using Cluster and TreeView software [34] with the following parameters: (1) standard deviation > 0.4 as the filtering cutoff point (1852 genes with marked changes selected among 35 arrays); (2) mean-centered genes and normalized genes; and (3) cluster analysis conducted using uncentered correlation of arrays. Cluster and TreeView programs were downloaded from http://bonsai.hgc.jp/~mdehoon/software/cluster. The Student's t-test, Mann–Whitney U-test and PCA were performed using MATLAB version 7.4 and Statistics Toolbox version 3.1 (The MathWorks, Boston, MA, USA). A volcano plot was constructed using MATLAB to identify changes in replicate microarray data [35]. Specifically, the negative log of the p value ($-\log10$[p value]) was plotted on the y-axis, and the log2 ratio of the fold change was plotted on the x-axis.

We evaluated genes that were differentially expressed following acupoint herbal plaster applications (T1, T2, T3, T4, T5, are compared with T0). Changes in specific gene expression before and after treatment could suggest potential immune mechanisms associated with acupoint herbal plaster application. RQLQ results were compared with gene expression differences in the final analysis.

Network visualization and analysis
The MetaCore analytical suite (GeneGo, St. Joseph, MI, USA) was used to compare differences in gene expression networks [36–39]. MetaCore evaluates systems biology and drug development at the computational level, enabling analyses of human protein–protein interactions and mechanisms using the database. This suite contributes to analyses of regulatory networks and signaling pathway gene groups. To perform a network analysis of gene groups, MetaCore can work from an input list of genes and can randomly assign genes to different nodes to assess the probability of an interacting network [37]. In this study, the list of genes represented on the Affymetrix Human U133 Plus2 array was used as a base gene list to calculate p values using MetaCore procedures. MetaCore uses a hypergeometric model to determine significance [38, 39].

Results
Clinical outcomes of acupoint herbal plaster treatment
An otolaryngologist screened 23 study participants with allergic rhinitis, and the GMRCL conducted oligonucleotide chip experiments. Each participant's diagnosis of perennial allergic rhinitis also was confirmed using anterior nasal endoscopy. Based on the results of an ImmunoCAP Phadiatop blood test of allergen-specific IgE, the 23 volunteers were classified as either Ph-positive (19 participants) or Ph-negative (4 participants) (Table 1). Assessments of clinical symptoms and IgE indices were performed before the first, third, and after the fourth acupoint herbal plaster application. The RQLQ was used to survey the patients, and the results were statistically analyzed for clinical symptoms [14] (Tables 2 and 3).

In the Ph-positive group, the RQLQ results were compared before the first and after the fourth acupoint herbal plaster treatment. We identified significant improvements in six of the seven domains (activity, non-hay fever symptoms, eye symptoms, practical problems, nasal symptoms, and emotional symptoms) examined by the RQLQ (Tables 2 and 3). In the Ph-negative group, only two categories (nasal symptoms, emotional symptoms) appeared to improve following acupoint treatment. These results suggest that acupoint herbal plaster applications evoke distinct physiological responses in these two patient groups. These findings are consistent with our previous studies regarding acupuncture treatment for allergic rhinitis [16, 17].

Total serum IgE values were compared before the first and after the fourth acupoint herbal plaster application

Table 1 Comparison of baseline characteristics between Ph-positive and Ph-negative patients before treatment

Variables	Ph-positive N = 19 Mean	SD	Ph-negative N = 4 Mean	SD	p Value
Gender					
Male	10		3		
Female	9		1		0.60^
Age	32.11	5.37	35	3.37	0.22
Duration of allergic rhinitis					
≥ 10 years	14		3		
< 10 years	5		1		0.96^
Activity	3.12	1.39	3.08	1.32	0.66
Sleep	1.65	1.09	1.58	0.92	0.64
Non-hay fever symptoms	2.39	1.14	2.25	1.08	0.58
Practical problems	2.84	1.42	2.33	1.61	0.38
Nasal symptoms	2.78	1.17	2.94	1.43	0.98
Eye symptoms	2.37	1.41	1.75	1.14	0.24
Emotional symptoms	2.08	1.15	1.38	0.92	0.15
Overall score	2.46	1.02	2.19	0.96	0.40
IgE (Baseline)	302.12	78.75	21.25	7.70	0.002**
IgE (Follow-up)	333.61	86.01	25.10*	10.44	0.005**

SD Standard Deviation
Note: *p < 0.05, **p < 0.01 (Mann–Whitney *U* test)
^Fisher's exact test

(Tables 4 and 5). Following the course of herbal plaster treatments, total IgE levels were unchanged in both the Ph-positive and -negative groups (Tables 4 and 5). This is consistent with previous short-term studies by our laboratory [16, 17] and others [40], which found that total serum IgE levels in allergic rhinitis patients treated with TCM did not change.

Table 2 Changes in RQLQ results following the third and fourth herbal plaster (hp) treatments in Ph-positive patients

Area of RQLQ	Baseline score	After 3rd hp score	P value (3rd hp vs. baseline)	After 4th hp score	P value (4th hp vs. baseline)
Activity	3.12	2.56	0.1322	2.09	0.0002**
Sleep	1.65	1.58	0.8488	1.35	0.0804
Non-hay fever symptoms	2.39	2.02	0.1465	1.64	0.0012**
Practical problems	2.84	2.39	0.1549	2.05	0.0018**
Nasal symptoms	2.78	2.30	0.1006	1.92	0.0000**
Eye symptoms	2.37	1.57	0.0330*	1.29	0.0066**
Emotional symptoms	2.08	1.62	0.0634	1.33	0.0010**
Overall score	2.46	2.00	0.0635	1.67	0.0000**

Paired Student's *t*-test; *n* = 19, *p < 0.05 **p < 0.01

Table 3 Changes in RQLQ results following the third and fourth herbal plaster (hp) treatments in Ph-negative patients

Area of RQLQ	Baseline score	After 3rd hp score	P value (3rd hp vs. baseline)	After 4th hp score	P value (4th hp vs. baseline)
Activity	3.08	1.58	0.0577	1.33	0.0800
Sleep	1.58	1.58	1.0000	1.17	0.3677
Non-hay fever symptoms	2.25	1.79	0.3477	1.21	0.0564
Practical problems	2.33	1.67	0.3994	1.33	0.1135
Nasal symptoms	2.94	2.06	0.1881	1.31	0.0065**
Eye symptoms	1.75	1.19	0.4338	1.19	0.4594
Emotional symptoms	1.38	1.06	0.5551	0.69	0.0486*
Overall score	2.19	1.56	0.1940	1.18	0.0371*

Paired Student's *t*-test; *n* = 4, *p < 0.05 **p < 0.01

Ph-positive and Ph-negative allergic rhinitis patients exhibit distinct gene expression profiles following acupoint herbal plaster treatment

Since Ph-positive and Ph-negative groups exhibited different clinical outcomes, we explored the gene expression profiles of these two patient groups following acupoint herbal plaster treatment. Total RNA was extracted from peripheral blood samples at each of the 6 time points analyzed (23 patients, 138 RNA samples total). Because of insufficient blood RNA quantities (1–2 μg/subject), we pooled sets of 2–3 RNA samples from subjects with similar clinical indices, resulting in seven pooled RNA samples for each of the six time points. The 42 pooled RNA samples were applied to GeneChip Human Genome U133 Plus 2.0 arrays. Patient and sample information are detailed in Table 6.

To estimate the effects of acupoint herbal plaster treatment, the gene expression level at each treatment point was subtracted from the first time point (T0; before herbal plaster treatment). After filtering the low-intensity non-significant genes (standard deviation < 0.4), 1852 genes remained for analysis with non-supervised hierarchical clustering methods. We identified distinct gene expression profiles in Ph-positive and -negative patients using a hierarchical approach (Fig. 1a). We further analyzed the correlation matrix for all 35 samples using a PCA [41]. The three-dimensional plot of the first three principal components by the matrix containing 80 % of the information

Table 4 Changes in total IgE levels following the fourth herbal plaster (hp) treatment in Ph-positive patients

	No.	Baseline Mean ± SD	Follow-up Mean ± SD	P value^
IgE	19	302.12 ± 78.75	333.61 ± 86.01	0.085

SD Standard Deviation
^Mann–Whitney *U*-test

Table 5 Changes in patient total IgE levels following the fourth herbal plaster (hp) treatment in Ph-negative patients

	No.	Baseline Mean ± SD	Follow-up Mean ± SD	P value^
IgE	4	21.25 ± 7.70	25.10 ± 10.44	0.63

SD Standard Deviation
^Mann–Whitney U-test

is shown in Fig. 1b. This analysis indicated that the Ph-positive and -negative groups were distinct in their responses to acupoint herbal plaster treatment. Because the hierarchical clustering and PCA suggested that the M4-2 and M4-4 samples were outliers in the Ph-positive group, these samples were excluded from further analysis.

Since, the clinical outcomes (RQLQ) after treatment in the Ph-positive and -negative groups differed, we explored the gene expression profiles for these two groups in response to acupoint herbal plaster application. We used a volcano plot to obtain an overview of the 1852 filtered genes (Fig. 2a), and we selected 89 genes that exhibited fold-changes exceeding $2^{0.75} = 1.682$ ($p < 0.01$, Student's t-test) between Ph-positive and -negative participants (Fig. 2b and Table 7). These genes were examined using MetaCore software (http://lsresearch.thomsonreuters.com/pages/solutions/1/metacore) for reaction pathway analysis, and the pathways "Immune response_IL-13 signaling via JAK-STAT (Janus kinase and signal transducers and activators of transcription)" and "Inflammation_Interferon signaling" were identified to correspond to the down- and up-regulated genes, respectively, in the Ph-positive group (Fig. 2b and Table 8).

Differentially expressed genes after acupoint herbal plaster treatment in Ph-positive patients

The RQLQ indicated that the clinical efficacy of herbal plaster treatment was different between Ph-positive patients and Ph-negative patients. Then we evaluated genes that were differentially expressed following acupoint herbal plaster applications (T1, T2, T3, T4, T5, are compared with T0)

in Ph-positive patients. Since the differentially expresse in Ph-positive group is less than Ph-positive group compared with Ph-negative group. We selected 47 genes that exhibited $p < 0.01$ (via Student's t-test) and fold changes (vs. T0) of $2^{0.4} = 1.320$ (Fig. 3 and Table 9). Globally, most genes were down-regulated (45/47) after herbal plaster treatment. This result was consistent with our previous report that most genes were down-regulated after acupuncture treatment in Ph-positive allergic rhinitis patients [17].

These 45 genes then were input to the MetaCore reaction pathways analysis. The data indicated that Ph-positive allergic rhinitis patients who received acupoint herbal plaster applications significantly induced several pathways ($p < 0.01$; Table 10). Among the 45 down-regulated genes, pathway analysis identified significant involvement of the "Oxidative phosphorylation pathway" ($p < 0.0001$). Network analysis also identified "Protein folding_Response to unfolded proteins," "Immune response Antigen presentation," and "Immune response Phagosome in antigen presentation" as significant ($p < 0.001$) relative to the 45 down-regulated genes.

Discussion

Allergic rhinitis likely results from an imbalance in the Th1 and Th2 cell-mediated inflammatory responses [20, 21]. In addition to the hygiene hypothesis causing deviation of the Th1 and Th2 balance and reduced immune suppression, investigators have implicated decreases in T-regulatory (Treg) activity in allergy diseases [42, 43]. People suffering from allergies, usually have a reduced Th1 reaction and a predominant Th2 response. Th1 cells tended to decrease in patients with allergic rhinitis, whereas Th2 cells were significantly increased. Significant deviations from the normal Th1/Th2 ratio may be associated with the incidence of allergic diseases [18, 20, 44]. A study examining allergic inflammation that focused on Th2 cytokines (IL-4, IL-5, IL-9, and IL-13) reported that these cytokines recruited cells that induced allergic inflammation via chemokine secretion [44]. Few reports have described human allergic inflammation with respect to cytokine antagonists [19, 21, 45].

Table 6 Pooling strategy for RNA samples. The first number in each cell indicates the group type, and the second indicates the time point (T0–T5 correspond to 1–6, respectively). A total of 42 chips were used. M, microarray chip

	Before 1st herbal plaster (hp) (T0)	After 1st hp 24 h (T1)	Before 3rd hp (T2)	After 3rd hp 24 h (T3)	Before 4th hp (T4)	After 4th hp 24 h (T5)
Ph(+)	M1-1	M1-2	M1-3	M1-4	M1-5	M1-6
Ph(+)	M2-1	M2-2	M2-3	M2-4	M2-5	M2-6
Ph(+)	M3-1	M3-2	M3-3	M3-4	M3-5	M3-6
Ph(+)	M4-1	M4-2	M4-3	M4-4	M4-5	M4-6
Ph(+)	M5-1	M5-2	M5-3	M5-4	M5-5	M5-6
Ph(+)	M6-1	M6-2	M6-3	M6-4	M6-5	M6-6
Ph(−)	M7-1	M7-2	M7-3	M7-4	M7-5	M7-6

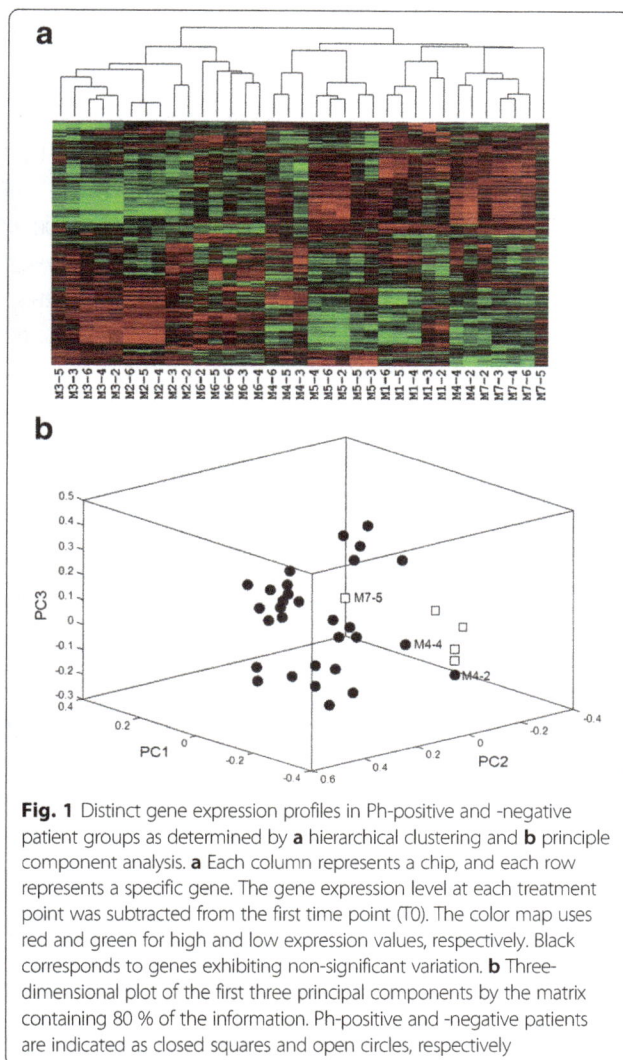

Fig. 1 Distinct gene expression profiles in Ph-positive and -negative patient groups as determined by **a** hierarchical clustering and **b** principle component analysis. **a** Each column represents a chip, and each row represents a specific gene. The gene expression level at each treatment point was subtracted from the first time point (T0). The color map uses red and green for high and low expression values, respectively. Black corresponds to genes exhibiting non-significant variation. **b** Three-dimensional plot of the first three principal components by the matrix containing 80 % of the information. Ph-positive and -negative patients are indicated as closed squares and open circles, respectively

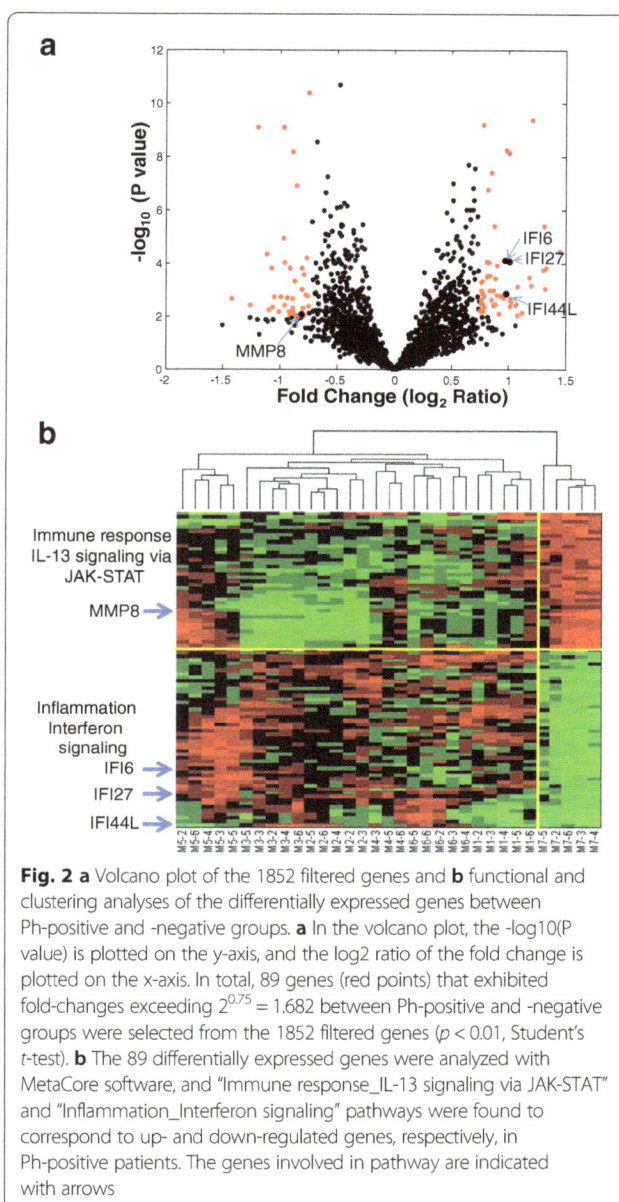

Fig. 2 a Volcano plot of the 1852 filtered genes and **b** functional and clustering analyses of the differentially expressed genes between Ph-positive and -negative groups. **a** In the volcano plot, the -log10(P value) is plotted on the y-axis, and the log2 ratio of the fold change is plotted on the x-axis. In total, 89 genes (red points) that exhibited fold-changes exceeding $2^{0.75} = 1.682$ between Ph-positive and -negative groups were selected from the 1852 filtered genes ($p < 0.01$, Student's t-test). **b** The 89 differentially expressed genes were analyzed with MetaCore software, and "Immune response_IL-13 signaling via JAK-STAT" and "Inflammation_Interferon signaling" pathways were found to correspond to up- and down-regulated genes, respectively, in Ph-positive patients. The genes involved in pathway are indicated with arrows

Although strengthening the Th1 response is regarded as a novel therapeutic approach for allergic rhinitis, this method has not been applied clinically [19, 21]. A restructuring of the Th1 and Th2 responses in patients with allergic rhinitis may be accomplished with acupuncture [16, 17]. Studies have shown that acupuncture treatment of allergic inflammation can maintain the equilibrium between Th1 and Th2 cells and between Tregs and Th2 cells [16, 17].

Many patients choose acupoint herbal plaster treatments for allergic rhinitis in Taiwan [3–5] and mainland China [6, 7]. We previously examined the efficacy of acupoint herbal plaster treatment for allergic rhinitis [13]. The present study is the first to apply the RQLQ to comprehensively assess the effects of acupoint herbal plaster on allergic rhinitis symptoms. Our results suggest that acupoint herbal plaster is a safe, effective, and convenient treatment for allergic rhinitis. A comparison

of baseline characteristics before treatment between Ph-positive and Ph-negative patients showed no differences, with the exception of total IgE levels (Table 1). The RQLQ results after the fourth treatment of 19 Ph-positive patients indicated symptom improvements in six of seven categories (activity, non-hay fever symptoms, practical problems, nasal symptoms, eye symptoms, emotional symptoms; Tables 2 and 3). In contrast, the four Ph-negative volunteers (−) reported symptom improvements in only two categories (nasal symptoms, emotional symptoms; Tables 2 and 3). These results are similar to those found in our previous report on acupuncture treatment for allergic rhinitis [16, 17]; however,

Table 7 The 89 genes that were differentially expressed between Ph-positive and Ph-negative patients with allergic rhinitis following treatment with acupoint herbal paste

ID	Gene Symbol	Gene Title	Fold change[a]	P value
1552288_at	CILP2	cartilage intermediate layer protein 2	1.45	3.4E-05
1556590_s_at	NA	NA	1.32	1.4E-04
1557195_at	NA	NA	1.31	8.8E-04
1557761_s_at	LOC400794	hypothetical LOC400794	1.31	3.9E-06
1562216_at	NA	NA	1.30	1.7E-04
1565913_at	NA	NA	1.21	4.2E-10
1566134_at	CARHSP1	Calcium regulated heat stable protein 1, 24 kDa	1.20	6.5E-04
1566964_at	NA	NA	1.18	3.4E-04
1567240_x_at	OR2L2	olfactory receptor, family 2, subfamily L, member 2	1.11	7.1E-03
1569482_at	NA	NA	1.08	8.8E-03
200038_s_at	RPL17	ribosomal protein L17	1.08	7.4E-04
200082_s_at	RPS7	ribosomal protein S7	1.06	3.7E-03
200705_s_at	EEF1B2	eukaryotic translation elongation factor 1 beta 2	1.02	2.6E-03
200986_at	SERPING1	serpin peptidase inhibitor, clade G (C1 inhibitor), member 1	1.02	2.0E-03
201699_at	PSMC6	proteasome (prosome, macropain) 26S subunit, ATPase, 6	1.01	4.0E-03
202086_at	MX1	myxovirus (influenza virus) resistance 1, interferon-inducible protein p78 (mous	1.01	7.2E-09
202411_at	IFI27	interferon, alpha-inducible protein 27	1.00	7.8E-05
202635_s_at	POLR2K	polymerase (RNA) II (DNA directed) polypeptide K, 7.0 kDa	0.99	1.4E-03
204286_s_at	PMAIP1	phorbol-12-myristate-13-acetate-induced protein 1	0.98	5.5E-09
204415_at	IFI6	interferon, alpha-inducible protein 6	0.97	7.6E-05
204439_at	IFI44L	interferon-induced protein 44-like	0.96	2.0E-03
204732_s_at	TRIM23	tripartite motif-containing 23	0.93	1.7E-03
205849_s_at	UQCRB	ubiquinol-cytochrome c reductase binding protein	0.91	7.7E-03
205914_s_at	GRIN1	glutamate receptor, ionotropic, N-methyl D-aspartate 1	0.90	1.5E-03
206584_at	LY96	lymphocyte antigen 96	0.90	1.2E-04
207723_s_at	KLRC3	killer cell lectin-like receptor subfamily C, member 3	0.88	3.6E-04
208792_s_at	CLU	clusterin	0.88	3.5E-03
209160_at	AKR1C3	aldo-keto reductase family 1, member C3 (3-alpha hydroxysteroid dehydrogenase, t	0.88	3.9E-06
209651_at	TGFB1I1	transforming growth factor beta 1 induced transcript 1	0.86	1.0E-03
209732_at	CLEC2B	C-type lectin domain family 2, member B	0.86	3.7E-03
209743_s_at	ITCH	itchy E3 ubiquitin protein ligase homolog (mouse)	0.85	2.3E-03
209795_at	CD69	CD69 molecule	0.85	3.9E-08
210103_s_at	FOXA2	forkhead box A2	0.84	9.9E-04
210432_s_at	SCN3A	sodium channel, voltage-gated, type III, alpha subunit	0.83	2.8E-04

Table 7 The 89 genes that were differentially expressed between Ph-positive and Ph-negative patients with allergic rhinitis following treatment with acupoint herbal paste *(Continued)*

210548_at	CCL23	chemokine (C-C motif) ligand 23	0.83	8.5E-05
210639_s_at	ATG5	ATG5 autophagy related 5 homolog (S. cerevisiae)	0.82	1.7E-07
210873_x_at	APOBEC3A	apolipoprotein B mRNA editing enzyme, catalytic polypeptide-like 3A	0.82	2.7E-04
211968_s_at	HSP90AA1	heat shock protein 90 kDa alpha (cytosolic), class A member 1	0.81	8.0E-05
212270_x_at	RPL17	ribosomal protein L17	0.81	2.9E-04
212537_x_at	RPL17	ribosomal protein L17	0.78	1.6E-03
213226_at	CCNA2	cyclin A2	0.78	4.2E-03
214070_s_at	ATP10B	ATPase, class V, type 10B	0.78	3.3E-03
215101_s_at	CXCL5	chemokine (C-X-C motif) ligand 5	0.78	6.0E-03
215394_at	PIK3C3	phosphoinositide-3-kinase, class 3	0.77	6.3E-10
215646_s_at	VCAN	versican	0.77	4.3E-04
216412_x_at	LOC100290557	similar to hCG91935	0.77	1.3E-03
216834_at	RGS1	regulator of G-protein signaling 1	0.76	2.3E-03
217915_s_at	RSL24D1	ribosomal L24 domain containing 1	0.76	9.8E-04
219519_s_at	SIGLEC1	sialic acid binding Ig-like lectin 1, sialoadhesin	0.76	4.7E-04
219551_at	EAF2	ELL associated factor 2	0.76	3.1E-03
220141_at	C11orf63	chromosome 11 open reading frame 63	0.75	5.8E-03
220184_at	NANOG	Nanog homeobox	−0.75	3.9E-03
220646_s_at	KLRF1	killer cell lectin-like receptor subfamily F, member 1	−0.75	3.9E-11
220827_at	NA	NA	−0.76	1.6E-03
222229_x_at	RPL26	ribosomal protein L26	−0.77	5.9E-05
222465_at	RSL24D1	ribosomal L24 domain containing 1	−0.78	1.5E-03
223963_s_at	IGF2BP2	insulin-like growth factor 2 mRNA binding protein 2	−0.79	2.5E-04
224293_at	TTTY10	testis-specific transcript, Y-linked 10 (non-protein coding)	−0.79	8.6E-03
225541_at	RPL22L1	ribosomal protein L22-like 1	−0.80	4.7E-03
226344_at	ZMAT1	zinc finger, matrin type 1	−0.81	1.4E-04
227454_at	TAOK1	TAO kinase 1	−0.81	9.4E-04
227766_at	LIG4	ligase IV, DNA, ATP-dependent	−0.82	9.9E-03
228174_at	SCAI	suppressor of cancer cell invasion	−0.83	8.5E-03
228439_at	BATF2	basic leucine zipper transcription factor, ATF-like 2	−0.83	9.6E-03
228970_at	ZBTB8OS	zinc finger and BTB domain containing 8 opposite strand	−0.86	1.1E-07
229431_at	RFXAP	regulatory factor X-associated protein	−0.86	8.8E-03
229437_at	MIR155HG	MIR155 host gene (non-protein coding)	−0.87	4.5E-04
229893_at	FRMD3	FERM domain containing 3	−0.89	7.0E-03
229910_at	SHE	Src homology 2 domain containing E	−0.89	2.0E-03
230153_at	NEK9	NIMA (never in mitosis gene a)-related kinase 9	−0.89	6.2E-09
231014_at	TRIM50	tripartite motif-containing 50	−0.89	4.8E-03
231038_s_at	NA	NA	−0.92	8.1E-03

Table 7 The 89 genes that were differentially expressed between Ph-positive and Ph-negative patients with allergic rhinitis following treatment with acupoint herbal paste (Continued)

231484_at	NA	NA	−0.92	1.5E-04
231688_at	MMP8	matrix metallopeptidase 8 (neutrophil collagenase)	−0.93	6.4E-03
231975_s_at	MIER3	mesoderm induction early response 1, family member 3	−0.94	1.9E-03
233015_at	MBNL1	muscleblind-like (Drosophila)	−0.96	3.7E-03
235762_at	TAS2R14	taste receptor, type 2, member 14	−0.97	8.7E-05
236495_at	NA	NA	−0.97	8.1E-10
236666_s_at	LRRC10B	leucine rich repeat containing 10B	−0.98	1.1E-05
237689_at	SARS	Seryl-tRNA synthetase	−1.00	1.8E-03
238174_at	NA	NA	−1.01	6.3E-03
238918_at	NA	NA	−1.06	1.7E-03
239655_at	NA	NA	−1.07	4.2E-03
239819_at	NA	NA	−1.08	1.4E-04
240145_at	NA	NA	−1.10	5.3E-03
240262_at	NA	NA	−1.11	4.2E-05
240652_at	NA	NA	−1.20	8.0E-10
240866_at	NA	NA	−1.26	3.8E-03
242625_at	RSAD2	radical S-adenosyl methionine domain containing 2	−1.43	2.0E-03

NA Not Available
[a]fold change (Log$_2$ ratio)

the herbal plaster treatment was noninvasive and easy to apply. The degree of symptom improvement among Ph-positive allergic rhinitis patients was different with the Ph-negative group, indicating that the acupoint herbal plaster treatment in these patient groups evoked distinct physiological responses. Due to its preliminary nature,

this study has some limitations including the lack of a control group or a safety assessment.

In this study, the average total serum IgE levels tended to increase in Ph-positive and -negative groups following the fourth herbal plaster treatment, but the changes were not statistically significant (Table 4 and 5). This

Table 8 Metacore process map for the 89 genes that were differentially expressed between Ph-positive and Ph-negative patients with allergic rhinitis following acupoint herbal paste treatment

Process map of down-regulated genes in Ph(+)			
Maps	*P* value	Filter Genes[a]	Map genes[b]
DNA damage_NHEJ mechanisms of DSBs repair	1.4E-02	1 (LIG4)	19
Neurophysiological process_Bitter taste signaling	2.0E-02	1 (TAS2R14)	28
Apoptosis and survival_Granzyme A signaling	2.1E-02	1 (LIG4)	30
Cell cycle_Role of Nek in cell cycle regulation	2.3E-02	1 (NEK9)	32
Development_Role of Activin A in cell differentiation and proliferation	2.9E-02	1 (NANOG)	40
Immune response_IL-13 signaling via JAK-STAT	3.1E-02	1 (MMP8)	44
Process map of up-regulated genes in Ph(+)			
Maps	*P* value	Filter Genes[a]	Map genes[b]
Inflammation_Interferon signaling	1.1E-02	3 (IFI6,IFI27, MX1)	110
Autophagy_Autophagy	2.3E-02	2 (PIK3C3,ATG5)	55
Cell cycle_S phase	2.6E-02	2 (HSP90AA1, CCNA2)	149

[a]Number of filter genes in the map
[b]Number of genes in the map

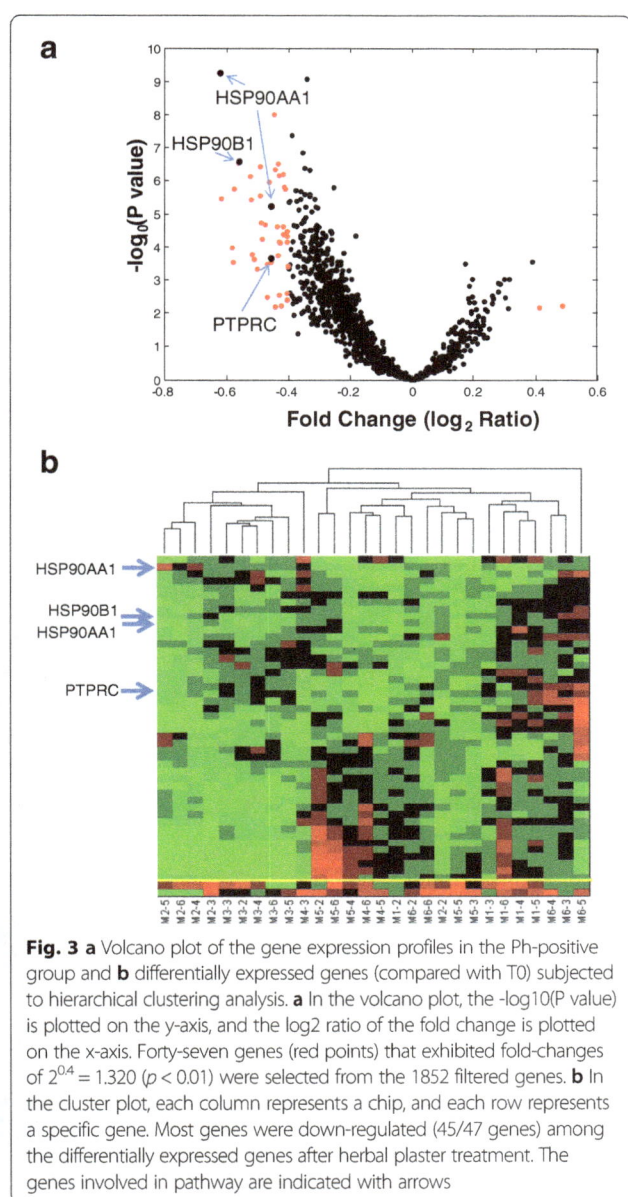

Fig. 3 a Volcano plot of the gene expression profiles in the Ph-positive group and **b** differentially expressed genes (compared with T0) subjected to hierarchical clustering analysis. **a** In the volcano plot, the -log10(P value) is plotted on the y-axis, and the log2 ratio of the fold change is plotted on the x-axis. Forty-seven genes (red points) that exhibited fold-changes of $2^{0.4} = 1.320$ ($p < 0.01$) were selected from the 1852 filtered genes. **b** In the cluster plot, each column represents a chip, and each row represents a specific gene. Most genes were down-regulated (45/47 genes) among the differentially expressed genes after herbal plaster treatment. The genes involved in pathway are indicated with arrows

genes, respectively, between Ph-positive and Ph-negative patients (Fig. 2b and Table 8). Since a Th1/Th2 cytokine imbalance contributes to the etiology and pathogenesis of allergic rhinitis, understanding the mechanisms of this disease will help to find novel targets for therapy. Th1 cells secrete primarily IL-2, IFNγ, IL-3, and GM-CSF, whereas Th2 cells secrete IL-3, IL-4, IL-5, IL-10, IL-13, and GM-CSF [22]. Cytokines released after activation of T-cell receptors interact with cytokine receptors on mononuclear cells and activate these cells via the JAK-STAT (Janus kinase and signal transducers and activators of transcription) pathway. The JAK-STAT pathway is involved in histamine-mediated regulation of the Th2 cytokines IL-5, IL-10, and IL-13, and of the Th1 cytokine IFNγ [22]. IL-13 plays a central role in the promotion of an allergic inflammatory eosinophilic reaction in allergic diseases via IgE isotype switching. IFNγ down-regulates the secretion of certain Th2 cytokines [22]. Local administration of IFNγ in mice prevented antigen-induced eosinophil infiltration into the trachea and normalized airway function. However, recombinant subcutaneous administration of IFNγ had no benefit in the treatment of steroid-dependent asthma [22]. Pathways that down-regulated IL-13 signaling via JAK-STAT and upregulated Interferon signaling pathways were differentially expressed between Ph-positive and Ph-negative patients with allergic rhinitis after acupoint herbal paste treatment; however, further studies are necessary to confirm these results.

Several pathways were significantly induced in Ph-positive allergic rhinitis patients who received acupoint herbal plaster applications. Phagosomal immune response in antigen presentation was noted due to an immune response to the herbal plater treatment (Table 10). Macrophages function to clear infectious particles, and this process involves engulfing microbes into phagosomes where they are lysed and degraded. Phagosomes are pivotal in linking both the innate and adaptive immune responses [46]. Phagosomal proteins regulated by IFNγ include proteins expected to alter phagosome maturation, enhance microbe degradation, trigger the macrophage immune response, and promote antigen loading on major histocompatibility complex (MHC) class I molecules [46]. IFNγ delays phagosomal acquisition of lysosomal hydrolases and peptidases to aid in antigen presentation, which is dependent on phagosomal networks of the actin cytoskeleton and vesicle-trafficking proteins, as well as Src kinases and calpain proteases [47].

In this preliminary study, Ph-positive patients with allergic rhinitis who received acupoint herbal plaster treatments manifested gene expression changes involved in the "Immune response_IL-13 signaling via JAK-STAT" pathway. These patients reported improved clinical

result is similar to that of our previous acupuncture study [16, 17] and may indicate that reducing total IgE synthesis is not the primary mechanism of acupoint herbal plaster treatment of allergic rhinitis.

The Ph-positive and -negative groups exhibited different gene expression trends after acupoint herbal plaster treatment (Fig. 2 and Table 7). This supports the results of the RQLQ, and indicates that the patient groups respond differently to acupoint herbal plaster.

Pathway analysis of the differentially expressed genes indicated that "Immune response_IL-13 signaling via JAK-STAT" and "Inflammation_Interferon signaling" pathways corresponded to down- and up-regulated

Table 9 The 47 genes that were differentially expressed as compared to the first time point (T0; before herbal plaster treatment in the Ph-positive group)

ID	Gene Symbol	Gene Title	Fold change[a]	P value
211969_at	HSP90AA1	heat shock protein 90 kDa alpha (cytosolic), class A member 1	−0.62	5.4E-10
224567_x_at	MALAT1	Metastasis associated lung adenocarcinoma transcript 1 (non-protein coding)	−0.62	3.3E-06
226675_s_at	MALAT1	Metastasis associated lung adenocarcinoma transcript 1 (non-protein coding)	−0.58	1.0E-04
216563_at	ANKRD12	Ankyrin repeat domain 12	−0.58	2.8E-04
222465_at	RSL24D1	ribosomal L24 domain containing 1	−0.58	1.6E-06
204732_s_at	TRIM23	tripartite motif-containing 23	−0.56	2.8E-07
201304_at	NDUFA5	NADH dehydrogenase (ubiquinone) 1 alpha subcomplex, 5, 13 kDa	−0.52	6.9E-07
203491_s_at	CEP57	centrosomal protein 57 kDa	−0.52	3.5E-06
235643_at	SAMD9L	sterile alpha motif domain containing 9-like	−0.52	1.7E-04
209662_at	CETN3	centrin, EF-hand protein, 3 (CDC31 homolog, yeast)	−0.51	2.3E-04
212417_at	SCAMP1	secretory carrier membrane protein 1	−0.50	4.5E-04
217915_s_at	RSL24D1	ribosomal L24 domain containing 1	−0.49	2.6E-06
200598_s_at	HSP90B1	heat shock protein 90 kDa beta (Grp94), member 1	−0.49	3.6E-07
242429_at	ZNF567	zinc finger protein 567	−0.49	1.8E-05
232958_at	NA	NA	−0.48	5.6E-05
222326_at	NA	NA	−0.48	2.0E-05
200026_at	RPL34	ribosomal protein L34	−0.47	3.1E-03
221765_at	UGCG	UDP-glucose ceramide glucosyltransferase	−0.47	3.1E-04
212794_s_at	KIAA1033	KIAA1033	−0.46	1.0E-06
200099_s_at	RPS3A	ribosomal protein S3A	−0.46	2.2E-04
203153_at	IFIT1	interferon-induced protein with tetratricopeptide repeats 1	−0.46	2.9E-04
211968_s_at	HSP90AA1	heat shock protein 90 kDa alpha (cytosolic), class A member 1	−0.45	5.6E-06
226800_at	EFCAB7	EF-hand calcium binding domain 7	−0.45	9.2E-09
225312_at	COMMD6	COMM domain containing 6	−0.44	6.1E-03
201699_at	PSMC6	proteasome (prosome, macropain) 26S subunit, ATPase, 6	−0.44	4.4E-07
222848_at	CENPK	centromere protein K	−0.44	2.4E-05
212587_s_at	PTPRC	protein tyrosine phosphatase, receptor type, C	−0.43	1.7E-04
219239_s_at	ZNF654	zinc finger protein 654	−0.43	3.0E-07
205849_s_at	UQCRB	ubiquinol-cytochrome c reductase binding protein	−0.43	2.7E-03
214453_s_at	IFI44	interferon-induced protein 44	−0.43	6.8E-05
227152_at	C12orf35	chromosome 12 open reading frame 35	−0.43	7.2E-05
200061_s_at	RPS24	ribosomal protein S24	−0.42	5.8E-03
205809_s_at	WASL	Wiskott-Aldrich syndrome-like	−0.42	4.0E-05
222616_s_at	USP16	ubiquitin specific peptidase 16	−0.42	6.0E-07
219356_s_at	CHMP5	chromatin modifying protein 5	−0.42	2.4E-05
244042_x_at	NA	NA	−0.41	4.0E-05

Table 9 The 47 genes that were differentially expressed as compared to the first time point (T0; before herbal plaster treatment in the Ph-positive group) *(Continued)*

205871_at	PLGLA	plasminogen-like A	−0.41	1.4E-06
235653_s_at	THAP6	THAP domain containing 6	−0.41	1.7E-06
219387_at	CCDC88A	coiled-coil domain containing 88A	−0.41	6.8E-05
202110_at	COX7B	cytochrome c oxidase subunit VIIb	−0.41	4.0E-03
209795_at	CD69	CD69 molecule	−0.41	4.5E-05
224786_at	SCOC	short coiled-coil protein	−0.40	2.4E-03
221728_x_at	XIST	X (inactive)-specific transcript (non-protein coding)	−0.40	3.2E-05
214218_s_at	XIST	X (inactive)-specific transcript (non-protein coding)	−0.40	3.9E-04
212391_x_at	RPS3A	ribosomal protein S3A	−0.40	3.6E-04
202411_at	IFI27	interferon, alpha-inducible protein 27	0.41	6.5E-03
228582_x_at	MALAT1	Metastasis associated lung adenocarcinoma transcript 1 (non-protein coding)	0.49	5.8E-03

NA Not Available
[a]fold change (Log$_2$ ratio)

symptoms of allergic rhinitis according to the RQLQ scale. Pathway analysis suggested that allergic rhinitis patients treated with acupoint herbal plaster improved their balance of Th1-derived pro-inflammatory cytokines versus Th2-derived anti-inflammatory cytokines. Our results indicate that acupoint herbal plaster application diminished allergic inflammation by maintaining an appropriate equilibrium between Th1 and Th2 cells.

Conclusions

RQLQ and gene expression profiles indicated that patients with Ph-positive and -negative allergic rhinitis exhibit distinct physiological responses after receiving acupoint herbal plaster treatments. Gene expression levels were compared before and after acupoint herbal plaster application and in Ph-positive versus Ph-negative participants. In this preliminary study, we find that the

IL-13 immune response via JAK-STAT signaling and interferon inflammation signaling were down- and upregulated, respectively, in the Ph-positive group. Further studies are required to verify these pathways in Ph-positive patients, and to determine the mechanism of such pathway dysregulation.

Acknowledgements
We thank the National Science Council NSC 97-3112-B-001-020 by the National Research Program for Genomic Medicine for assistance with statistical analyses, the Genomic Medicine Research Core Laboratory of Chang Gung Memorial Hospital provided technical assistance.

Funding
This study was supported by Chang Gung Medical Research Project CMRPG 380661 and CMRPG 380662, and by CMU under the Aim for Top University Plan of the Ministry of Education, Taiwan and is supported in part by Taiwan Ministry of Health and Welfare Clinical Trial and Research Center of Excellence (MOHW105-TDU-B-212-133019) .

Table 10 Metacore process map for the 45 genes that were down-regulated in Ph-positive patients with allergic rhinitis following acupoint herbal paste treatment

Process map of down-regulated genes in Ph(+)			
Maps	*P* value	Filter Genes[a]	Map genes[b]
Protein folding_Response to unfolded proteins	2.3E-04	2 (HSP90AA1, HSP90B1)	69
Immune response_Antigen presentation	3.3E-04	3 (PTPRC, HSP90AA1, HSP90B1)	197
Immune response_ Phagosome in antigen presentation	7.4E-04	3 (WASL, HSP90AA1, HSP90B1)	243

[a]Number of filter genes in the map
[b]Number of genes in the map

Authors' contributions
SHS, LYS, and CHH conceived the study and designed the study protocol. SHS and LYS wrote the manuscript. CHH and TCN revised study protocols and wrote several sections of the manuscript. CHH and SHS coordinated and directed study implementation. LYS and TCN helped to develop study measures as well as data analysis and interpretation. All authors contributed to drafting the manuscript and have read and approved the final manuscript.

Competing interests
The authors declare that they have no competing interest.

Author details
[1]Chang Gung Memorial Hospital and Chang Gung University College of Medicine, Taoyuan, Taiwan. [2]Department of Biotechnology, Ming Chuan University, Taoyuan, Taiwan. [3]School of Post-Baccalaureate Chinese Medicine, and Research Center for Chinese Medicine and Acupuncture, China Medical University, Taichung, Taiwan. [4]Departments of Chinese Medicine, China Medical University Hospital, Taichung, Taiwan.

References

1. Swartzman LC, Harshman RA, Burkell J, Lundy ME. What Accounts for the Appeal of Complementary/Alternative Medicine, and What Makes Complementary/Alternative Medicine "Alternative"? Med Decis Making. 2002;22(5):431–50.

2. Passalacqua G, Bousquet PJ, Carlsen KH, Kemp J, Lockey RF, Niggemann B, Pawankar R, Price D, Bousquet J. ARIA update: I–Systematic review of complementary and alternative medicine for rhinitis and asthma. J Allergy Clin Immunol. 2006;117(5):1054–62.

3. Tai CJ, Chien LY. The treatment of allergies using Sanfujiu: A method of applying Chinese herbal medicine paste to acupoints on three peak summer days. Am J Chin Med. 2004;32(6):967–76.

4. Tai CJ, Chang CP, Huang CY, Chien LY. Efficacy of sanfujiu to treat allergies: patient outcomes at 1 year after treatment. Evid Based Complement Alternat Med. 2007;4(2):241–6.

5. Hsu WH, Ho TJ, Huang CY, Ho HC, Liu YL, Liu HJ, Lai NS, Lin JG. Chinese medicine acupoint herbal patching for allergic rhinitis: a randomized controlled trial. Am J Chin Med. 2010;38(4):661–73.

6. Wu X, Peng J, Li G, Zhang W, Liu G, Liu B. Efficacy evaluation of summer acupoint application treatment on asthma patients: a two-year follow-up clinical study. J Tradit Chin Med. 2015;35(1):21–7.

7. Zhou F, Yang D, Lu J-y, Li Y-f, Gao K-y, Zhou Y-j, Yang R-x, Cheng J, Qi X-x, Lai L, et al. Characteristics of clinical studies of summer acupoint herbal patching: a bibliometric analysis. BMC Complement Altern Med. 2015;15(1):1–10.

8. China association of Acupuncture-Moxibustion, Guideline of application of 'Winter diseases treated in summer' Herbal patch(draf). Chin Acupunct Moxibustion. 2009;07:541–2.

9. Wen CY, Liu YF, Zhou L, Zhang HX, Tu SH. A Systematic and Narrative Review of Acupuncture Point Application Therapies in the Treatment of Allergic Rhinitis and Asthma during Dog Days. Evid Based Complement Alternat Med. 2015;2015:846851.

10. Chen X, Lu C, Stålsby-Lundborg C, Li Y, Li X, Sun J, Ouyang W, Li G, et al. Efficacy and Safety of Sanfu Herbal Patch at Acupoints for Persistent Allergic Rhinitis: Study Protocol for a Randomized Controlled Trial. Evid Based Complement Altern Med. 2015;2015:10.

11. Zhou F, Yan LJ, Yang GY, Liu JP. Acupoint herbal patching for allergic rhinitis: a systematic review and meta-analysis of randomised controlled trials. Clin Otolaryngol. 2015;40(6):551–68.

12. Xue CC, Li CG, Hugel HM, Story DF. Does acupuncture or Chinese herbal medicine have a role in the treatment of allergic rhinitis? Curr Opin Allergy Clin Immunol. 2006;6(3):175–9.

13. Chang Y-C, Shiue H-S, Chang H-H, Chang C-H, Yang Y-L, Yen H-R. The therapeutic effect of appllying herbal paste onto acupoints for allergic rhinitis during dog days - a preliminary study. J Chin Med. 2006;17(1–2):15–24.

14. Juniper EF, Guyatt GH. Development and testing of a new measure of health status for clinical trials in rhinoconjunctivitis. Clin Exp Allergy. 1991;21(1):77–83.

15. Wang TH, Lee YS, Chen ES, Kong WH, Chen LK, Hsueh DW, Wei ML, Wang HS. Establishment of cDNA microarray analysis at the Genomic Medicine Research Core Laboratory (GMRCL) of Chang Gung Memorial Hospital. Chang Gung Med J. 2004;27(4):243–60.

16. Shiue HS, Lee YS, Tsai CN, Hsueh YM, Sheu JR, Chang HH. DNA microarray analysis of the effect on inflammation in patients treated with acupuncture for allergic rhinitis. J Altern Complement Med. 2008;14(6):689–98.

17. Shiue HS, Lee YS, Tsai CN, Hsueh YM, Sheu JR, Chang HH. Gene expression profile of patients with phadiatop-positive and -negative allergic rhinitis treated with acupuncture. J Altern Complement Med. 2010;16(1):59–68.

18. Skoner DP. Allergic rhinitis: definition, epidemiology, pathophysiology, detection, and diagnosis. J Allergy Clin Immunol. 2001;108(1 Suppl):S2–8.

19. Valenta R. The future of antigen-specific immunotherapy of allergy. Nat Rev Immunol. 2002;2(6):446–53.

20. Benson M, Adner M, Cardell LO. Cytokines and cytokine receptors in allergic rhinitis: how do they relate to the Th2 hypothesis in allergy? Clin Exp Allergy. 2001;31(3):361–7.

21. Holgate ST, Broide D. New targets for allergic rhinitis–a disease of civilization. Nat Rev Drug Discov. 2003;2(11):902–14.

22. Packard KA, Khan MM. Effects of histamine on Th1/Th2 cytokine balance. Int Immunopharmacol. 2003;3(7):909–20.

23. Benson M, Carlsson B, Carlsson LM, Mostad P, Svensson PA, Cardell LO. DNA microarray analysis of transforming growth factor-beta and related transcripts in nasal biopsies from patients with allergic rhinitis. Cytokine. 2002;18(1):20–5.

24. Zhang JH, Cao XD, Lie J, Tang WJ, Liu HQ, Fenga XY. Neuronal specificity of needling acupoints at same meridian: a control functional magnetic resonance imaging study with electroacupuncture. Acupunct Electrother Res. 2007;32(3–4):179–93.

25. Benson M, Jansson L, Adner M, Luts A, Uddman R, Cardell LO. Gene profiling reveals decreased expression of uteroglobin and other anti-inflammatory genes in nasal fluid cells from patients with intermittent allergic rhinitis. Clin Exp Allergy. 2005;35(4):473–8.

26. Eriksson NE. Allergy screening with Phadiatop and CAP Phadiatop in combination with a questionnaire in adults with asthma and rhinitis. Allergy. 1990;45(4):285–92.

27. Liu YH, Chou HH, Jan RL, Lin HJ, Liang CC, Wang JY, Wu YC, Shieh CC. Comparison of two specific allergen screening tests in different patient groups. Acta Paediatr Taiwan. 2006;47(3):116–22.

28. Group IRMW. International Consensus Report on the diagnosis and management of rhinitis. International Rhinitis Management Working Group. Allergy. 1994;49(19 Suppl):1–34.

29. Bousquet J, Van Cauwenberge P, Khaltaev N. Allergic rhinitis and its impact on asthma. J Allergy Clin Immunol. 2001;108(5 Suppl):S147–334.

30. Bachert C, van Cauwenberge P, Khaltaev N. Allergic rhinitis and its impact on asthma. In collaboration with the World Health Organization. Executive summary of the workshop report. 7–10 December 1999, Geneva, Switzerland. Allergy. 2002;57(9):841–55.

31. Juniper EF, Stahl E, Doty RL, Simons FE, Allen DB, Howarth PH. Clinical outcomes and adverse effect monitoring in allergic rhinitis. J Allergy Clin Immunol. 2005;115(3 Pt 2):S390–413.

32. Benson M, Svensson PA, Carlsson B, Jernas M, Reinholdt J, Cardell LO, Carlsson L. DNA microarrays to study gene expression in allergic airways. Clin Exp Allergy. 2002;32(2):301–8.

33. Quackenbush J. Computational analysis of microarray data. Nat Rev Genet. 2001;2(6):418–27.

34. Eisen MB, Spellman PT, Brown PO, Botstein D. Cluster analysis and display of genome-wide expression patterns. Proc Natl Acad Sci U S A. 1998;95(25):14863–8.

35. Cui X, Churchill GA. Statistical tests for differential expression in cDNA microarray experiments. Genome Biol. 2003;4(4):210.

36. Nikolsky Y, Ekins S, Nikolskaya T, Bugrim A. A novel method for generation of signature networks as biomarkers from complex high throughput data. Toxicol Lett. 2005;158(1):20–9.

37. Mason CW, Swaan PW, Weiner CP. Identification of interactive gene networks: a novel approach in gene array profiling of myometrial events during guinea pig pregnancy. Am J Obstet Gynecol. 2006;194(6):1513–23.

38. Winn ME, Zapala MA, Hovatta I, Risbrough VB, Lillie E, Schork NJ. The effects of globin on microarray-based gene expression analysis of mouse blood. Mamm Genome. 2010;21(5–6):268–75.

39. Falcon S, Gentleman R. Using GOstats to test gene lists for GO term association. Bioinformatics. 2007;23(2):257–8.

40. Xue CC, Thien FC, Zhang JJ, Da Costa C, Li CG. Treatment for seasonal allergic rhinitis by Chinese herbal medicine: a randomized placebo controlled trial. Altern Ther Health Med. 2003;9(5):80–7.

41. Raychaudhuri S, Stuart JM, Altman RB. Principal components analysis to summarize microarray experiments: application to sporulation time series. Pac Symp Biocomput. 2000;455–466.

42. Romagnani S. Immunologic influences on allergy and the TH1/TH2 balance. J Allergy Clin Immunol. 2004;113(3):395–400.
43. Jabri B, Kasarda DD, Green PH. Innate and adaptive immunity: the yin and yang of celiac disease. Immunol Rev. 2005;206:219–31.
44. Romagnani S. Th1 and Th2 in human diseases. Clin Immunol Immunopathol. 1996;80(3 Pt 1):225–35.
45. Rengarajan J, Szabo SJ, Glimcher LH. Transcriptional regulation of Th1/Th2 polarization. Immunol Today. 2000;21(10):479–83.
46. Jutras I, Houde M, Currier N, Boulais J, Duclos S, LaBoissiere S, Bonneil E, Kearney P, Thibault P, Paramithiotis E, et al. Modulation of the phagosome proteome by interferon-gamma. Mol Cell Proteomics. 2008;7(4):697–715.
47. Trost M, English L, Lemieux S, Courcelles M, Desjardins M, Thibault P. The phagosomal proteome in interferon-gamma-activated macrophages. Immunity. 2009;30(1):143–54.

9

Feasibility study of transfer function model on electrocardiogram change caused by acupuncture

Haebeom Lee[1] (iD), Hyunho Kim[2], Jungkuk Kim[3], Hwan-Sup Oh[1,4], Young-Jae Park[1,2] and Young-Bae Park[1,2]*

Abstract

Background: Acupuncture treatments that regulate the heart are used to treat various clinical disorders and conditions. Although many studies have been conducted to measure quantitatively the effects of acupuncture, thus far, models that describe these effects have not been established. The purpose of this study was to derive a transfer function model of acupuncture stimulation within the electrocardiograms based on the periods before, during, and after acupuncture.

Methods: Fourteen healthy subjects were included in this clinical trial. Five-minute electrocardiograms were captured before, during, and after acupuncture at HT7. For each period, signal-averaged electrocardiograms were created from all of the subjects' 5-min electrocardiograms for that period. Individual transfer functions, which has the highest average goodness of fit, were derived for each period pair. By averaging individual transfer functions, generalized transfer functions were derived.

Results: The transfer function with the highest average goodness of fit was a fraction with 4th order numerator and 5th order denominator. Fourteen individual transfer functions were derived separately for each pair of periods: before and during acupuncture, during and after acupuncture, and before and after acupuncture. Three generalized transfer functions were derived by averaging individual transfer functions for each period pair.

Conclusion: The three generalized transfer functions that were derived may reflect the electrocardiogram changes caused by acupuncture. However, this clinical trial included only 14 subjects. Further studies with control groups and more subjects are needed.

This clinical trial has been registered on the Clinical Research Information Service, Republic of Korea (No. KCT0001944). The first enrolment of subject started at 2 June 2015 and this trial was retrospectively registered at 14 June 2016

Keywords: Acupuncture, Transfer function, ECG, TCM, Korean medicine

Background

Acupuncture can have local, segmental, extrasegmental, and central regulatory effects [1]. Thus, acupuncture is known to affect not only the somatic nervous system but also the autonomic nervous system (ANS). Acupuncture can be used to treat various clinical disorders or conditions related to the ANS, such as insomnia [2] and hypertension [3]. HT7 (*Shenmen*) is a commonly used acupuncture point used to treat these symptoms [4–6].

To measure effects of acupuncture quantitatively, many studies were conducted by using blood tests, positron emission tomography (PET) [7, 8], functional MRI (fMRI) [9–12], or heart rate variability (HRV) [13, 14]. Acupuncture can reduce heart rate and change HRV by activating the parasympathetic nervous system in the ANS [15, 16]. However, these previous studies lacked quantitative assessments and specific models to describe changes.

In mechanical engineering and electrical engineering, when a known system model is not available, a system

---

* Correspondence: bmppark@khu.ac.kr
[1]Department of Human Informatics of Korean Medicine, Interdisciplinary Programs, Kyung Hee University, Seoul, South Korea
[2]Department of Biofunctional Medicine & Diagnostics, College of Korean Medicine, Kyung Hee University, Seoul, South Korea
Full list of author information is available at the end of the article

identification method is often used. Since transfer function (TF) is a well-known system identification technique to derive a model from an input and output signal, it is widely used in automobile engineering [17], acoustics engineering [18], and electronic circuit engineering [19]. In the biosignal field, TF models are used to analyze EEGs and vibration systems in vehicles [20], human acoustic systems [21], and vascular systems [22–24]. However, much is still unknown about the physiological mechanism or model of electrocardiogram (ECG) changes caused by acupuncture. Therefore, a mathematical model cannot be derived from the previous studies, and simulation of ECG after acupuncture stimulation is not possible.

In this study, to derive a mathematical model, we applied an acupuncture treatment at HT7 (*Shenmen*) on the dominant hand and conducted 5-min ECGs before, during, and after acupuncture to the healthy subjects. After individual TF (ITF) models were derived from each pair of periods, generalized TF (GTF) models were derived by averaging all subjects' ITFs for each pair of periods. By this method, ECG changes caused by acupuncture could be expressed as a GTF. If the error of the GTF and the ITF are similar, the acupuncture stimulus, as well as the personal characteristics, may have a specific effect on the ECG. Therefore, GTF is a mathematical model that can reflect the characteristics of acupuncture stimulation. We try to develop a mathematical model that reflects the general characteristics of acupuncture stimulus by the clinical trial.

Methods
Subjects
All subjects participated voluntarily. The inclusion criteria were as follows: (1) age between 20 and 49 years; (2) ability to communicate adequately about his or her physical condition with a clinical researcher and fill out the questionnaires; and (3) willingness to participate in this clinical trial and sign a written informed consent form. The following subjects were excluded from the study: (1) subjects having an abnormal heart beat period; (2) subjects practicing Qigong or who were athletes; (3) subjects with a cardiovascular disease history including hypertension, arrhythmia, or ischemic heart disease; (4) subjects who had taken cardiovascular-related medicines in the past month; and (5) subjects judged inappropriate by the researcher.

From June 2 to 25 in 2015, 14 subjects were recruited; none was excluded. Sample size 14 was decided by 12 participants from "rule of 12" with 20% marginal window that considering possible drop out [25]. Ultimately, 14 healthy subjects were included in this clinical trial (4 males, 10 females; age, 24–32 years; mean age, 27.07 ± 2.67 years). All subjects were allocated to single intervention group and there is no drop-out subject. Data

from all subject were used for this study. The CONSORT flowchart of this trial is shown in Fig. 1.

ECG instrument and questionnaire
We used an LXC3203 (Laxtha, INC., Daejon, South Korea) and Telescan (Laxtha Inc., Daejon, Republic of Korea) to measure a 4-lead ECG. The sampling frequency was 1024 Hz. Only the lead II signal from the ECG was analyzed in this study.

Subjects were asked to fill out the Korean language version of the Massachusetts General Hospital Acupuncture Sensation Scale (MASS) questionnaire [26] and assess their sensations with the intensity of *de qi* scale [27]. *De qi* is the sensation caused by acupuncture and is an important aspect of acupuncture treatment [26]. To confirm that *de qi* occurred during the acupuncture treatment, we used the MASS index from MASS questionnaire and the scores from the intensity of *de qi* scale. The MASS questionnaire has 13 questions about sensations during the needle-manipulating phase and stationary phase. The intensity of *de qi* scale is a visual analogue scale for *de qi* intensity. One value was missing for one subject; we substituted it with the mean of the other subjects' responses.

Procedure
The procedure of this trial is shown in Fig. 2. Before each subject was included in this clinical trial, we received written consent from him or her after he or she had received a written description of this trial. The clinical trial was conducted in a quiet, designated room at Kyung Hee University Korean Medicine Hospital. ECGs were obtained from the standard 4 leads on the extremities.

After 5 min of relaxation in a comfortable supine position, the pre-acupuncture ECG was recorded for another 5 min. The acupuncture ECG was recorded for 5 min after inserting and twirling an acupuncture needle for 1 min at HT7 of subject's dominant hand. After withdrawing the acupuncture needle, post-acupuncture ECG was recorded for 5 min. After the withdrawal of acupuncture needle, subjects were asked to fill out the MASS questionnaires and *de qi* intensity questionnaire. After a doctor of Korean medicine confirmed that the subject did not have bleeding or other side effects, that subject was considered to have completed the trial. Incentives was given after the completion of the trial.

This clinical trial was approved and supervised by Kyung Hee University Korean Medicine Hospital's Institutional Review Board (No. KOMCIRB-150420-HR-015). The authors confirm that all ongoing and related trials for this intervention are registered.

Acupuncture intervention
All of the acupuncture treatments were performed by the same doctor of Korean medicine, who had 2 years'

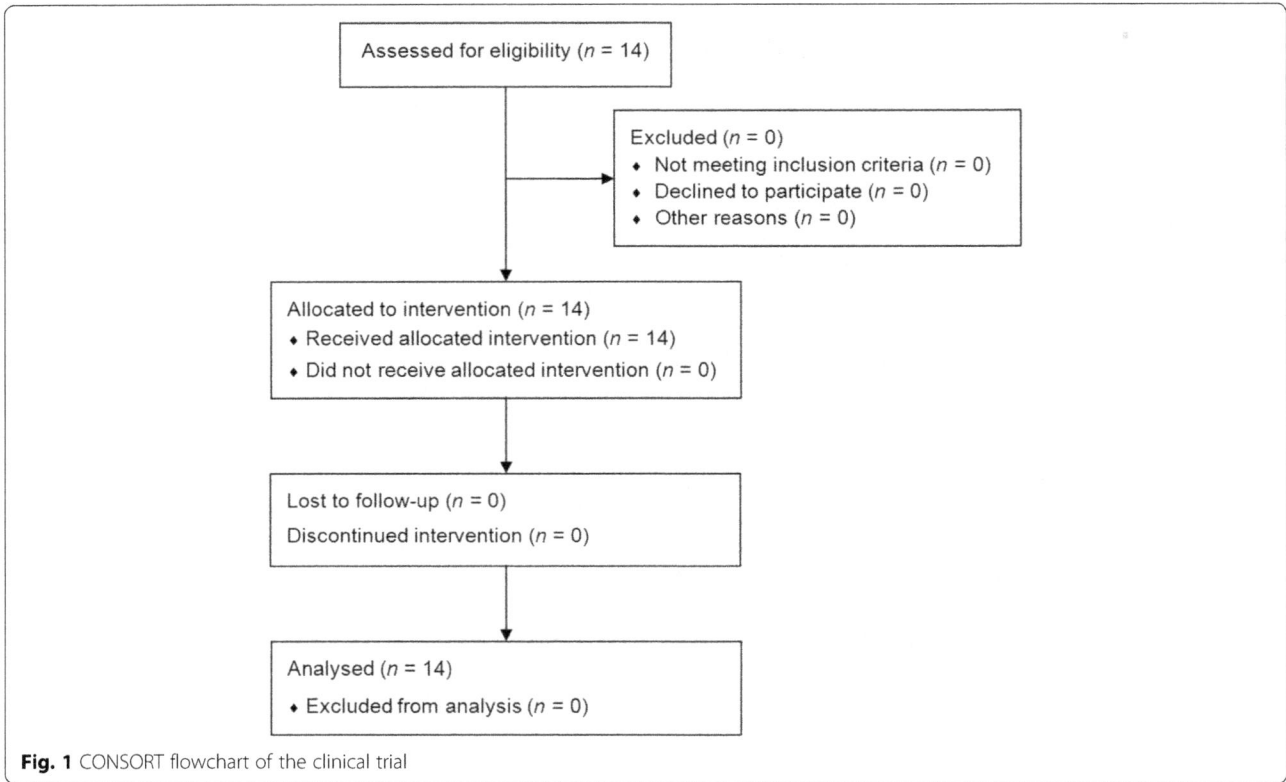

Fig. 1 CONSORT flowchart of the clinical trial

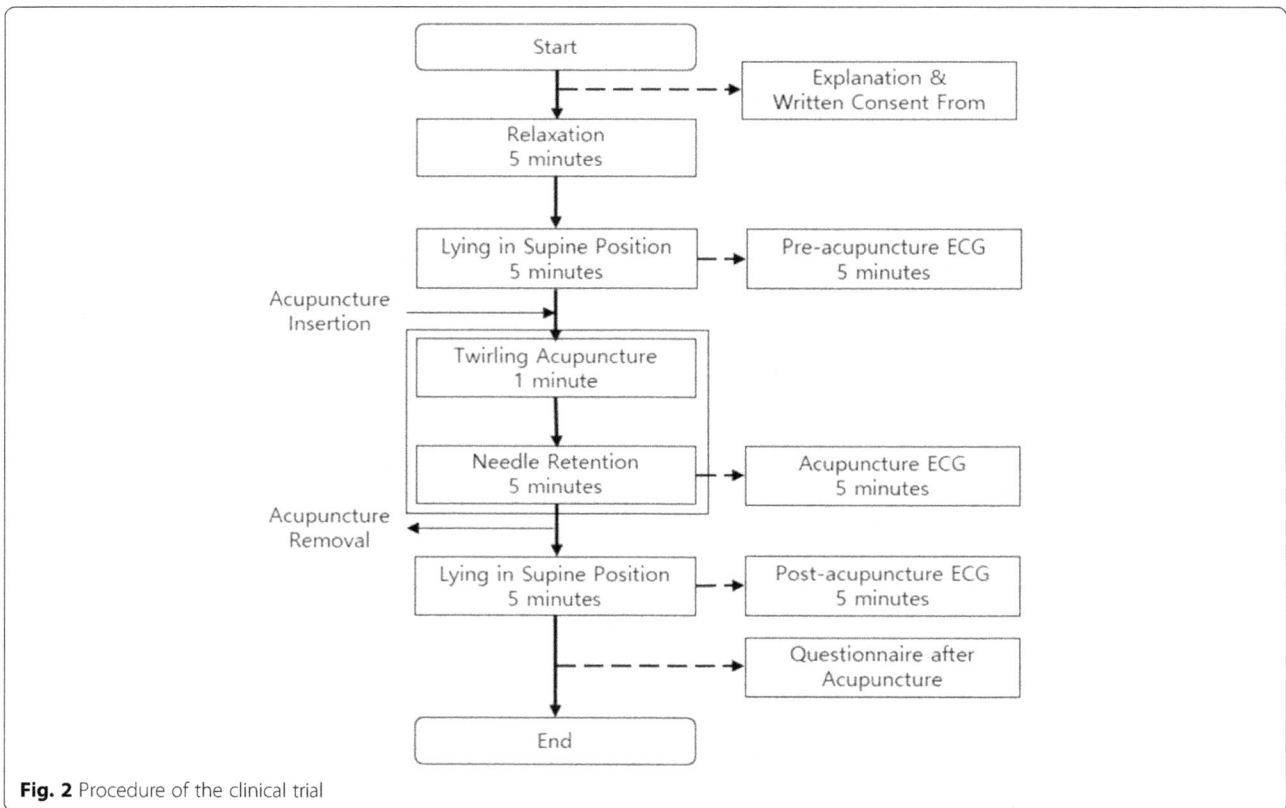

Fig. 2 Procedure of the clinical trial

clinical experience. Subjects received treatment at HT7 (*Shenmen*) on the dominant hand. HT7 is a commonly used acupuncture point for observing HRV [28, 29]. The location of HT7 was determined by using the general guidelines in the World Health Organization Standard Acupuncture Point Locations in the Western Pacific Region [30]. We selected the dominant hand for the acupuncture treatment to be consistent with previous acupuncture studies [31, 32]. The skin near the HT7 acupuncture point was sterilized with 79% alcohol before needle insertion. A 0.30×40 mm acupuncture needle (DongBang Medical, Gyeonggi-do, South Korea) was inserted to a depth of 5–10 mm with a disposable guide tube (DongBang Medical, Gyeonggi-do, South Korea). After the needle was inserted, the guide tube was removed. The twirling method was used to generate a needle sensation. The needle was manipulated for 1 min with 2 Hz and then retained for 5 min without any stimulation. Immediately after 5 min of needle retention, the needle was withdrawn.

Data analysis
Excel 2010 (Microsoft, Redmond, WA, USA) and SPSS Statistics 18 (SPSS, Inc., Chicago, IL, USA) were used for data preprocessing and statistical calculations. Matlab R2015a (Mathworks, Inc., Natick, MA, USA) was used to analyze signal processing.

The lead II signal from the standard 4-lead ECG was used. Signal was filtered with a 0.5–45 Hz band-pass filter. The 5-min ECG signal from lead II was divided into several single ECGs (SECGs) with average heart rate. After reviewing every SECG, all abnormal SECGs that have 2 times higher amplitude than the average SECG of the subject were removed for data cleansing. A single averaged ECG (SAECG) was derived by averaging all SECGs except abnormal SECGs and by aligning the R peaks of SECGs. Consequently, for each subject, an SAECG was obtained at 3 time points: before acupuncture, during acupuncture, and after acupuncture.

The TF, G(z), is a function that can show a relation between the input signal, X(z), and the output signal, Y(z) when z means discrete-time signal in a complex frequency domain: G(z) = Y(z)/X(z). Generally, the TF of a discrete signal comprises a fraction including the n-th order polynomial numerator and m-th order polynomial denominator when b is the coefficient of numerator and a is the coefficient of denominator (Eq. 1).

$$Gz = \frac{b_n z^n + b_{n-1} z^{n-1} + \cdots + b_0}{a_m z^m + a_{m-1} z^{m-1} + \cdots + a_0} \quad (1)$$

The TF was derived by using the tfest function in Matlab for the SAECGs of 3 pairs of periods (before and during acupuncture [BDA], during and after acupuncture

[DAA], and before and after acupuncture [BAA] as the former is the input and the latter is the output) and by aligning the R peaks of the SAECGs within each pair. To use the tfest function in Matlab, m should be ≥ n [33]. As we supposed that our TF model would not have feed-through, eventually we derived n-1th numerator order by the *tfest* function that made the leading coefficient of numerator to 0 [33].

If y_m is a measured signal and y_s is a signal simulated by TF, then the goodness of fit (GF) can be calculated by Eq. 2 using the *compare* function in Matlab [34, 35]. || indicates the 2-norm of a vector. If GF goes to 100, it means that the simulated signal has high similarity to the measured signal.

$$\text{Goodness of Fit} = 100 \times \left(1 - \frac{\|y_m - y_s\|}{\|y_m - \overline{y_m}\|}\right) \quad (2)$$

For the best fit, we explored the GFs of ITFs with 1st–5th order polynomial denominators to find a simple model. An ITF was derived for each subject and for each BDA, DAA, and BAA; the GF for each ITF was then determined. After collecting every GF of ITFs for each period pair, the order of the numerator and the order of the denominator that have highest average GF were used to determine the optimized order. A GTF was derived by averaging each subject's ITF on this optimized order [36, 37]. The process of averaging TF is to average every subject's coefficient on each order and on a specific period pair.

Results
De qi intensity
The MASS index results were as follows: the average was 6.2 out of 10; the standard deviation (SD) was ±1.80; the minimum was 2.48; and the maximum was 8.49. The results for *de qi* intensity were as follows: the average was 5.6 out of 10; the SD was ±1.76; the minimum was 2.0; and the maximum was 8.0. These results indicate that sufficiently intense *de qi* sensations were provided in this trial.

Goodness of fit from all subjects
Table 1 shows the average GFs from all subject's GFs for 1st-5th denominator order of TF for each period pair. The TF with 4th order polynomial numerator and 5th order polynomial denominator has the highest average GF, 94.48. The average GF seems to be saturated under 95, 97, and 94, respectively.

GTFs and ITFs
Each order's coefficient of every subject's ITFs (circle) and GTF (star and line) for BDA, DAA, and BAA pairs are shown in Fig. 3.

Table 1 Averaged goodness of fit for each transfer function for each subject

ON/OD	GF of BDA	GF of DAA	GF of BAA	Mean GF
0/1	92.48	94.07	90.64	92.40
0/2	87.72	95.77	91.46	91.65
1/2	93.56	95.83	92.05	93.81
0/3	87.84	89.12	82.69	86.55
1/3	94.21	96.25	92.35	94.27
2/3	93.43	96.38	92.78	94.20
0/4	42.37	53.79	45.00	47.05
1/4	84.56	86.03	77.63	82.74
2/4	87.84	95.35	92.87	92.02
3/4	93.85	96.21	93.05	94.37
0/5	16.59	30.57	16.97	21.38
1/5	76.49	80.97	48.41	68.62
2/5	83.13	96.41	87.08	88.87
3/5	92.01	96.26	88.18	92.15
4/5	94.91	95.73	92.81	94.48

ON order of numerator, *OD* order of denominator, *GF* goodness of fit, *BDA* periods before and during acupuncture, *DAA* periods during and after acupuncture, *BAA* periods before and after acupuncture

$G_{BD}(z)$ is the GTF for BDA, $G_{DA}(z)$ for DAA, and $G_{BA}(z)$ for BAA. The functions showed as Eqs. 3, 4, and 5.

$$G_{BD}(z) = \frac{2.1655z^4 - 7.1340z^3 + 8.7569z^2 - 4.7618z + 0.9737}{z^5 - 2.7147z^4 + 2.4578z^3 - 0.7302z^2 - 0.0416z + 0.0292}$$

$$(3)$$

$$G_{DA}(z) = \frac{2.7395z^4 - 8.4351z^3 + 96060z^2 - 4.8410z + 0.9312}{z^5 - 2.3208z^4 + 1.8338z^3 - 0.8285z^2 + 0.4626z - 0.1466}$$

$$(4)$$

$$G_{BA}(z) = \frac{2.1861z^4 - 6.5264z^3 + 7.2857z^2 - 3.6988z + 0.7536}{z^5 - 2.3920z^4 + 1.9120z^2 - 0.5381z^2 - 0.0529z + 0.0713}$$

$$(5)$$

For example, Fig. 4a shows a diagram for 3 SAECGs that are used for TF of BDA in Fig. 4b. The measured pre-acupuncture ECG is used as the input signal for the ITF and GTF. The measured acupuncture SAECG is used for calculating GF. Figure 4b shows the 3 acupuncture-phase SAECGs of subject 11. The line is a measured SAECG, the dashed line is the simulated SAECG by ITF for the acupuncture phase, and the dash-dot line is the simulated SAECG by GTF for the acupuncture phase. In the ideal case, the 3 SAECGs would be identical, but differences were seen between the measured acupuncture SAECG,

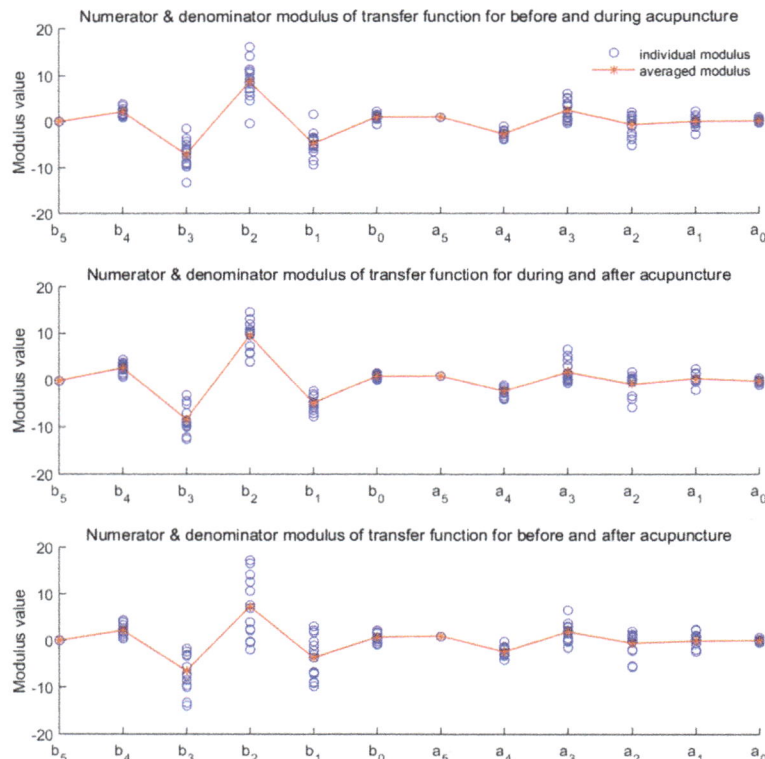

Fig. 3 Coefficients of numerator and denominator of generalized transfer function

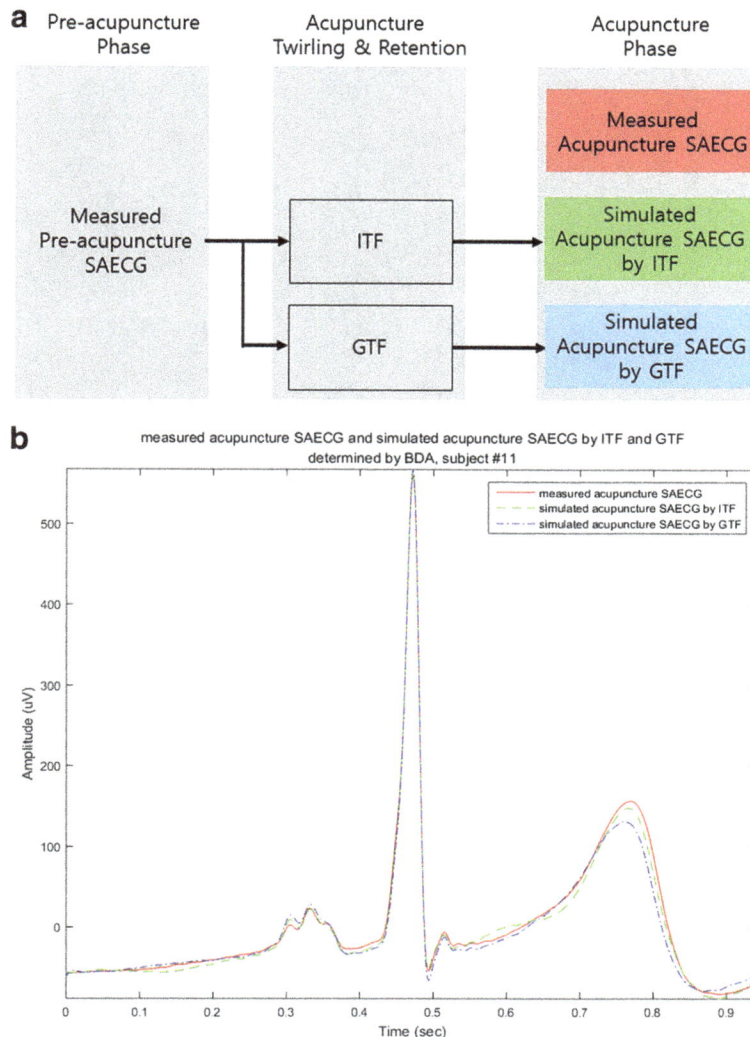

Fig. 4 Three SAECGs and simulated results. **a** Three SAECGs; measured SAECG, simulated SAECG by individual, and generalized transfer function. **b** Example of 3 acupuncture SAECGs: a measured SAECG, a simulated SAECG by individual transfer function, and a simulated SAECG by generalized transfer function. ITF, individual transfer function; GTF, generalized transfer function; SAECG, signal-averaged electrocardiogram; BDA, before and during acupuncture

the acupuncture SAECG estimated by ITF, and the acupuncture SAECG estimated by GTF.

Table 2 shows GFs by ITF and GTF. The average GF differences between ITF and GTF were 0.23, 1.47, and 0.98 for before and during acupuncture, during and after acupuncture, and before and after acupuncture, respectively.

Discussion
Transfer function analysis
To quantify the ECG changes caused by acupuncture, we considered the system identification method. In the field of biomedical engineering, not only is TF model used, but also impulse response model [38] and state space model [39] are widely used as well. The advantage of the TF model is that the system can be easily

expressed. Because of this, we chose to use the TF model over other system identification methods.

The previous studies in which the TF model was used addressed the phase of TF [24, 40]. We did not derive the phase of TF, because the SAECG is not a periodically repeated signal, unlike ECGs used in the previous studies [36, 37]. What we have derived is the TF for an ECG magnitude change from SAECG for a certain period to the SAECG for another period. For example, the acupuncture SAECG can be predicted when pre-acupuncture SAECG is used as the input signal for the TF of BDA.

We derived 3 GTFs from the SAECG changes caused by acupuncture stimulation. These mathematical functions indicate that acupuncture can cause changes in the

Table 2 Goodness of fit of individual and generalized transfer function model

ID	Before and during acupuncture		During and after acupuncture		Before and after acupuncture	
	GF of ITFM	GF of GTFM	GF of ITFM	GF of GTFM	GF of ITFM	GF of GTFM
1	94.03	94.35	97.95	95.34	95.62	94.47
2	97.53	95.90	94.71	92.98	90.41	90.27
3	98.01	97.23	94.19	93.59	93.78	92.49
4	98.44	98.03	97.96	97.33	98.15	97.85
5	96.16	94.30	97.68	96.44	94.75	91.71
6	96.06	95.71	98.31	97.79	96.03	95.62
7	90.90	88.93	90.89	88.10	82.35	76.95
8	92.65	92.94	97.16	96.57	95.66	93.88
9	93.02	91.76	96.68	96.02	91.02	88.24
10	83.03	96.42	98.48	97.72	94.01	94.43
11	92.95	87.80	97.65	96.82	91.32	84.31
12	92.42	90.16	96.93	96.60	94.03	93.50
13	94.47	93.76	97.51	97.44	92.98	92.02
14	94.03	93.19	98.91	98.60	89.08	92.88
Avg	93.84	93.61	96.79	95.81	92.80	91.33
SD	3.857	3.074	2.157	2.712	3.894	5.282

ID subject identification number, *GF* goodness of fit, *ITFM* individual transfer function model, *GTFM* generalized transfer function model, *Avg* average, *SD* standard deviation

heart's electrical system, and they explain the general ECG changes in subjects as well. These 3 GTFs demonstrate different phenomena. In this clinical trial, the TF of BDA reflects acupuncture insertion, twirling, and retention. The TF of DAA reflects acupuncture twirling, retention, and removal. The TF of BAA reflects acupuncture insertion, twirling, and retention. In future studies, 1 or 2 TFs related to a specific type of stimulation can be derived from the result of pairing 2 periods (BDA, DAA, or BAA).

Because this study was a feasibility study, we tried to find the differences and tendencies among the 3 GTFs. We tried to find the same optimized TF order that has the highest GF under the order to be ≤ 5th order denominator for the 3 GTFs. To find the optimized order, we made 15 TFs and calculated 15 GFs per subject and period pair (Table 1). For 14 subjects and 3 period pairs, 630 TFs were needed. To find the optimized TF order ≤ 10th order denominator, we need 2310 TFs. Since 2310 TFs can be too large to probe, we had limited the maximum degree of denominator to 5th order. In this study, we decided 4th order numerator and 5th order denominator as the optimized order, because that TF with optimized orders has the highest average GF under the limit we set.

If a further study were carried out only for a specific period pair, the optimized order might be different. For example, the optimized order for only a BAA is a 3th order numerator and 4th order denominator.

Further study and limitations
From these TFs, we derived models of ECG changes caused by acupuncture stimulation. From these TFs, a SAECG during acupuncture or after acupuncture can be predicted from an arbitrary SAECG before acupuncture, and a SAECG after acupuncture can be predicted from an arbitrary SAECG during acupuncture with a high GF. In previous studies, signal changes caused by acupuncture were hard to predict. HRV was mainly analyzed statistically and it can be influenced by individual differences in the ANS and daily activity patterns [41]. Among the many studies using ECG, there have been a lot of studies that used statistical methods to test the difference of the changes, but the methods of quantitatively predicting the changes were rarely used. The method we used can be used to predict a post-stimulation signal from a specific model with a high GF. In addition 5-min SAECG is widely used because it is also robust against small errors by averaging the signals while 20-min of ECG recording recommended for HRV [42–44].

In this study, we found that the TF method can represent the difference between before, during, and after acupuncture stimulation as a mathematical function. Based on this, it is possible to identify quantitative differences between mathematical models of acupuncture points after finding the mathematical function of ECG changes by acupuncture points in acupuncture stimulation. In addition, the change of ECG according to the needle stimulation technique can be quantitatively expressed as the difference of the mathematical function, so that a quantitative comparison can be made as to which technique changes a lot of ECG. The optimal acupuncture points and techniques for ECG and autonomic control can be found and used in clinically. In addition, this method can be used to make a model that explains the signal changes between a pre-intervention and a post-intervention period. As a result, this method can be useful to evaluate and quantify acupuncture interventions, because an exclusive or singular model related for acupuncture has not established yet.

In the aspect of study design, this study does not include any control group, but only compare the ECG signals before, during, and after acupuncture. There is a disadvantage that it is not known what type of needle stimulation due to the ECG, i.e. whether it is specific to HT7 or needle twirling.

This study was a feasibility study, and the sample size was 14 subjects. Because of this small size, the GTF can be sensitive to outlier subject. To generalize our results, a larger sample size and comparative studies are needed, but we tried to find a feasibility of TF model for acupuncture in this study.

Conclusions

There is no known system model that can describe the ECG changes caused by acupuncture stimulation. We took ECGs before, during, and after acupuncture. For each subject, we made 3 SAECGs: 1 for each period. ITFs were derived from BDA, DAA, and BAA SAECG pairs. By averaging the ITFs, GTFs were derived for each period pair. As a result of prediction of BDA, DAA and BAA with GTF, average GF was 93.6, 95.8, 91.3. The GTF was slightly lower than the ITF, but the difference was small. This means that acupuncture stimulation has a common characteristic to the ECG, and it can be represented by this mathematical model.

Abbreviations

ANS: Autonomic nervous system; BAA: Before and after acupuncture; BDA: Before and during acupuncture; DAA: During and after acupuncture; ECG: Electrocardiogram; fMRI: Functional MRI; GF: Goodness of fit; GTF: Generalized TF; HRV: Heart rate variability; ITF: Individual TF; MASS: Massachusetts General Hospital Acupuncture Sensation Scale; PET: Positron emission tomography; SD: Standard deviation; SECG: Single ECG; TF: Transfer function

Funding
This study did not receive any fund.

Authors' contributions
HL performed the clinical trial, data analysis, and manuscript preparation. HK conceived the clinical trial design, data collection, and manuscript preparation. JK conceived the analysis method and the interpretation. HO participated in result analysis and discussion. YJP conceived the clinical interpretation. YBP conceived the idea of this study. All authors read and approved the final manuscript.

Competing interests
The authors declare that they have competing interests.

Author details
[1]Department of Human Informatics of Korean Medicine, Interdisciplinary Programs, Kyung Hee University, Seoul, South Korea. [2]Department of Biofunctional Medicine & Diagnostics, College of Korean Medicine, Kyung Hee University, Seoul, South Korea. [3]Department of Electronics Engineering, Myongji University, Gyeonggi-do, South Korea. [4]Department of Mechanical Engineering, Kyung Hee University, Gyeonggi-do, South Korea.

References
1. White A, Cummings M, Filshie J. An introduction to western medical acupuncture, 1e. 1st ed. London: Churchill Livingstone; 2008. p. 320.
2. Shergis JL, Ni X, Jackson ML, Zhang AL, Guo X, Li Y, et al. A systematic review of acupuncture for sleep quality in people with insomnia. Complement Ther Med. 2016;26:11–20.
3. Liu Y, Park J-E, Shin K-M, Lee M, Jung HJ, Kim A-R, et al. Acupuncture lowers blood pressure in mild hypertension patients: a randomized, controlled, assessor-blinded pilot trial. Complement Ther Med. 2015;23(5):658–65.
4. Yeung W-F, Chung K-F, Poon MM-K, Ho FY-Y, Zhang S-P, Zhang Z-J, et al. Prescription of Chinese herbal medicine and selection of acupoints in pattern-based traditional Chinese medicine treatment for insomnia: a systematic review. Evid-Based Complement Altern Med Evid-Based Complement Altern Med. 2012;2012:902578.
5. Cevik C, Işeri SO. The effect of acupuncture on high blood pressure of patients using antihypertensive drugs. Acupunct Electrother Res. 2013;38(1–2):1–15.
6. Chae Y, Park HJ, Kang OS, Lee HJ, Kim SY, Yin CS, Lee H. Acupuncture attenuates autonomic responses to smoking-related visual cues. Complement Ther Med. 2011;19 Suppl 1:S1–7.
7. Scheffold BE, Hsieh C-L, Litscher G. Neuroimaging and neuromonitoring effects of electro and manual acupuncture on the central nervous system: a literature review and analysis. Evid Based Complement Alternat Med. 2015; 2015:641742.
8. Shen J. Research on the neurophysiological mechanisms of acupuncture: review of selected studies and methodological issues. J Altern Complement Med N Y N. 2001;7 Suppl 1:S121–7.
9. He T, Zhu W, Du S-Q, Yang J-W, Li F, Yang B-F, et al. Neural mechanisms of acupuncture as revealed by fMRI studies. Auton Neurosci. 2015;190:1–9.
10. Chae Y, Chang DS, Lee SH, Jung WM, Lee IS, Jackson S, Kong J, Lee H, Park HJ, Lee H, Wallraven C. Inserting needles into the body: a meta-analysis of brain activity associated with acupuncture needle stimulation. J Pain. 2013; 14(3):215–22.
11. Huang W, Pach D, Napadow V, Park K, Long X, Neumann J, Maeda Y, Nierhaus T, Liang F, Witt CM. Characterizing acupuncture stimuli using brain imaging with FMRI–a systematic review and meta-analysis of the literature. PLoS One. 2012;7(4):e32960.
12. Chae Y. Acupuncture and brain imaging: what do we have to consider? Acupunct Med. 2012;30(4):250–1.
13. Lee S, Lee MS, Choi J-Y, Lee S-W, Jeong S-Y, Ernst E. Acupuncture and heart rate variability: a systematic review. Auton Neurosci. 2010;155(1–2):5–13.
14. Chung JWY, Yan VCM, Zhang H. Effect of acupuncture on heart rate variability: a systematic review. Evid Based Complement Alternat Med. 2014;2014:819871.

15. Wang J, Kuo TB, Yang CC. An alternative method to enhance vagal activities and suppress sympathetic activities in humans. Auton Neurosci. 2002;100(1–2):90–5.

16. da Silva MAH, Dorsher PT. Neuroanatomic and clinical correspondences: acupuncture and vagus nerve stimulation. J Altern Complement Med. 2014; 20(4):233–40.

17. Thiene M, Ghajari M, Galvanetto U, Aliabadi MH. Effects of the transfer function evaluation on the impact force reconstruction with application to composite panels. Compos Struct. 2014;114:1–9.

18. Elliott S, Stothers I, Nelson P. A multiple error LMS algorithm and its application to the active control of sound and vibration. IEEE Trans Acoust Speech Signal Process. 1987;35(10):1423–34.

19. Yin Y, Zane R, Glaser J, Erickson RW. Small-signal analysis of frequency-controlled electronic ballasts. IEEE Trans Circuits Syst Fundam Theory Appl. 2003;50(8):1103–10.

20. Broman H, Pope M, Hansson T. A mathematical model of the impact response of the seated subject. Med Eng Phys. 1996;18(5):410–9.

21. Aibara R, Welsh JT, Puria S, Goode RL. Human middle-ear sound transfer function and cochlear input impedance. Hear Res. 2001;152(1–2):100–9.

22. O'Rourke MF, Avolio AP. Arterial transfer functions: background, applications and reservations. J Hypertens. 2008;26(1):8–10.

23. Meel-van den Abeelen ASS, van Beek AHEA, Slump CH, Panerai RB, Claassen JAHR. Transfer function analysis for the assessment of cerebral autoregulation using spontaneous oscillations in blood pressure and cerebral blood flow. Med Eng Phys. 2014;36(5):563–75.

24. Chen C-H, Nevo E, Fetics B, Pak PH, Yin FCP, Maughan WL, et al. Estimation of central aortic pressure waveform by mathematical transformation of radial tonometry pressure validation of generalized transfer function. Circulation. 1997;95(7):1827–36.

25. Charity M, Rickey C, Paul N, Paul S. Recommendations for planning pilot studies in clinical and translational research. Clin Transl Sci. 2011;4(5):332–7.

26. Kong J, Gollub R, Huang T, Polich G, Napadow V, Hui K, et al. Acupuncture De Qi, from qualitative history to quantitative measurement. J Altern Complement Med. 2007;13(10):1059–70.

27. Oh HJ, Lee ES, Lee YJ, Lee SD, Kim KS, Kim EJ. The clinical study about qualitative and quantitative characteristics of acupuncture sensation according to the body parts. The Acupuncture. 2013;30(5):65–76.

28. Huang H, Zhong Z, Chen J, Huang Y, Luo J, Wu J, et al. Effect of acupuncture at HT7 on heart rate variability: an exploratory study. Acupunct Med. 2015;33(1):30–5.

29. Litscher G, Liu C-Z, Wang L, Wang L-P, Li Q-Q, Shi G-X, et al. Improvement of the dynamic responses of heart rate variability patterns after needle and laser acupuncture treatment in patients with burnout syndrome: a transcontinental comparative study. Evid Based Complement Alternat Med. 2013;2013:128721.

30. WHO western pacific region. WHO standard acupuncture point locations in the western pacific region. In: WHO standard acupuncture point locations in the western pacific region. Manila: WHO western pacific region; 2008. p. 85.

31. Pfab F, Huss-Marp J, Gatti A, Fuqin J, Athanasiadis GI, Irnich D, et al. Influence of acupuncture on type I hypersensitivity itch and the wheal and flare response in adults with atopic eczema - a blinded, randomized, placebo-controlled, crossover trial: effect of acupuncture on allergen-induced itch in atopic eczema. Allergy. 2009;65(7):903–10.

32. Xu M, Zhou S-J, Jiang C-C, Wu Y, Shi W-L, Gu H-H, et al. The effects of P6 electrical acustimulation on postoperative nausea and vomiting in patients after infratentorial craniotomy. J Neurosurg Anesthesiol. 2012;24(4):312–6.

33. Mathworks, Transfer function estimation. http://www.mathworks.com/help/ident/ref/tfest.html. Accessed 4 Apr 2016.

34. Mathworks, Compare model output and measured output. http://www.mathworks.com/help/ident/ref/compare.html. Accessed 15 Dec 2016.

35. Mathworks, Goodness of fit between test and reference data. http://www.mathworks.com/help/ident/ref/goodnessoffit.html. Accessed 4 Apr 2016.

36. Saul JP, Berger RD, Albrecht P, Stein SP, Chen MH, Cohen RJ. Transfer function analysis of the circulation: unique insights into cardiovascular regulation. Am J Physiol. 1991;261(4 Pt 2):H1231–45.

37. Berger RD, Saul JP, Cohen RJ. Transfer function analysis of autonomic regulation. I. Canine atrial rate response. Am J Physiol. 1989;256(1 Pt 2): H142–52.

38. Ehlert FA, Korenstein D, Steinberg JS. Evaluation of P wave signal-averaged electrocardiographic filtering and analysis methods. Am Heart J. 1997;134(6): 985–93.

39. Fojt O, Holcik J. Applying nonlinear dynamics to ECG signal processing. Two approaches to describing ECG and HRV signals. IEEE Eng Med Biol Mag Q Mag Eng Med Biol Soc. 1998;17(2):96–101.

40. Karamanoglu M, O'Rourke MF, Avolio AP, Kelly RP. An analysis of the relationship between central aortic and peripheral upper limb pressure waves in man. Eur Heart J. 1993;14(2):160–7.

41. Grossman P. Respiratory sinus arrhythmia, cardiac vagal control, and daily activity. AJP Heart Circ Physiol. 2004;287(2):H728–34.

42. Schneider MAE, Plewan A, Schmitt C, Meinertz T. The signal-averaged ECG obtained by a New digital holter recording system. Ann Noninvasive Electrocardiol. 1996;1(4):379–85.

43. Goldberger JJ, Challapalli S, Waligora M, Kadish AH, Johnson DA, Ahmed MW, et al. Uncertainty principle of signal-averaged electrocardiography. Circulation. 2000;101(25):2909–15.

44. Electrophysiology TF o. t. ES o. C t. NAS. Heart rate variability : standards of measurement, physiological interpretation, and clinical use. Circulation. 1996;93(5):1043–65.

Antidepressant-like effects of acupuncture involved the ERK signaling pathway in rats

Xuhui Zhang[1], Yingzhou Song[1], Tuya Bao[1*], Miao Yu[1], Mingmin Xu[1], Yu Guo[1], Yu Wang[1], Chuntao Zhang[1,2] and Bingcong Zhao[1]

Abstract

Background: The extracellular signal-regulated kinase (ERK) signaling pathway is considered to be associated with the pathogenesis and treatment of depression. Acupuncture has been demonstrated to ameliorate depression-related behavior and promote neurogenesis. In this study, we explored the role of the ERK signaling pathway in the antidepressant-like effects of acupuncture in rats exposed to chronic unpredictable mild stress (CUMS).

Methods: Eighty male Sprague–Dawley rats were randomly divided into eight groups: control group, model group, model + Acupuncture group (Acu group), model + fluoxetine group (FLX group), model + DMSO group (DMSO group), model + PD98059 group (PD group), model + Acupuncture + PD98059 group (Acu + PD group) and model + fluoxetine + PD98059 group (FLX + PD group). Except for the control group, all rats were subjected to 3 weeks of CUMS protocols to induce depression. Acupuncture was carried out for 10 min at acupoints of Baihui (GV-20) and Yintang (GV-29) each day during the experimental procedure. The ERK signaling pathway was inhibited using PD98059 through intracerebroventricular injection. The depression-like behaviors were evaluated using the sucrose intake and open-field tests. The protein levels of ERK1/2, phosphor (p)-ERK1/2, cAMP response element-binding protein (CREB), p-CREB and brain-derived neurotrophic factor (BDNF) in the hippocampus were examined using western blot.

Results: Acupuncture ameliorated the depression-like behaviors and dysfunction of the ERK signaling pathway in the hippocampus of CUMS rats. PD98059 pretreatment inhibited the improvements brought about by acupuncture on the ERK signaling pathway.

Conclusions: Taken together, our results indicated that acupuncture had a significant antidepressant-like effect on CUMS-induced depression model rats, and the ERK signaling pathway was implicated in this effect.

Keywords: Acupuncture, Depression, Extracellular signal-regulated kinase (ERK), Chronic unpredictable mild stress (CUMS), Neurogenesis

Background

Depression is a common mental disorder and a leading cause of disability throughout the world [1, 2]. Antidepressants remain the main clinical treatment for depression [3, 4]; however, antidepressants cannot completely meet the needs of depression patients [5]. Acupuncture, an important part of traditional Chinese medicine, has been shown promising effects in alleviating the progression of depression [6, 7]. However, the underlying mechanism is poorly understood.

In the last few years, studies have found that a decline in neurogenesis might be an etiological factor in depression [8, 9]. Brain-derived neurotrophic factor (BDNF) has been shown to mediate neurogenesis and synaptic plasticity, which is implicated in depression pathogenesis [10]. The extracellular signal-regulated kinase (ERK) 1/2, a downstream target of BDNF, is activated by the binding of BDNF to tyrosine kinase receptor-B (Trk-B) via the Ras-dependent cascade, including phosphorylation (p) of transcription factors such as cAMP response element-binding protein (CREB) [11] (Fig. 1). Some studies have proved that a decrease in ERK1/2 expression leads to depression-like behaviors in model rats

* Correspondence: tuyab_tcm@163.com
[1]Beijing University of Chinese Medicine, Beijing, Beijing 100029, China
Full list of author information is available at the end of the article

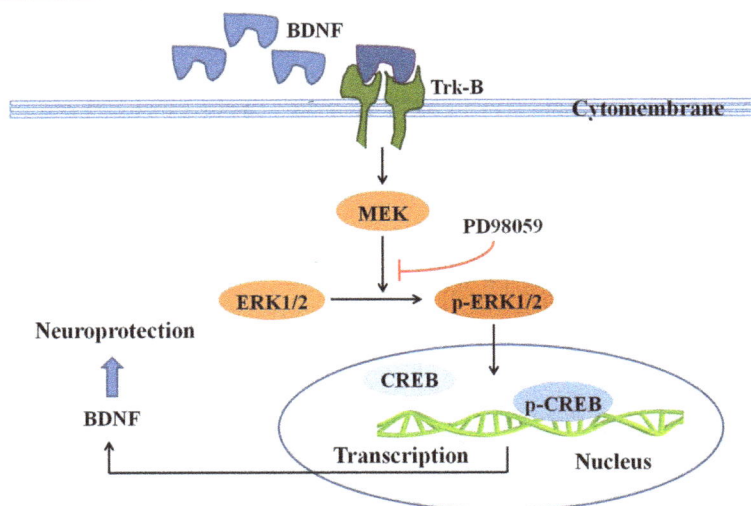

Fig. 1 The ERK signaling pathway. BDNF combines with its specific receptor Trk-B and the compound object can activate the Ras-dependent cascade. The Ras-dependent cascade is Ras-Raf-MEK-ERK signaling pathway. Phosphorylated ERK1/2 (p-ERK1/2) can further phosphorylate CREB and promote the transcription of BDNF mRNA. PD98059 prevents the ERK1/2 from being phosphorylated. Activating reactions were depicted by an *arrow* with a *black* color and the inhibiting effect of PD98059 was depicted by a *line* with a *red* color. The proteins involved in the present study were marked by a *rectangle box* with a *black* color. *BDNF* brain-derived neurotrophic factor, *CREB* cAMP response element-binding protein, *ERK1/2* extracellular signal-regulated kinase 1/2, *MEK* ERK1/2 kinase, *p-CREB* phosphor-CREB, *p-ERK1/2* phosphor-ERK 1/2, *Trk-B* tyrosine receptor kinase B

[12–14]. Antidepressants can alleviate the symptoms of depression by increasing ERK1/2 [15] and p-ERK1/2 expression [16–19].

Recent studies showed that acupuncture produced the neuroprotective effects in many neurological disorders [20], including up regulating the gene and protein expression of BDNF in hippocampus [21, 22], reducing neural apoptosis and promoting adult neuron neurogenesis [23, 24]. Additionally, our previous study found that acupuncture activated the proteins expression of phosphor (p)-ERK1/2 and p-CREB in the hippocampus and prefrontal cortex in depression model rats [25]. Therefore, we had a hypothesis that the antidepressant-like effect of acupuncture might via modulation of the ERK signaling pathway [25, 26].

The aim of the present study was to investigate the regulation of acupuncture on the depressive-like behaviors and the ERK signaling pathway as well as BDNF protein expression in chronic unpredictable mild stress (CUMS)-induced depression model rats. We used PD98059 pretreatment to inhibit the activity of p-ERK1/2; then, we evaluated the behavioral activities by the sucrose intake and open field tests, as well as the protein levels of ERK1/2, p-ERK1/2, CREB, p-CREB and BDNF in the hippocampus by western blot analysis.

Methods
Animals
Eighty male Sprague–Dawley rats aged 8 weeks old and weighing 180~200 g each were obtained from Vital River

Laboratory Animal Technology Co. Ltd, China (license number SCXK [Jing] 2012-0001). The experimental procedures were conducted in compliance with the *Guidance Suggestions for the Care and Use of Laboratory Animal*, issued by the Ministry of Science and Technology of China [27] and received approval from the Animal Ethics Committee of Beijing University of Chinese Medicine (permission No. Kj-dw-18-20140923-01).

Overall research design
All animals were fed ad libitum, and housed at 23–25 °C on a 12 h light/dark cycle (lights on between 7:00 A.M. and 7:00 P.M.). They were randomly divided into eight groups ($n = 10$ per group) as follows: (1) The control rats were not subjected to any stress except general handling for 3 weeks. (2) The CUMS group rats were exposed to CUMS for 3 weeks. (3) The Acu group rats received acupuncture stimulation and CUMS for 3 weeks. (4) The FLX group rats received fluoxetine treatment and CUMS for 3 weeks. (5) The DMSO group or (6) PD98059 group (PD group) rats were exposed to CUMS and intracerebroventricular injection of either dimethylsulfoxide (DMSO) or PD98059, respectively, for 3 weeks. Then, the groups in which PD98059 was administered were treated in the same manner as the PD group except (7) acupuncture (Acu + PD group) or (8) fluoxetine (FLX + PD group) was also administered. One rat in the Acu + PD group died during stereotactic surgery; thus, 79 rats were involved in the final analysis. The overall research design is shown in Fig. 2.

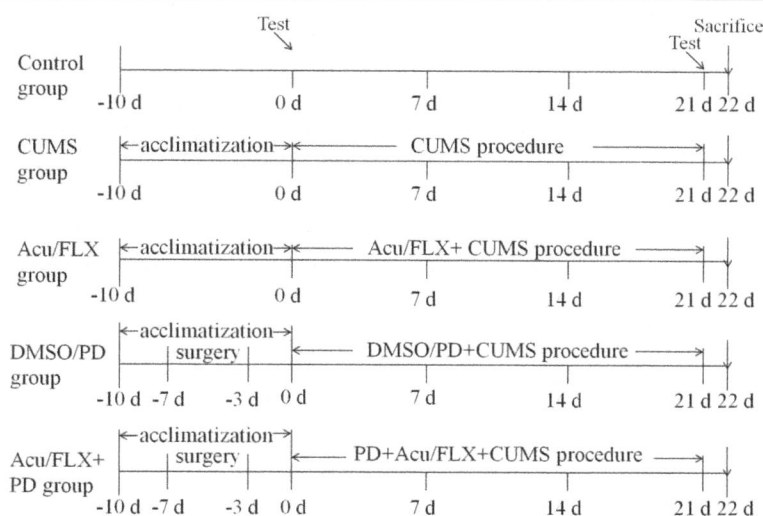

Fig. 2 Overall research design

Fluoxetine is a classic antidepressant that belongs to selective serotonin reuptake inhibitor medication. The recent study demonstrated that fluoxetine-induced the increase in BDNF protein level was accompanied by activating the ERK signaling pathway [28]. So we chose fluoxetine as the positive medication to evaluate the effect of acupuncture on the ERK signaling pathway. PD98059 is dissolved in DMSO to meet the concentration that can inhibit the ERK signaling pathway [29, 30]. DMSO is characteristic of anti-inflammation, analgesic and promoting blood circulation. Besides, the placement of cannula is an invasive surgery. So we set the DMSO group and compared it with the CUMS and PD groups respectively to eliminate the interferences of DMSO and the surgery to the behavior tests and the indexes.

Chronic unpredictable mild stress procedure

The chronic unpredictable mild stress (CUMS) model was modified from the methods previously described [31] and has been validate as one of the most relevant models of depression. Except for the control group, all rats were exposed to CUMS after 10 d of acclimatization under the housing conditions. Seven different stressors were used to model a state of depression as follows: food deprivation (24 h), water deprivation (24 h), wet bedding (24 h), overnight illumination (12 h), using a restraining device (2 h), shaking the cage on a rocking bed (30 min), and clamping the middle of tail with a binder clip (3 min). The CUMS procedure was carried out for 3 weeks and a different stressor was administered randomly each day.

Intracerebroventricular injection

Rats were anesthetized with 350 mg/kg 10 % chloral hydrate i.p. and placed in a rat brain stereotactic frame (RWD, Shenzhen, China) with the incisor bar positioned 4 mm below the interaural zero. A burr hole (0.9 mm posterior to the bregma; 1.5 mm lateral to the midline) was drilled through the parietal bone and a stainless-steel guide cannula (RWD; 0.58 mm outside diameter [OD], 0.38 mm inside diameter [ID], 3.5 mm under the dura [L]) was positioned in the lateral ventricle and secured with screws and dental acrylic onto the skull, serving as a guide for the accurate insertion of a internal cannula (RWD; 0.36 mm OD, 0.20 mm ID, aligning to the tip of the guide cannula). A cap (RWD; 0.36 mm diameter, aligning to the tip of the guide cannula) was always placed in the guide cannula and removed during the injection to prevent clogging or infection in the brain tissue. Reflux of cerebrospinal fluid from the guide cannula verified the correct placement of the intracerebroventricular cannula. The rats were given 3 d to recover after the surgery. After recovery, either 5 μL PD98059 (100 μM, dissolved in DMSO) or 5 μL DMSO was delivered by micro-injection with a pressure equalizer tube connected to the internal cannula. After injection, the internal cannula was left in the guide cannula for 1 min to ensure proper delivery.

Acupuncture and drug treatment

Acupuncture was performed at the acupoints of Baihui (GV-20) and Yintang (GV-29) in Acu group and Acu + PD group each day during the experimental procedure. Sterilized disposable stainless steel needles of 0.3 mm diameter were inserted as deep as 2–3 mm. GV-20 is located above the apex auriculate, on the midline of the head. GV-29 is located at the midpoint of the two eyes. The acupuncture treatment was manually delivered by twisting the acupuncture needles at a frequency of twice per second for 1 min, and then the needles were retained for 10 min [25]. The FLX group and FLX + PD group were treated with 2.5 mg kg^{-1} d^{-1} fluoxetine (intragastric administration) each day during the experimental procedure.

Behavior tests

The sucrose intake test (SIT) is used as a measure of anhedonia [32]. Before the first SIT, the rats were habituated to consume 1 % sucrose solution for 24 h without any water and then deprived of water for 24 h. The rats were then given a 2-h window for SIT between 12:00 and 14:00 h. The amount of sucrose consumed was measured by comparing the bottle weight before and after the 2-h window. The SIT was performed at beginning (0 d) and at end (21 d) of the experiment.

The open-field test (OFT) is commonly used to measure general locomotor activity and willingness to explore in rodents [33]. In the OFT, the rat was gently placed at the center of a square arena, which was a four-sided $80 \times 80 \times 40$ cm^3 box with the floor and walls painted black. The arena was divided into 16×16 equal squares that had been drawn on the floor. Each rat was allowed to freely explore the arena for 5 min. The activity of the rat was recorded by a video camera installed on top of the lateral high wall, similar to our previous experiment [34]. Two observers, blind to the experiment, counted the crossing number (defined as at least three paws in a square) and the rearing number (defined as the rat standing upright on its hind legs). After each animal was tested, the box was cleaned with a 10 % ethanol solution to remove any olfactory cues. The OFT was also performed at beginning (0 d) and at end (21 d) of the experiment.

Western blotting analysis

Hippocampal tissue from rats was collected, immediately placed on dry ice, and stored at −80 °C until assay. Samples were homogenized in a standard lysis buffer supplemented with protease or phosphatase inhibitor cocktail, incubated on ice for 20 min, and centrifuged at 13,000 rpm for 20 min. The protein concentration was determined using a bicinchoninic acid (BCA) protein assay kit (Cwbio, Beijing, China). Proteins (24 μg) were separated on a 10 % sodium dodecyl sulfate-polyacrylamide gel electrophoresis gel (120 V, 60 min) and blotted (300 mA, 100 min) onto a polyvinylidene fluoride membrane. The membranes were blocked in 5 % bull serum albumin (BSA) tris-buffered saline plus Tween (BSA-TBST) for 1 h at room temperature (RT) and incubated at 4 °C overnight with the following primary antibodies: anti-ERK1/2 (catalogue NO.: 4965), anti-phosphor (p)-ERK1/2 (catalogue NO.: 4377), anti-response element binding protein (CREB) (catalogue NO.: 4820), anti-p-CREB

(catalogue NO.: 9198), and anti-BDNF (catalogue NO.: ab46176) (1:1000 in 5 % BSA-TBST; Cell Signaling Technology, Danvers, MA, USA). Equal loading was confirmed using anti-β-actin (catalogue NO.: TA-09) (1:1000 in 5 % BSA-TBST; ZSGB-BIO, Beijing, China). Membranes were washed with TBST and incubated for 60 min at RT with horseradish peroxidase conjugated to goat anti-rabbit/mouse IgG (catalogue NO.: 111-035-003/115-035-003) (1:10,000 in 5 % BSA-TBST; Jackson ImmunoResearch Laboratories, Inc., West Grove, PA, USA). Immunoreactivity was visualized using enhanced chemiluminescence (Merck Millipore, USA).

Statistical analysis

Data are presented as the mean ± SD. The comparisons of sucrose intake and western blot analysis between groups within the same time point were examined by one-way analysis of variance (ANOVA) method after the test of normal distribution and homogeneity of variance, followed by the LSD *post hoc* test. Since the crossing number and rearing number were not normally distributed, Kruskal-Wallis test was used, followed by the Mann–Whitney U-test. Statistical significance was defined as $P < 0.05$.

Results

Changes in sucrose intake

At the beginning (0 d), there was no significant difference among groups [$F_{(7,71)} = 0.862$, $P > 0.05$]. At the end of the experiment (21 d), the sucrose intake was significantly different among groups [$F_{(7,71)} = 26.302$, $P < 0.01$] (Fig. 3 and Table 1). It was markedly reduced in the CUMS group compared to that in the control group ($P < 0.01$). Both acupuncture and fluoxetine treatment increased the sucrose intake ($P < 0.01$ for both), and fluoxetine treatment showed more effectiveness than acupuncture in the sucrose intake test ($P < 0.05$). However, they were still lower than those in the control group ($P < 0.01$ and $P < 0.05$, respectively). The difference between the CUMS and DMSO groups was not significant ($P > 0.05$), and the difference between the DMSO and PD groups was also not significant ($P > 0.05$); however, the sucrose intake in the PD group was lower than that in the CUMS group ($P < 0.05$). PD98059 pretreatment obviously inhibited the increase induced by acupuncture or fluoxetine ($P < 0.01$ for both).

Comparison of crossing and rearing numbers

There was no significant difference among groups in crossing [chi-square = 3.424, $P > 0.05$] (Fig. 4 and Table 2) and rearing numbers [chi-square = 8.831, $P > 0.05$] (Fig. 5 and Table 2) at 0 d. After the 21-d stress procedure, the crossing number (chi-square = 63.461, $P < 0.01$) (Fig. 4) and rearing number [chi-square = 61.099, $P < 0.01$] (Fig. 5)

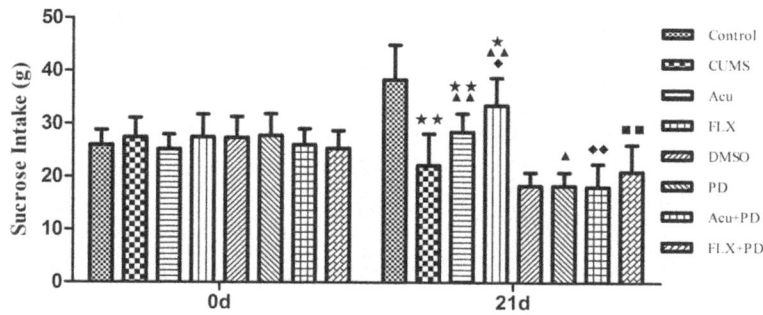

Fig. 3 Sucrose intake at 0 d and 21 d. ★$P < 0.05$, ★★$P < 0.01$ versus control group; ▲$P < 0.05$, ▲▲$P < 0.01$ versus CUMS group; ♦$P < 0.05$, ♦♦$P < 0.01$ versus Acu group; ■■$P < 0.01$ versus FLX group. (mean ± SD, $n = 9$–10)

differed significantly among groups. Compared to the control group, CUMS rats showed a significant reduction in crossing and rearing numbers ($P < 0.01$ for both); however, both acupuncture treatment and fluoxetine treatment improved both crossing ($P < 0.01$ for both) and rearing numbers ($P < 0.01$ for both). There was no difference among the CUMS, DMSO and PD groups in crossing ($P > 0.05$) or rearing numbers ($P > 0.05$). The increase in rearing numbers induced by both acupuncture and fluoxetine was inhibited by PD98059 pretreatment ($P < 0.01$ for both); however, the increase in crossing numbers induced by acupuncture or fluoxetine was not affected by PD98059 pretreatment ($P > 0.05$ for both).

Western blot analysis of ERK1/2 and p-ERK1/2 in the hippocampus

There was no significant difference in ERK1/2 protein expression in the hippocampus [$F_{(7,40)} = 0.598$, $P > 0.05$] among the groups; however, p-ERK1/2 expression different significantly among the groups [$F_{(7,40)} = 6.804$, $P < 0.01$] (Fig. 6 and Table 3). The p-ERK1/2 levels were down-regulated in the CUMS group ($P < 0.01$) compared to that in the control group, and acupuncture or fluoxetine treatment markedly increased these levels ($P < 0.05$ for both). The expression of p-ERK1/2 decreased more

in the PD group than that in the CUMS group ($P < 0.05$) and the DMSO group ($P < 0.01$); however, there was no difference between the CUMS and DMSO groups ($P > 0.05$). The expression of p-ERK1/2 in the Acu + PD group was lower than that in the Acu group ($P < 0.05$). There was no significant difference in p-ERK1/2 between the FLX + PD and FLX groups, but the P value was close to the critical point ($P = 0.067$).

Western blot analysis of CREB and p-CREB in the hippocampus

There was a significant difference in CREB [$F_{(7.40)} = 3.323$, $P < 0.01$] and p-CREB [$F_{(7,40)} = 5.368$, $P < 0.01$] expression among the groups (Fig. 7 and Table 4). The expression of both proteins was significantly down-regulated in the CUMS group ($P < 0.05$ and $P < 0.01$, respectively) compared to that in the control group. Acupuncture markedly increased CREB and p-CREB protein expressions ($P < 0.05$ for both). Fluoxetine also increased CREB and p-CREB protein expressions ($P < 0.05$ for both). There was no significant difference in the expression of CREB ($P > 0.05$) and p-CREB ($P > 0.05$) proteins among the CUMS, DMSO and PD groups; however, CREB and p-CREB protein expressions in the Acu + PD group were lower than those in the Acu group ($P < 0.05$ for both). Additionally, CREB and p-CREB protein expressions in the FLX + PD group were lower than those in the FLX group ($P < 0.01$ and $P < 0.05$, respectively).

Western blot analysis of BDNF in the hippocampus

There was a significant difference in BDNF expression among the groups [$F_{(7.40)} = 2.842$, $P < 0.05$] (Fig. 8 and Table 5). It was significantly down-regulated in the CUMS group ($P < 0.01$) compared to that in the control group, and acupuncture or fluoxetine treatment markedly increased these levels ($P < 0.05$ for both). There was no significant difference in the expression of BDNF protein among the CUMS, CUMS and PD groups ($P > 0.05$). Additionally, the increase in BDNF protein induced by acupuncture or

Table 1 Sucrose intake at 0 d and 21 d

Group	Sucrose intake (g)	
	0 d	21 d
Control	25.96 ± 2.83	38.31 ± 6.63
CUMS	27.44 ± 3.68	22.17 ± 5.96★★
Acu	25.20 ± 2.77	28.49 ± 3.47★★▲▲
FLX	27.47 ± 4.29	33.51 ± 5.17★▲▲
DMSO	27.37 ± 3.95	18.35 ± 2.54
PD	27.77 ± 4.13	17.43 ± 3.96▲
Acu+PD	26.03 ± 3.02	18.15 ± 4.38♦♦
FLX+PD	25.37 ± 3.31	21.06 ± 5.10■■

★$P < 0.05$, ★★$P < 0.01$ vs. control group; ▲$P < 0.05$, ▲▲$P < 0.01$ vs. CUMS group; ♦♦$P < 0.01$ vs. Acu group; ■■$P < 0.01$ vs. FLX group. (mean ± SD, $n = 9$–10)

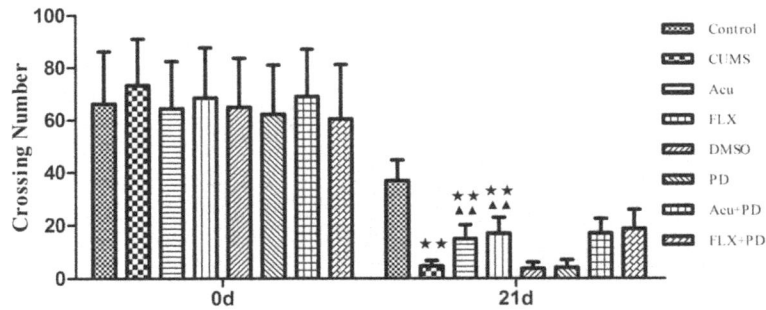

Fig. 4 Crossing number at 0 d and 21 d. $\star\star P < 0.01$ versus control group; $\blacktriangle\blacktriangle P < 0.01$ versus CUMS group. (mean ± SD, $n = 9$–10)

fluoxetine was not affected by PD98059 pretreatment ($P > 0.05$ for both).

Discussion

Depression-like behaviors induced by CUMS

Chronic unpredictable mild stress (CUMS) can be used as a valid and reliable method by which to build an animal model of depression [35–37]. There are various methods to evaluate the model behaviors including the sucrose intake test (SIT), the open-field test (OFT) and the forced-swim test (FST). The decrease in sucrose consumption is considered as the inhibition of the brain reward system [38]. The OFT has been used widely to assess the anxiety behaviors [39]; however, it also can be used to evaluate the spontaneous activity in rodents [34, 40, 41]. Increased immobility in the FST is often anthropomorphized as an expression of despair; however, it can also be understood as a successful and adaptive behavioral response that functions to conserve energy [42]. Additionally, it was not recommended that the rats which received the surgery to perform the FST. As a result, we chose the SIT and OFT to analyze the depressive state of the model rats. The present study showed that CUMS induced an obvious decrease in sucrose intake and locomotion. The results suggested that CUMS decreased the sensitivity of model rats to sucrose and

exploration, which were similar to the depressive symptoms, such as anhedonia and behavioral and cognitive dysfunction.

Chronic unpredictable mild stress made the hippocampal extracellular signal-regulated kinase signaling pathway dysfunction

The ERK signaling pathway participates in neural proliferation, differentiation and neurogenesis and plays an important role in learning and memory [11, 43, 44]. A growing body of study demonstrates that the ERK signaling pathway is involved in the potential target for depression therapy [45–47], and inhibiting the ERK signaling pathway can block antidepressant medications activities [46, 48]. Furthermore, activated ERK protein can regulate transcription by controlling the phosphorylation of cyclic adenosine monophosphate response element binding protein (CREB) [12], which mediates the transcription of its target genes, such as BDNF mRNA and Bcl-2 mRNA. An early study found that the expression of CREB and p-CREB was decreased in the postmortem orbitofrontal cortex of patients with major depression disorder [49]. Another study found that CRE-DNA complexes, CREB protein, and CREB mRNA were reduced in the prefrontal cortex of depression patients who committed suicide [50]. Therefore, CREB also plays an important role in the physiology and pathology of depression [51] and treatment with antidepressants [52]. However, our early study showed that p-ERK1/2 and p-CREB, but not ERK1/2 and CREB, proteins decreased in the hippocampus and prefrontal cortex of rats exposed to CUMS [25]. Thus, in the present study, phosphorylated signaling proteins were tested in conjunction with their counterparts. Interesting, our finding showed that p-ERK1/2, CREB and p-CREB, but not ERK1/2, proteins reduced in the hippocampus of rats exposed to CUMS. It is known that only phosphorylated proteins exhibit full enzymatic activity; therefore, CUMS only reduced the expression of p-ERK1/2. Nevertheless, the depression-like behaviors were associated with the reductions of both CREB and p-CREB in the hippocampus.

Table 2 Numbers of crossing and rearing at 0 d and 21 d

Group	Crossing number		Rearing number	
	0 d	21 d	0 d	21 d
Control	66.2 ± 20.0	36.9 ± 7.8	18.4 ± 5.9	15.0 ± 5.2
CUMS	73.3 ± 17.6	4.7 ± 2.1**	13.5 ± 2.3	2.5 ± 1.7**
Acu	64.4 ± 18.0	15.0 ± 5.1$^{\star\star\blacktriangle\blacktriangle}$	14.8 ± 3.7	8.9 ± 2.5$^{\blacktriangle\blacktriangle}$
FLX	68.5 ± 19.1	16.9 ± 6.0$^{\star\star\blacktriangle\blacktriangle}$	15.9 ± 3.8	9.5 ± 2.1$^{\blacktriangle\blacktriangle}$
DMSO	64.9 ± 18.6	3.8 ± 2.3	14.3 ± 3.6	1.5 ± 1.4
PD	62.2 ± 18.8	4.1 ± 2.9	12.8 ± 3.0	1.4 ± 1.3
Acu+PD	69.0 ± 18.0	17.0 ± 5.5	14.3 ± 3.1	4.2 ± 2.0**
FLX+PD	60.4 ± 20.8	18.7 ± 7.2	13.4 ± 3.9	3.7 ± 2.2$^{\blacksquare\blacksquare}$

$\star\star P < 0.01$ vs. control group; $\blacktriangle\blacktriangle P < 0.01$ vs. CUMS group; $\star\star P < 0.01$ vs. Acu group; $\blacksquare\blacksquare P < 0.01$ vs. FLX group. (mean ± SD, $n = 9$–10)

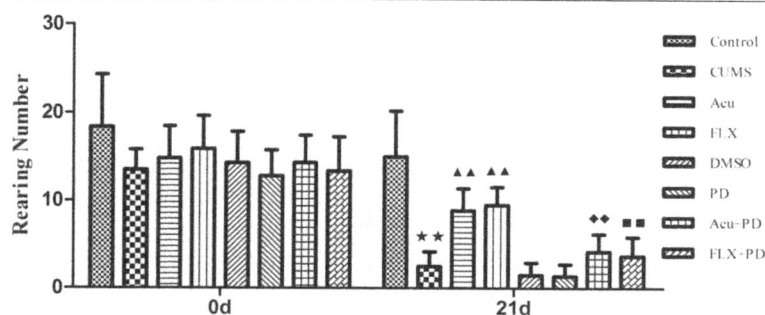

Fig. 5 Rearing number at 0 d and 21 d. ★★$P < 0.01$ versus control group; ▲▲$P < 0.01$ versus CUMS group; ✦✦$P < 0.01$ versus Acu group; ■■$P < 0.01$ versus FLX group. (mean ± SD, $n = 9$–10)

Effect of CUMS on expression of BDNF protein in the hippocampus

Previous studies have confirmed that hippocampal neurogenesis plays an important role in cognitive and emotional control [53] and that an increase in neural apoptosis can lead to mental disorders [54]. Additionally, a recent study gave direct evidence that the decreased neurogenesis was implicated in the pathogenesis of anxiety and depression [55]. Furthemore, research increasingly suggests that antidepressants can promote hippocampal neuron proliferation and differentiation [56–60]. BDNF is associated with neuroprotective and synaptic plasticity in the central nervous system [61], especially in the hippocampus [62, 63]. An early study proved that a reduction in BDNF in the hippocampus affects several behaviors related to depression [64]. Consistent with the previous studies, our results showed that the expression of BDNF protein decreased in rats exposed to CUMS, which demonstrated that the depression-like behaviors induced by CUMS were associated with BDNF protein in the hippocampus. Moreover, BDNF protein can activate the ERK signaling pathway by combining with its specific receptor tyrosine receptor kinase-B (Trk-B) [11]. Thus, reduction of BDNF protein might lead to a negative feedback to the ERK signaling pathway.

Effect of PD98059 pretreatment on the behavior of CUMS rats and the ERK signaling pathway

Intracerebroventricular injection of PD98059, an inhibitor of ERK1/2, had no marked effect on the OFT and the expression of ERK1/2, CREB, p-CREB and BDNF in model rats; however, PD98059 pretreatment aggravated the

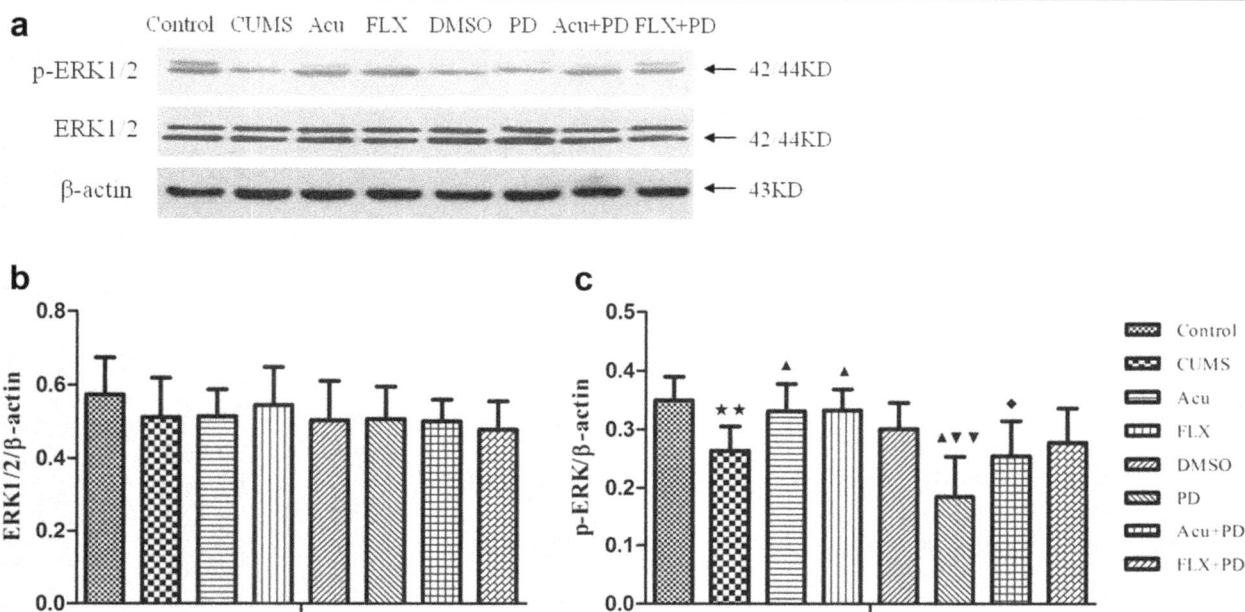

Fig. 6 Western blot analysis of ERK1/2 and p-ERK1/2. **a** The representative immunoblot made from hippocampal tissue of rats. **b** The quantification of ERK1/2/β-actin ratio levels. **c** The quantification of p-ERK1/2/β-actin ratio levels. ★★$P < 0.01$ vs. control group; ▲$P < 0.05$ vs. CUMS group; ▼▼$P < 0.01$ vs. DMSO group; ✦$P < 0.05$ vs. Acu group. (mean ± SD, $n = 6$)

Table 3 Western blot analysis of ERK1/2 and p-ERK1/2

Group	ERK1/2/β-actin	p-ERK1/2/β-actin
Control	0.573 ± 0.101	0.350 ± 0.040
CUMS	0.512 ± 0.108	0.264 ± 0.041**
Acu	0.515 ± 0.073	0.332 ± 0.046▲
FLX	0.546 ± 0.104	0.333 ± 0.036▲
DMSO	0.505 ± 0.107	0.301 ± 0.045
PD	0.508 ± 0.089	0.185 ± 0.069▲▼▼
Acu+PD	0.502 ± 0.059	0.255 ± 0.060♦
FLX+PD	0.480 ± 0.077	0.278 ± 0.059

**P < 0.01 vs. control group; ▲P < 0.05 vs. CUMS group; ▼▼P < 0.01 vs. DMSO group; ♦P < 0.05 vs. Acu group. (mean ± SD, n = 6)

decrease in the sucrose intake and the expression of p-ERK1/2 protein compared to those in the CUMS or DMSO group. The results were consistent with the property of PD98059 that prevents ERK1/2 from being phosphorylated without affecting the total protein, and suggested that inhibiting the expression of p-ERK1/2 protein in the hippocampus might lead to anhedonia. Additionally, there was no significant difference between the CUMS and DMSO groups in the SIT and OFT as well as the expressions of above proteins, which eliminated the disturbance of the surgery and DMSO.

Acupuncture ameliorated depression-like behaviors and activated the ERK signaling pathway in the hippocampus

Acupuncture has been extensively used to treat depression in East Asian countries and has exhibited effective results in clinics. According to traditional Chinese medicine, Baihui (GV-20) and Yintang (GV-29) are points pertaining to Governor Meridian [34] and Governor Meridian has a direct contact with brain through channels and collaterals [41]. Thus, the acupoints of Baihui (GV-20) and Yintang (GV-29) are commonly used for treating depression [65]. In early studies, stimulation at Baihui (GV-20) and Yintang (GV-29) with electro-acupuncture (EA) exhibited antidepressant-like efficacy on in the SIT and OFT [34, 41]. In the present study, manual acupuncture performed at these acupoints also increased sucrose intake in the SIT and numbers of crossing and rearing in the OFT compared to the model rats, which proved that acupoint specificity can also play a significant role, independent of the electrical stimulus [25, 66, 67]. However, acupuncture was not as effective as fluoxetine in increasing sucrose intake in our study. In animals, the administration of acupuncture treatment is also a stimulation that is not as controllable as intragastric injection administration of a drug. Although the acupuncture has no effect on rats having a normal physiological state [25], the stimulation might influence the antidepressant-like effects of acupuncture on CUMS rats.

In the last few years, some studies indicated that the ERK signaling pathway was implicated in the antidepressant-like effects of acupuncture (manual acupuncture or EA). We previous found that manual acupuncture stimulation at Baihui (GV-20) and Neiguan (PC-6) increased the ratio of p-ERK1/2 to ERK1/2 and the ratio of p-CREB to CREB in the hippocampus and prefrontal cortex in CUMS rats [25].

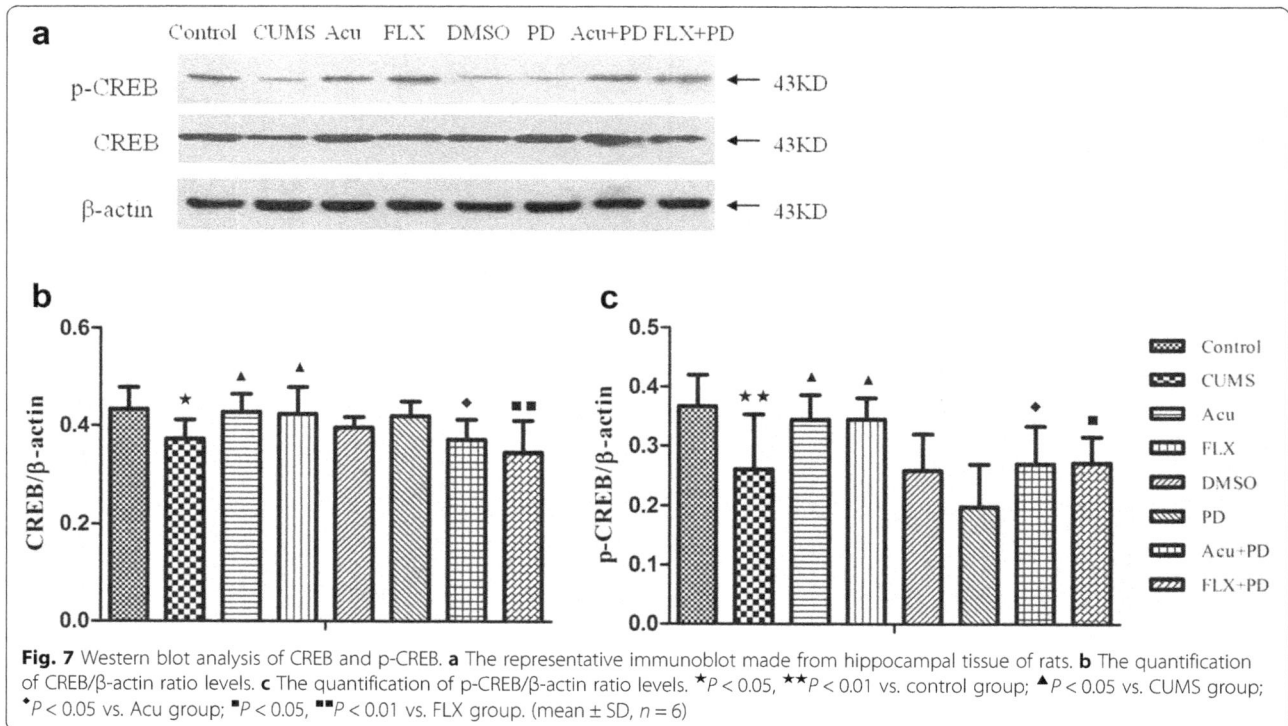

Fig. 7 Western blot analysis of CREB and p-CREB. **a** The representative immunoblot made from hippocampal tissue of rats. **b** The quantification of CREB/β-actin ratio levels. **c** The quantification of p-CREB/β-actin ratio levels. ★P < 0.05, ★★P < 0.01 vs. control group; ▲P < 0.05 vs. CUMS group; ♦P < 0.05 vs. Acu group; ■P < 0.05, ■■P < 0.01 vs. FLX group. (mean ± SD, n = 6)

Table 4 Western blot analysis of CREB and p-CREB

Group	CREB/β-actin	p-CREB/β-actin
Control	0.434 ± 0.045	0.367 ± 0.053
CUMS	0.371 ± 0.039*	0.261 ± 0.092**
Acu	0.427 ± 0.037▲	0.344 ± 0.042▲
FLX	0.423 ± 0.055▲	0.345 ± 0.036▲
DMSO	0.394 ± 0.022	0.259 ± 0.061
PD	0.419 ± 0.030	0.198 ± 0.072
Acu+PD	0.371 ± 0.041♦	0.270 ± 0.063♦
FLX+PD	0.345 ± 0.065■■	0.272 ± 0.043■

*$P < 0.05$, **$P < 0.01$ vs. control group; ▲$P < 0.05$ vs. CUMS group; ♦$P < 0.05$ vs. Acu group; ■$P < 0.05$, ■■$P < 0.01$ vs. FLX group. (mean ± SD, $n = 6$)

In addition, Liu et al. showed that EA stimulation at Baihui (GV-20) and Yang-ling-quan (GB-34) mitigated depressive-like behaviors through increasing the p-ERK1/2 level in the hippocampus [26]. One research also found that EA stimulation at Baihui (GV-20) and Yintang (GV-29) acted on depression by enhancing the p-ERK1/2 in the hippocampus [68]. In the present study, we found that manual acupuncture performed at acupoints of Baihui (GV-20) and Yintang (GV-29) increased levels of p-ERK1/2, CREB, and p-CREB in the hippocampus. Pretreatment with PD98059 inhibited these improvements as well as the increase in sucrose intake and numbers of crossing and rearing. These results provided the direct evidence that the ERK signaling pathway was involved in the antidepressant-like effects of acupuncture.

Effect of acupuncture on the expression of BDNF protein in the hippocampus

Recent research on depression focuses on neuroprotection, and an increasing number of studies support the

Table 5 Western blot analysis of BDNF

Group	BDNF/β-actin
Control	0.334 ± 0.076
CUMS	0.217 ± 0.018**
Acu	0.301 ± 0.066▲
FLX	0.319 ± 0.069▲
DMSO	0.222 ± 0.043
PD	0.231 ± 0.054
Acu+PD	0.245 ± 0.088
FLX+PD	0.250 ± 0.090

**$P < 0.01$ vs. control group; ▲$P < 0.05$ vs. CUMS group. (mean ± SD, $n = 6$)

notion that acupuncture is a rescuer of impaired neurogenesis [69]. It has been reported that acupuncture acts on depression by enhancing neuropeptide Y (NYP) in the hypothalamus [70] and amplifying neural progenitors (ANPs) proliferation, as well as preserving quiescent neural progenitors (QNPs) from apoptosis [71]. In our study, acupuncture markedly increased BDNF protein level, which provided further evidence to support the positive results. An early study found that inhibiting ERK1/2 phosphorylation can block the antidepressant-like consequences produced by infusing BDNF into the dentate gyrus [72]. Thus, we speculated that the ERK signaling pathway was implicated in acupuncture's regulation of BDNF protein; however, the results showed that pretreatment with PD98059 did not abolish the effect of acupuncture on the BDNF protein. It is well known that CREB is an intersection of several signaling pathways. In addition to the ERK signaling pathway, cAMP-PKA and Ca^{2+}/CaMK can also phosphorylate CREB and promote the transcription of BDNF mRNA. So an inhibited ERK

signaling pathway can not suppress acupuncture on the regulation of BDNF protein. In addition, acupuncture's neuroprotective effects may associate with the enhancement of p-p38 [68] and inhibition of pro-inflammatory cytokines [34, 73] and NF-kB signaling pathway [74] in the hippocampus. Moreover, in our previous study, it was found that acupuncture decreased the protein expressions of phosphor-Jun N-terminal kinase (p-JNK) and c-Jun, two important proteins in the JNK signaling pathway, and inhibited neural apoptosis mediated by caspases (data not published). Thus, the ERK signaling pathway is involved in the effects of acupuncture on neurotrophy and neurogenesis. However, the neuroprotective effect of acupuncture is not limited to the ERK signaling pathway.

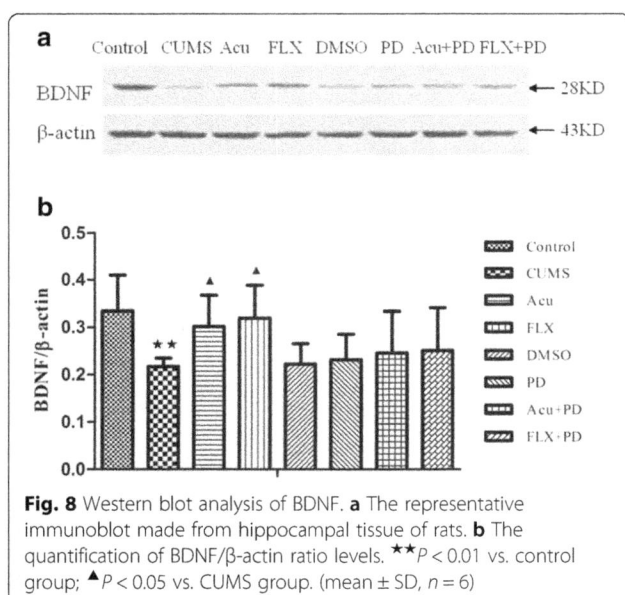

Fig. 8 Western blot analysis of BDNF. **a** The representative immunoblot made from hippocampal tissue of rats. **b** The quantification of BDNF/β-actin ratio levels. **$P < 0.01$ vs. control group; ▲$P < 0.05$ vs. CUMS group. (mean ± SD, $n = 6$)

Conclusions

In conclusion, the present study demonstrated that depression-like behaviors of rats induced by CUMS were associated with the dysfunction of the ERK signaling pathway in the hippocampus. Importantly, our findings indicated that acupuncture treatment effectively mitigated depressive behaviors and the ERK signaling pathway was involved in the antidepressant-like effects of this treatment.

Acknowledgements

We would like to express our thanks to all teachers form the Scientific Research Experiment Center, Beijing University of Chinese Medicine for their guidance in the molecular biology experiment.

Funding

This work was made possible by the funding from National Natural Science Foundation of China (No. 81173334).

Author's contributions

TB was responsible for the study concept and design. XZ conducted animal experiment and wrote the manuscript. YS, MY, MX, YW, YG, CZ, BZ conducted the experiments and collected the data. YS helped to analyze the data. All authors approved the final version of the manuscript.

Competing interests

The authors declare that they have no competing interests.

Author details

[1]Beijing University of Chinese Medicine, Beijing, Beijing 100029, China.
[2]Shanxi University of Chinese Medicine, Xianyang, Shanxi 712046, China.

References

1. Kupfer DJ, Frank E, Phillips ML. Major depressive disorder: new clinical, neurobiological, and treatment perspectives. Lancet. 2012;379(9820):1045–55.
2. Ferrari AJ, Charlson FJ, Norman RE, Patten SB, Freedman G, Murray CJ, Vos T, Whiteford HA. Burden of depressive disorders by country, sex, age, and year: findings from the global burden of disease study 2010. PLoS Med. 2013; 10(11):e1001547.
3. Cipriani A, Santilli C, Furukawa TA, Signoretti A, Nakagawa A, McGuire H, Churchill R, Barbui C. Escitalopram versus other antidepressive agents for depression. Cochrane Database Syst Rev. 2009;2:CD006532.
4. Arroll B, Macgillivray S, Ogston S, Reid I, Sullivan F, Williams B, Crombie I. Efficacy and tolerability of tricyclic antidepressants and SSRIs compared with placebo for treatment of depression in primary care: a meta-analysis. Ann Fam Med. 2005;3(5):449–56.
5. Preston TC, Shelton RC. Treatment resistant depression: strategies for primary care. Curr Psychiatry Rep. 2013;15(7):370.
6. Ma S, Qu S, Huang Y, Chen J, Lin R, Wang C, Li G, Zhao C, Guo S, Zhang Z. Improvement in quality of life in depressed patients following verum acupuncture or electroacupuncture plus paroxetine: a randomized controlled study of 157 cases. Neural Regen Res. 2012;7(27):2123–9.
7. Arvidsdotter T, Marklund B, Taft C. Six-month effects of integrative treatment, therapeutic acupuncture and conventional treatment in alleviating psychological distress in primary care patients–follow up from an open, pragmatic randomized controlled trial. BMC Complement Altern Med. 2014;14:210.
8. Galecki P, Talarowska M, Anderson G, Berk M, Maes M. Mechanisms underlying neurocognitive dysfunctions in recurrent major depression. Med Sci Monit. 2015;21:1535–47.
9. Malberg JE. Implications of adult hippocampal neurogenesis in antidepressant action. J Psychiatry Neurosci. 2004;29(3):196–205.
10. Groves JO. Is it time to reassess the BDNF hypothesis of depression? Mol Psychiatry. 2007;12(12):1079–88.
11. Mazzucchelli C, Brambilla R. Ras-related and MAPK signalling in neuronal plasticity and memory formation. Cell Mol Life Sci. 2000;57(4):604–11.
12. Guan L, Jia N, Zhao X, Zhang X, Tang G, Yang L, Sun H, Wang D, Su Q, Song Q, et al. The involvement of ERK/CREB/Bcl-2 in depression-like behavior in prenatally stressed offspring rats. Brain Res Bull. 2013;99:1–8.
13. Leem YH, Yoon SS, Kim YH, Jo SA. Disrupted MEK/ERK signaling in the medial orbital cortex and dorsal endopiriform nuclei of the prefrontal cortex in a chronic restraint stress mouse model of depression. Neurosci Lett. 2014;580:163–8.
14. Kuo JR, Cheng YH, Chen YS, Chio CC, Gean PW. Involvement of extracellular signal regulated kinases in traumatic brain injury-induced depression in rodents. J Neurotrauma. 2013;30(14):1223–31.
15. Liu D, Wang Z, Gao Z, Xie K, Zhang Q, Jiang H, Pang Q. Effects of curcumin on learning and memory deficits, BDNF, and ERK protein expression in rats exposed to chronic unpredictable stress. Behav Brain Res. 2014;271:116–21.
16. Huang W, Zhao Y, Zhu X, Cai Z, Wang S, Yao S, Qi Z, Xie P. Fluoxetine upregulates phosphorylated-AKT and phosphorylated-ERK1/2 proteins in neural stem cells: evidence for a crosstalk between AKT and ERK1/2 pathways. J Mol Neurosci. 2013;49(2):244–9.
17. First M, Gil-Ad I, Taler M, Tarasenko I, Novak N, Weizman A. The effects of fluoxetine treatment in a chronic mild stress rat model on depression-related behavior, brain neurotrophins and ERK expression. J Mol Neurosci. 2011;45(2):246–55.
18. Qi X, Lin W, Li J, Li H, Wang W, Wang D, Sun M. Fluoxetine increases the activity of the ERK-CREB signal system and alleviates the depressive-like behavior in rats exposed to chronic forced swim stress. Neurobiol Dis. 2008;31(2):278–85.
19. Gourley SL, Wu FJ, Kiraly DD, Ploski JE, Kedves AT, Duman RS, Taylor JR. Regionally specific regulation of ERK MAP kinase in a model of antidepressant-sensitive chronic depression. Biol Psychiatry. 2008;63(4):353–9.
20. Lin D, De La Pena I, Lin L, Zhou SF, Borlongan CV, Cao C. The neuroprotective role of acupuncture and activation of the BDNF signaling pathway. Int J Mol Sci. 2014;15(2):3234–52.
21. Liang J, Lu J, Cui SF, Wang JR, Tu Y. [Effect of acupuncture on expression of brain-derived neurotrophic factor gene and protein in frontal cortex and hippocampus of depression rats]. Zhen ci yan jiu = Acupuncture research/ [Zhongguo yi xue ke xue yuan Yi xue qing bao yan jiu suo bian ji]. 2012;37(1):20–4.
22. Lin D, Wu Q, Lin X, Borlongan CV, He ZX, Tan J, Cao C, Zhou SF. Brain-derived neurotrophic factor signaling pathway: modulation by acupuncture in telomerase knockout mice. Altern Ther Health Med. 2015;21(6):36–46.
23. Nam MH, Ahn KS, Choi SH. Acupuncture: a potent therapeutic tool for inducing adult neurogenesis. Neural Regen Res. 2015;10(1):33–5.
24. Ho TJ, Chan TM, Ho LI, Lai CY, Lin CH, Macdonald I, Harn HJ, Lin JG, Lin SZ, Chen YH. The possible role of stem cells in acupuncture treatment for neurodegenerative diseases: a literature review of basic studies. Cell Transplant. 2014;23(4–5):559–66.
25. Lu J, Liang J, Wang JR, Hu L, Tu Y, Guo JY. Acupuncture activates ERK-CREB pathway in rats exposed to chronic unpredictable mild stress. Evid Based Complement Alternat Med. 2013;2013:469765.
26. Yang L, Yue N, Zhu X, Han Q, Liu Q, Yu J, Wu G. Electroacupuncture upregulates ERK signaling pathways and promotes adult hippocampal neural progenitors proliferation in a rat model of depression. BMC Complement Altern Med. 2013;13:288.
27. China TMoSaTotPsRo. Guidance suggestion for the care and use of laboratory animals. In; 2006-9-30
28. Ubhi K, Inglis C, Mante M, Patrick C, Adame A, Spencer B, Rockenstein E, May V, Winkler J, Masliah E. Fluoxetine ameliorates behavioral and neuropathological deficits in a transgenic model mouse of alpha-synucleinopathy. Exp Neurol. 2012;234(2):405–16.

29. Ryan JA, Eisner EA, DuRaine G, You Z, Reddi AH. Mechanical compression of articular cartilage induces chondrocyte proliferation and inhibits proteoglycan synthesis by activation of the ERK pathway: implications for tissue engineering and regenerative medicine. J Tissue Eng Regen Med. 2009;3(2):107–16.

30. Davies SP, Reddy H, Caivano M, Cohen P. Specificity and mechanism of action of some commonly used protein kinase inhibitors. Biochem J. 2000; 351(Pt 1):95–105.

31. Willner P, Towell A, Sampson D, Sophokleous S, Muscat R. Reduction of sucrose preference by chronic unpredictable mild stress, and its restoration by a tricyclic antidepressant. Psychopharmacology. 1987;93(3):358–64.

32. Forbes NF, Stewart CA, Matthews K, Reid IC. Chronic mild stress and sucrose consumption: validity as a model of depression. Physiol Behav. 1996;60(6):1481–4.

33. Stanford SC. The open field test: reinventing the wheel. J Psychopharmacol. 2007;21(2):134–5.

34. Guo T, Guo Z, Yang X, Sun L, Wang S, Yingge A, He X, Ya T. The alterations of IL-1Beta, IL-6, and TGF-beta levels in hippocampal CA3 region of chronic restraint stress rats after electroacupuncture (EA) pretreatment. Evid Based Complement Alternat Med. 2014;2014:369158.

35. Willner P. Validity, reliability and utility of the chronic mild stress model of depression: a 10-year review and evaluation. Psychopharmacology. 1997;134(4):319–29.

36. Tanti A, Belzung C. Open questions in current models of antidepressant action. Br J Pharmacol. 2010;159(6):1187–200.

37. Willner P. Chronic mild stress (CMS) revisited: consistency and behavioural-neurobiological concordance in the effects of CMS. Neuropsychobiology. 2005;52(2):90–110.

38. Strekalova T, Spanagel R, Bartsch D, Henn FA, Gass P. Stress-induced anhedonia in mice is associated with deficits in forced swimming and exploration. Neuropsychopharmacology. 2004;29(11):2007–17.

39. Prut L, Belzung C. The open field as a paradigm to measure the effects of drugs on anxiety-like behaviors: a review. Eur J Pharmacol. 2003;463(1–3):3–33.

40. Liu RP, Fang JL, Rong PJ, Zhao Y, Meng H, Ben H, Li L, Huang ZX, Li X, Ma YG, et al. Effects of electroacupuncture at auricular concha region on the depressive status of unpredictable chronic mild stress rat models. Evid Based Complement Alternat Med. 2013;2013:789674.

41. Mo Y, Yao H, Song H, Wang X, Chen W, Abulizi J, Xu A, Tang Y, Han X, Li Z. Alteration of behavioral changes and hippocampus galanin expression in chronic unpredictable mild stress-induced depression rats and effect of electroacupuncture treatment. Evid Based Complement Alternat Med. 2014;2014:179796.

42. Krishnan V, Nestler EJ. Animal models of depression: molecular perspectives. Curr Top Behav Neurosci. 2011;7:121–47.

43. Einat H, Yuan P, Gould TD, Li J, Du J, Zhang L, Manji HK, Chen G. The role of the extracellular signal-regulated kinase signaling pathway in mood modulation. J Neurosci Off J Soc Neurosci. 2003;23(19):7311–6.

44. Sweatt JD. The neuronal MAP kinase cascade: a biochemical signal integration system subserving synaptic plasticity and memory. J Neurochem. 2001;76(1):1–10.

45. Chen YH, Zhang RG, Xue F, Wang HN, Chen YC, Hu GT, Peng Y, Peng ZW, Tan QR. Quetiapine and repetitive transcranial magnetic stimulation ameliorate depression-like behaviors and up-regulate the proliferation of hippocampal-derived neural stem cells in a rat model of depression: the involvement of the BDNF/ERK signal pathway. Pharmacol Biochem Behav. 2015;136:39–46.

46. Li J, Luo Y, Zhang R, Shi H, Zhu W, Shi J. Neuropeptide trefoil factor 3 reverses depressive-like behaviors by activation of BDNF-ERK-CREB signaling in olfactory bulbectomized rats. Int J Mol Sci. 2015;16(12):28386–400.

47. Reus GZ, Vieira FG, Abelaira HM, Michels M, Tomaz DB, dos Santos MA, Carlessi AS, Neotti MV, Matias BI, Luz JR, et al. MAPK signaling correlates with the antidepressant effects of ketamine. J Psychiatr Res. 2014;55:15–21.

48. Li E, Deng H, Wang B, Fu W, You Y, Tian S. Apelin-13 exerts antidepressant-like and recognition memory improving activities in stressed rats. Eur Neuropsychopharmacol. 2016;26(3):420–30.

49. Yamada S, Yamamoto M, Ozawa H, Riederer P, Saito T. Reduced phosphorylation of cyclic AMP-responsive element binding protein in the postmortem orbitofrontal cortex of patients with major depressive disorder. J Neural Transm. 2003;110(6):671–80.

50. Pandey GN, Dwivedi Y, Ren X, Rizavi HS, Roberts RC, Conley RR. Cyclic AMP response element-binding protein in post-mortem brain of teenage suicide victims: specific decrease in the prefrontal cortex but not the hippocampus. Int J Neuropsychopharmacol. 2007;10(5):621–9.

51. Thome J, Henn FA, Duman RS. Cyclic AMP response element-binding protein and depression. Expert Rev Neurother. 2002;2(3):347–54.

52. D'Sa C, Duman RS. Antidepressants and neuroplasticity. Bipolar Disord. 2002;4(3):183–94.

53. Vadodaria KC, Jessberger S. Functional neurogenesis in the adult hippocampus: then and now. Front Neurosci. 2014;8:55.

54. Arantes-Goncalves F, Coelho R. Depression and treatment. Apoptosis, neuroplasticity and antidepressants. Acta Med Port. 2006;19(1):9–20.

55. Snyder JS, Soumier A, Brewer M, Pickel J, Cameron HA. Adult hippocampal neurogenesis buffers stress responses and depressive behaviour. Nature. 2011;476(7361):458–61.

56. Perera TD, Dwork AJ, Keegan KA, Thirumangalakudi L, Lipira CM, Joyce N, Lange C, Higley JD, Rosoklija G, Hen R, et al. Necessity of hippocampal neurogenesis for the therapeutic action of antidepressants in adult nonhuman primates. PLoS One. 2011;6(4):e17600.

57. Mori M, Murata Y, Matsuo A, Takemoto T, Mine K. Chronic treatment with the 5-HT1A receptor partial agonist tandospirone increases hippocampal neurogenesis. Neurol Ther. 2014;3(1):67–77.

58. Walker AK, Rivera PD, Wang Q, Chuang JC, Tran S, Osborne-Lawrence S, Estill SJ, Starwalt R, Huntington P, Morlock L, et al. The P7C3 class of neuroprotective compounds exerts antidepressant efficacy in mice by increasing hippocampal neurogenesis. Mol Psychiatry. 2015;20(4):500–8.

59. Tyler CR, Solomon BR, Ulibarri AL, Allan AM. Fluoxetine treatment ameliorates depression induced by perinatal arsenic exposure via a neurogenic mechanism. Neurotoxicology. 2014;44:98–109.

60. Rayen I, van den Hove DL, Prickaerts J, Steinbusch HW, Pawluski JL. Fluoxetine during development reverses the effects of prenatal stress on depressive-like behavior and hippocampal neurogenesis in adolescence. PLoS One. 2011;6(9):e24003.

61. Autry AE, Monteggia LM. Brain-derived neurotrophic factor and neuropsychiatric disorders. Pharmacol Rev. 2012;64(2):238–58.

62. Harrisberger F, Smieskova R, Schmidt A, Lenz C, Walter A, Wittfeld K, Grabe HJ, Lang UE, Fusar-Poli P, Borgwardt S. BDNF Val66Met polymorphism and hippocampal volume in neuropsychiatric disorders: a systematic review and meta-analysis. Neurosci Biobehav Rev. 2015;55:107–18.

63. Waterhouse EG, An JJ, Orefice LL, Baydyuk M, Liao GY, Zheng K, Lu B, Xu B. BDNF promotes differentiation and maturation of adult-born neurons through GABAergic transmission. J Neurosci Off J Soc Neurosci. 2012;32(41):14318–30.

64. Taliaz D, Stall N, Dar DE, Zangen A. Knockdown of brain-derived neurotrophic factor in specific brain sites precipitates behaviors associated with depression and reduces neurogenesis. Mol Psychiatry. 2010;15(1):80–92.

65. Duan DM, Tu Y, Chen LP, Wu ZJ. Efficacy evaluation for depression with somatic symptoms treated by electroacupuncture combined with Fluoxetine. J Tradit Chin Med. 2009;29(3):167–73.

66. Jung WM, Lee IS, Wallraven C, Ryu YH, Park HJ, Chae Y. Cortical activation patterns of bodily attention triggered by acupuncture stimulation. Sci Rep. 2015;5:12455.

67. Feng Y, Johansson J, Shao R, Manneras-Holm L, Billig H, Stener-Victorin E. Electrical and manual acupuncture stimulation affect oestrous cyclicity and neuroendocrine function in an 5alpha-dihydrotestosterone-induced rat polycystic ovary syndrome model. Exp Physiol. 2012;97(5):651–62.

68. Xu J, She Y, Su N, Zhang R, Lao L, Xu S. Effects of electroacupuncture on chronic unpredictable mild stress rats depression-like behavior and expression of p-ERK/ERK and p-P38/P38. Evid Based Complement Alternat Med. 2015;2015:650729.

69. Nam MH, Ahn KS, Choi SH. Acupuncture stimulation induces neurogenesis in adult brain. Int Rev Neurobiol. 2013;111:67–90.

70. Lee B, Shim I, Lee HJ, Yang Y, Hahm DH. Effects of acupuncture on chronic corticosterone-induced depression-like behavior and expression of neuropeptide Y in the rats. Neurosci Lett. 2009;453(3):151–6.

71. Yang L, Yue N, Zhu X, Han Q, Li B, Liu Q, Wu G, Yu J. Electroacupuncture promotes proliferation of amplifying neural progenitors and preserves quiescent neural progenitors from apoptosis to alleviate depressive-like and anxiety-like behaviours. Evid Based Complement Alternat Med. 2014;2014:872568.

72. Shirayama Y, Chen AC, Nakagawa S, Russell DS, Duman RS. Brain-derived neurotrophic factor produces antidepressant effects in behavioral models of depression. J Neurosci Off J Soc Neurosci. 2002;22(8):3251–61.

73. Lu J, Shao RH, Hu L, Tu Y, Guo JY. Potential antiinflammatory effects of acupuncture in a chronic stress model of depression in rats. Neurosci Lett. 2016;618:31–8.

74. Shao RH, Jin SY, Lu J, Hu L, Tu Y. [Effect of acupuncture intervention on expression of NF-kappaB signal pathway in the hippocampus of chronic stress-induced depression rats]. Zhen ci yan jiu = Acupuncture research/[Zhongguo yi xue ke xue yuan Yi xue qing bao yan jiu suo bian ji]. 2015;40(5):368–72.

11

Effect of transcutaneous acupoint electrical stimulation on propofol sedation: an electroencephalogram analysis of patients undergoing pituitary adenomas resection

Xing Liu[1], Jing Wang[2], Baoguo Wang[1*], Ying Hua Wang[3,4], Qinglei Teng[1], Jiaqing Yan[5], Shuangyan Wang[1] and You Wan[6*]

Abstract

Background: Transcutaneous acupoint electrical stimulation (TAES) as a needleless acupuncture has the same effect like traditional manual acupuncture. The combination of TAES and anesthesia has been proved valid in enhancing the anesthetic effects but its mechanisms are still not clear.

Methods: In this study, we investigated the effect of TAES on anesthesia with an electroencephalogram (EEG) oscillation analysis on surgery patients anesthetized with propofol, a widely-used anesthetic in clinical practice. EEG was continuously recorded during light and deep propofol sedation (target-controlled infusion set at 1.0 and 3.0 μg/mL) in ten surgery patients with pituitary tumor excision. Each concentration of propofol was maintained for 6 min and TAES was given at 2–4 min. The changes in EEG power spectrum at different frequency bands (delta, theta, alpha, beta, and gamma) and the coherence of different EEG channels were analyzed.

Results: Our result showed that, after TAES application, the EEG power increased at alpha and beta bands in light sedation of propofol, but reduced at delta and beta bands in deep propofol sedation ($p < 0.001$). In addition, the EEG oscillation analysis showed an enhancement of synchronization at low frequencies and a decline in synchronization at high frequencies between different EEG channels in either light or deep propofol sedation.

Conclusions: Our study showed evidence suggested that TAES may have different effects on propofol under light and deep sedation. TAES could enhance the sedative effect of propofol at low concentration but reduce the sedative effect of propofol at high concentration.

Keywords: Anesthesia, Transcutaneous acupoint electrical stimulation (TAES), Electroencephalogram (EGG), Power spectrum, Pituitary adenoma

Background

Transcutaneous acupoint electric stimulation (TAES), or "needleless acupuncture", is an easy and non-invasive alternative to needle-based electro-acupuncture (EA). It combines the advantages of both acupuncture and transcutaneous electrical nerve stimulation by pasting electrode pads on the acupoints instead of piercing the skin with needles. Several studies indicated that intraoperative TAES could enhance the sedative effect of propofol, a widely-used sedative anesthetic [1–3], In addition, it could reduce the opioids consumption and the incidence of anesthesia-related side-effects, while improve the quality of recovery from anesthesia [4, 5]. Our recent study also suggested that TAES may exert analgesic effect, and the sufentanil consumption was significantly reduced during craniotomy [6]. Electroacupuncture stimulation at ST36 and PC6 has been reported to significantly deepen the sedation level of general anaesthesia [7]. These results

* Correspondence: baoguowang766@163.com; ywan@hsc.pku.edu.cn
[1]Department of Anesthesiology, Beijing Sanbo Brain Hospital, Capital Medical University, Beijing 100093, China
[6]Neuroscience Research Institute, Key Lab for Neuroscience, Peking University Health Science Center, Beijing 100191, China
Full list of author information is available at the end of the article

suggested that acupuncture and related techniques may have both analgesic and sedative effects. Nevertheless, the combination of TAES and anesthetic has been reported to be benefit, but it is still unclear how acupuncture works in propofol-induced deep or light sedation.

Electroencephalography (EEG) is a sensitive method for measuring the brain activities and is widely applied to monitor the depth of anesthesia. Previous researches showed that activity of EEG changed under anesthesia, power of alpha frequency band (8–12 Hz), especially the frontal alpha, was increased under propofol [8, 9] and beta, gamma frequency band was varies [8]. In addition, disrupted coherence of EEG activity was considered as the leading underlying mechanism of anesthesia [10, 11]. Evidence indicates that TAES or acupuncture could induce the changes of EEG activity. During acupuncture, activity of alpha and theta oscillations of EEG in human being increased [12]. After TAES, the power of theta frequency band was decreased [13]. These results suggested that TAES may modulate the activity and coherence of EEG to improve the sedition under anesthesia [13, 14]. In the present study, we investigated the effect of TAES on propofol anesthesia with an EEG oscillation analysis in patients undergoing pituitary adenoma resection.

Methods
Patient selection and clinical procedures
This study was approved by the ethics review board of the Beijing Sanbo Brain Hospital (2013121101) and registered in the Chinese Clinical Trial Registry (registration number: ChiCTR-TRC-13004051). All participants provided their written informed consent and consent to publish the individual and identifiable patient details before being enrolled in this study. Inclusion criteria were as follows: (1) The age of patients should range from 18 to 65 years; (2) Patients without gender limited; (3) The Body Mass Index (BMI) of patients should range from 18 to 30 Kg/m^2; (4) Patients meet the standard of American Society of Anesthesiology (ASA), Physical Status matain ASA I-II; (5) All patients signed their written informed consent. Exclusion criteria included: (1) Patients had a history of needleless acupuncture within 6 months; (2) Patients in lactation or pregnant; (3) Patients involved in other clinical trial within nearly 4 weeks; (4) Patients took sedatives and analgesics for a long-term, and have been addicted or alcoholics; (6) Patients with extreme anxiety fear, non-cooperation or communication barriers during the test. A total of ten patients scheduled for pituitary tumor excision and met with all above criteria were enrolled in this study during October 2013 to June 2014. All participants received standard pre-anesthesia assessments, and were tested with normal hearing and urine toxicology to exclude

other potential factors, which might interact with propofol or confound the EEG adversely.

Participants were fasted for at least 8 h before the procedure. The heart rate of patients was monitored with an electrocardiogram, oxygen saturation through pulse oximetry, respiration and expiratory carbon dioxide with capnography, and blood pressure through non-invasive cuff to ensure the patients' safety. There were at least three anesthesiologists involved in each study: one was in charge of the medical management of the subject during the study, the second handled the propofol administration, and the third accomplished EEG recording. When the patient became apneic, the first anesthesiologist assisted breathing with bag/mask ventilation. A phenylephrine infusion was applied to maintain mean arterial pressure above the specific level determined from the patients' baseline measurement.

Experimental design and procedure
The experiment paradigm was shown in Fig. 1. Before propofol infusion was started, we recorded the EEG for about 5 min as a baseline when the patient was kept in a conscious, eye-closed and calm situations, this phase was named as phase 0. Then we used a computer-controlled infusion to achieve propofol target effect-site concentrations of 1 μg/mL and then up to 3 μg/mL. Propofol was administered as target-controlled infusion (TCI) based on the pharmacokinetic model by Marsh et al. [15], and the target plasma concentration of sufentanil was set at a certain value (1 or 3 μg/mL) during the whole anesthesia. The concentration level on each target effect-site was maintained for 6 min, then divided each 6 min into three phases (2 min/phase): phase 1–3 (1 μg/mL propofol), and phase 4–6 (3 μg/mL propofol), respectively. TAES were applied in the phase two and phase five.

TAES
TAES was applied to the acupoints of Hégǔ (LI 4), Wàiguān (TE 5), Zúsānlǐ (ST 36) and Qiūxū (GB 40) on the left side of patient in phase two and five, respectively. The stimulation was applied by the HANS acupoint nerve stimulator (HANS 200A, Nanjing Jisheng Medical Technology Co., Ltd., Nanjing, China) with a dense-disperse frequency of 2/100 Hz (alternated once every 3 s; 0.6 ms at 2 Hz and 0.2 ms at 100 Hz). EEG was recorded in the whole procedure. We defined the whole procedure into three states: state one represents the basal state including phase 0; state two represents low-concentration of propofol (1 μg/mL) including phases one, two, and three (phase 1 is the basal state of phases 2 and 3); state three represents high-concentrationμg/mL of propofol (3 μg/mL) including

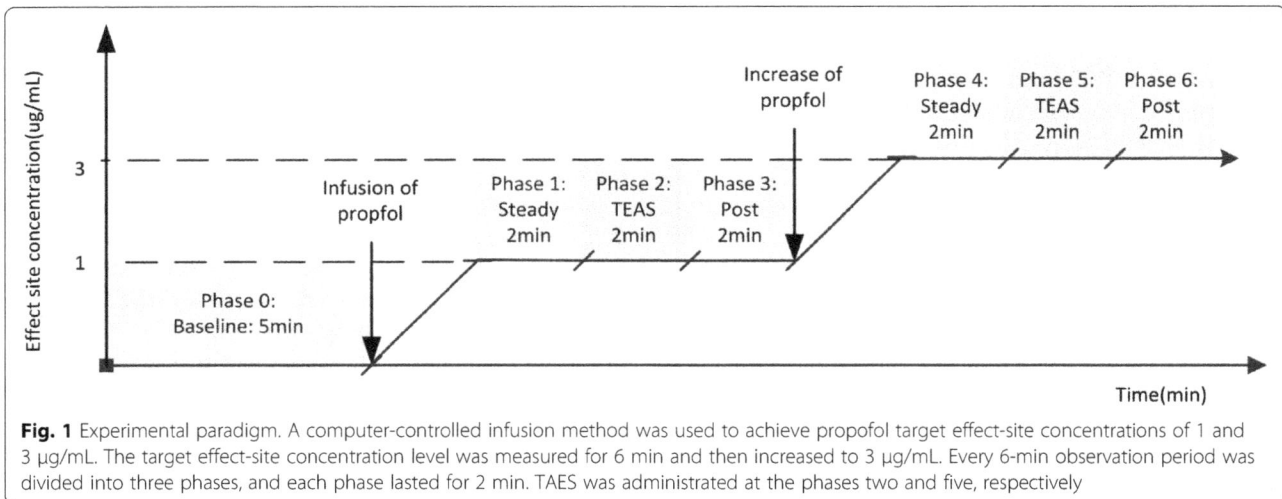

Fig. 1 Experimental paradigm. A computer-controlled infusion method was used to achieve propofol target effect-site concentrations of 1 and 3 μg/mL. The target effect-site concentration level was measured for 6 min and then increased to 3 μg/mL. Every 6-min observation period was divided into three phases, and each phase lasted for 2 min. TAES was administrated at the phases two and five, respectively

phases four, five, six (phase 4 is the basal state of phases 5 and 6).

EEG recordings

Scalp EEG electrodes were positioned at Fp1, Fp2, Fz3, F4, C3, C4, Cz, P3, P4, O1, O2, F7, F8, T3, T4, T5, and T6 (EEG, international 10–20 system); all channels were referenced to A1, A2 (bilateral Mastoid). Electrode impedances were reduced to below 5 kΩ prior to data collection. EEG signals were collected using the Nicolet One EEG-64 device (Nicolet Corp., USA) with a sampling frequency of 1024 Hz. The signals were band-passed at 1.6–45 Hz to avoid baseline drift and high frequency noise.

Power spectrum analysis

The power spectrum of EEG signals was estimated with a customized procedure as our previous reports [16, 17]. Considering the EEG spectrum should be relatively stable during the short time of each phase (2 min), we used the following method to reduce the abnormal variance in the power spectrum:

1. EEG data were segmented into epochs of 12 s;
2. For each epoch, (1) Perform the Morlet wavelet transform with the wavelet central angle frequency of 6 ($\omega 0 = 6$) at frequency band 2.0 Hz to 45 Hz, with a frequency resolution of 0.5 Hz; (2) EEG could have little chance of sudden change during anesthesia. Therefore, we reasonably treat the abrupt change in EEG energy as induced by artifacts. A common fluctuation range of wavelet energy at a particular frequency is within 1 uV. So in this study 1 uV is chosen as the threshold for removing artifacts. Then for each frequency, outliers in corresponding wavelet coefficients which has a

standard deviation (SD) larger than 1 μV was removed with a threshold of mean ± SD; (3) For each frequency, repeat step 2.2 with remaining coefficient, until the SD is less than 1 μV, or removed values exceeds a ratio of 20 %;
3. For each frequency, the mean coefficients of all epochs are considered as the power of that frequency.

EEG coherence analysis

We estimated the magnitude squared coherence between each pair of channels using Welch's overlapped averaged phaseogram method [18]. The method was described as follows:

For two time series x(n) and y(n), estimate the power spectral density (PSD) by the discrete Fourier transform

$$P_{xx}(\omega) = \frac{1}{2\pi} \sum_{m=-\infty}^{\infty} R_{xx}(m)e^{-j\omega m}$$

and

$$P_{yy}(\omega) = \frac{1}{2\pi} \sum_{m=-\infty}^{\infty} R_{yy}(m)e^{-j\omega m}$$

Then the magnitude-squared coherence between the two signals is given by

$$C_{xy}(\omega) = \frac{\left| P_{xx}(\omega)P_{yy}^*(\omega) \right|^2}{P_{xx}(\omega)P_{yy}(\omega)}$$

where $*$ denotes the conjugate of a complex number.

$$(\omega) = \frac{1}{2\pi} \sum_{m=-\infty}^{\infty} R_{xx}(m)e^{-j\omega m}$$

and

$$P_{yy}(\omega) = \frac{1}{2\pi} \sum_{m=-\infty}^{\infty} R_{yy}(m)e^{-j\omega m}$$

Then the magnitude-squared coherence between the two signals is given by

$$C_{xy}(\omega) = \frac{\left| P_{xx}(\omega)P_{yy}^*(\omega) \right|^2}{P_{xx}(\omega)P_{yy}(\omega)}$$

where * denotes the conjugate of a complex number.

We calculated the coherence index of every channel before and after TAES at each band.

Statistical analysis

Statistical analysis was performed using SAS 9.0 software (SAS Institute Inc., Cary, NC, USA). The power spectral data before and after TAES were analyzed by paired-sample t-test. And the power spectral data from different concentration level of propofol were analyzed by One-Way ANOVA. The further analysis used Dunnett-t test, and phase 0 as a control group. Paired-sample t-test was also applied to analyze the coherence index before and after TAES at each band for the same channel. A p value of < 0.05 was considered to be statistically significant.

Results

Effect of propofol on the EEG power

To investigate the effect of propofol on the ongoing brain activities, we calculated the averaged absolute spontaneous EEG powers at each frequency band for each recording session (Fig. 2). One-way ANOVA analysis showed significant difference at delta ($F_{(2, 158)} = 187.411$, $p < 0.001$), theta ($F_{(2, 158)} = 130.379$, $p < 0.001$), alpha ($F_{(2, 158)} = 742.112$, $p < 0.001$), and beta ($F_{(2, 158)} = 243.857$, $p < 0.001$) bands, but not at gamma band ($F_{(2, 158)} = 0.528$,

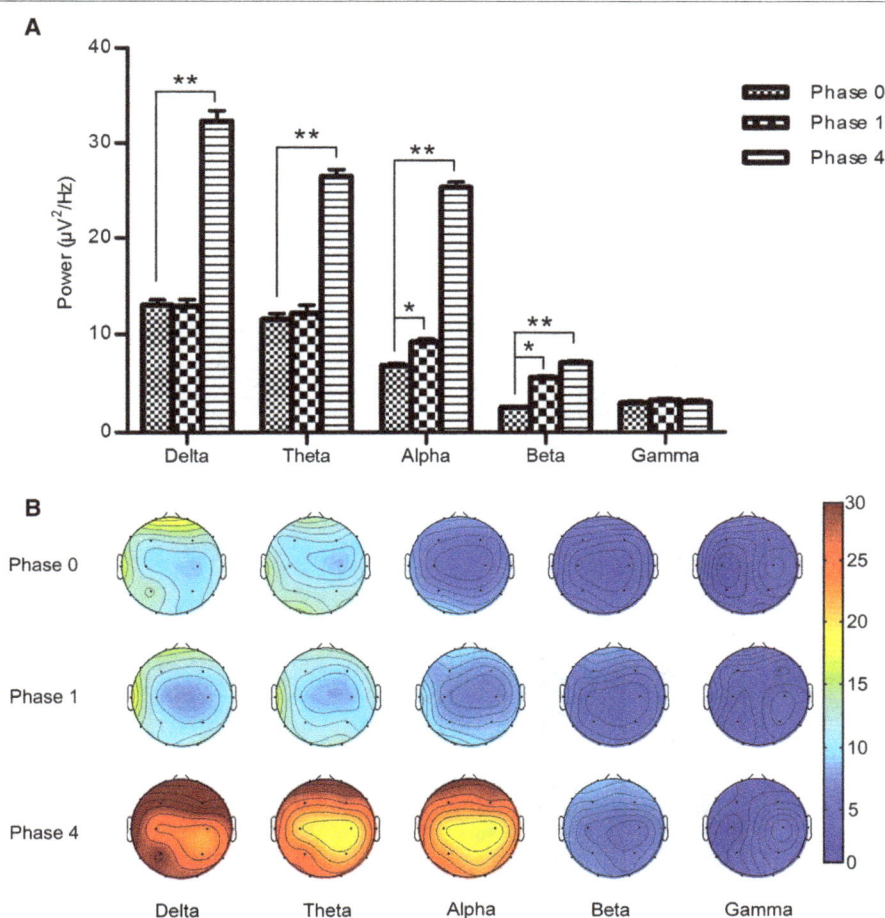

Fig. 2 Effect of propofol concentration on the EEG power at different frequency bands. **a**. The EEG power spectrum at each frequency band. **b**. Topoplot of EEG power at each frequency band. Phase 0: before propofol infusion, phase 1: 1 µg/mL propofol, phase 4: 3 µg/mL propofol. Data were color-coded and plotted at the corresponding position on the scalp. ** $p < 0.001$, and * $p < 0.05$ vs the phase 0

$p = 0.59$). Further analysis with Dunnett t-test revealed that the power of both alpha and beta frequency oscillations increased significantly at phase one compared with phase 0 ($p < 0.001$), while the power of other bands showed no significant change. In addition, the powers of all of alpha, beta, delta, and theta bands increased significantly at phase four ($p < 0.001$), while the power of gamma band showed no significant changes compared with phase 0.

Furthermore, we analyzed the power changes of different bands in each channel of different phases. Compared with the powers of each band in the corresponding channel of phase 0, the power of alpha band in channels O2 and P4 increased significantly (alpha band: $F_{(2, 8)} = 121.778$, $p < 0.05$), and the power of beta band in all channels increased significantly in phase 1 ($F_{(2,8)} = 46.388$, $p < 0.001$,). And the power of delta, theta, alpha, and beta bands in all channels increased significantly in

phase four (delta band: $F_{(2, 8)} = 187.411$, $p < 0.001$; theta band: $F_{(2, 8)} = 130.379$, $p < 0.001$; alpha band: $F_{(2,8)} = 742.112$, $p < 0.001$; beta band: $F_{(2,8)} = 243.857$, $p < 0.001$).

Effect of TAES on EEG power at different concentrations of propofol

We compared and analyzed the averaged absolute power changes of EEG at each frequency band in different phases. Figure 3 showed the effect of TAES on the changes of EEG power in different frequency bands at different concentrations of propofol, we can see an increase at low frequency bands in deep propofol sedation. To observe the main effects of TAES on the propofol-induced EEG power changes, we summarize the EEG power changes in phase one and three and phase four and six, respectively (Fig. 4a and b). Compared with those in phase one, the powers of alpha and beta bands increased significantly ($t = 7.324$, $p < 0.001$; $t =$

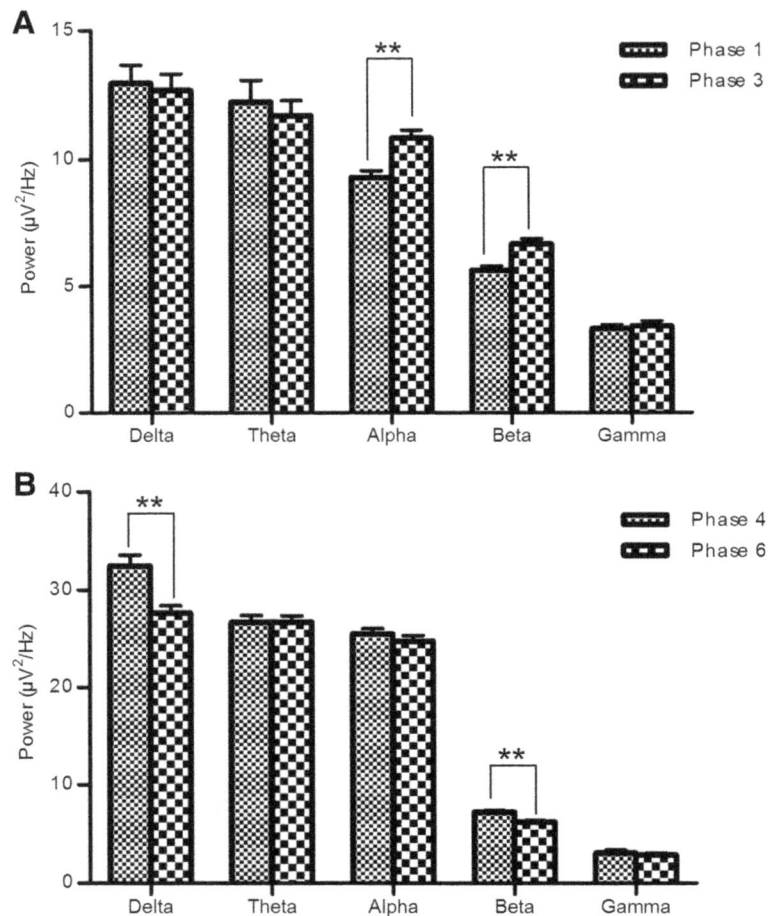

Fig. 3 Effect of TAES on the changes of EEG power induced at different propofol concentrations. **a**. EEG power spectrum at propofol concentration of 1 μg/mL; **b**. EEG power spectrum at propofol concentration of 3 μg/mL. In phase two and phase five, TAES were applied. ** $p < 0.001$ vs the phase one or four

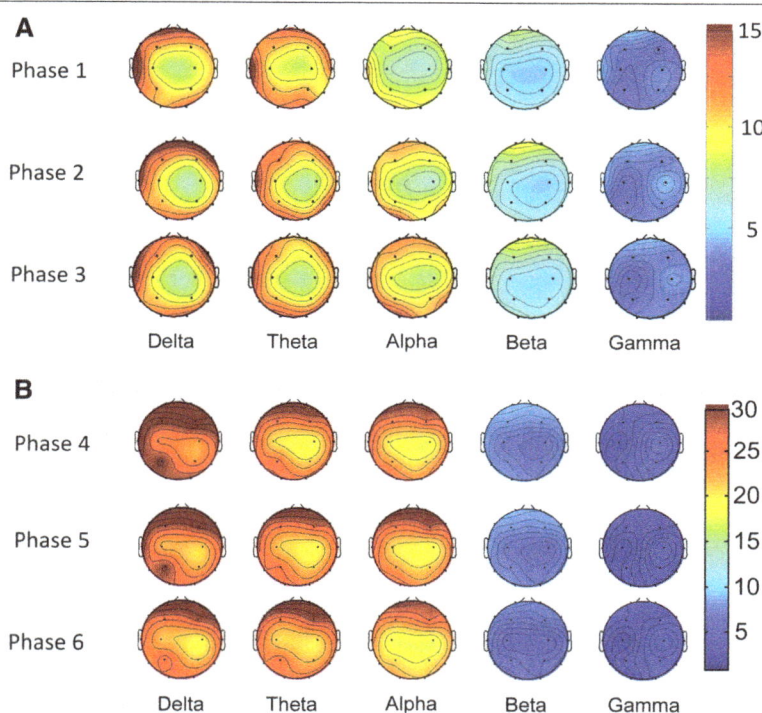

Fig. 4 Topoplot of EEG power at different frequency bands during the different phases. **a**: Topoplot of EEG power at the propofol concentration of 1 μg/mL; **b**: Topoplot of EEG power at the propofol concentration of 3 μg/mL TAES was applied in phase two and phase five. Data were color-coded and plotted at the corresponding position on the scalp

9.302, $p < 0.001$) at phase three, whereas the powers of the other bands did not show any significant changes. Compared with those in phase four, the powers of delta and beta bands in phase six showed significant decrease ($t = 7.819$, $p < 0.001$; $t = 17.312$, $p < 0.001$), whereas the powers of the other bands did not show any significant changes.

Furthermore, we analyzed the power changes of each band in different phases at each channel (Fig. 5). Compared with that in phase one, the power of alpha band in phase three was among 12 of 16 channels, and the power of beta band was among eight of 16 channels, both of them increased significantly ($p < 0.001$, $t = 9.457$), but the power of other bands did not show any significant changes. Compared with that in phase four, the power of beta band in all channels decreased significantly in phase six, except for channel Fp2. The power of theta band in channels O1 and O2, and the power of delta bands in channel T3, T6 and C4 increased significantly ($p < 0.001$, $t = 7.331$). The power of other bands did not show any significant changes in phase 6. The channels that TAES had significant influences on the EEG power at low- and high-concentrations of propofol were summarized in Table 1.

Effects of TAES on EEG coherence among different channels at different concentrations of propofol

We used magnitude squared coherence to estimate the correlation index between different EEG channels in each band before and after TAES at propofol target effect-site concentrations of 1 μg/mL and 3 μg/mL. Then we used paired-t test to analyze the changes of the correlation indices. The discrepancy and the extent of coherence changes of different channels in each band at different propofol concentrations were presented in Fig. 6. The following effects can been seen : Firstly, the synchronization between each pair of channels increased in low-frequency oscillations (delta, theta and alpha), but the synchronism in high-frequency oscillations (beta and gamma) decreased at 1 μg/mL propofol. The synchronization increased in theta and alpha bands at 3 μg/mL propofol, while decreased in beta band, and did not show any significant changes in the rest of the bands; Secondly, the synchronization in ipsilateral hemisphere was stronger than that in bilateral hemispheres at 1 μg/mL propofol. However, it did not show any significant discrepancies between two hemispheres; Thirdly, the synchronization in right hemisphere was stronger than that in left hemisphere at 3 μg/mL propofol.

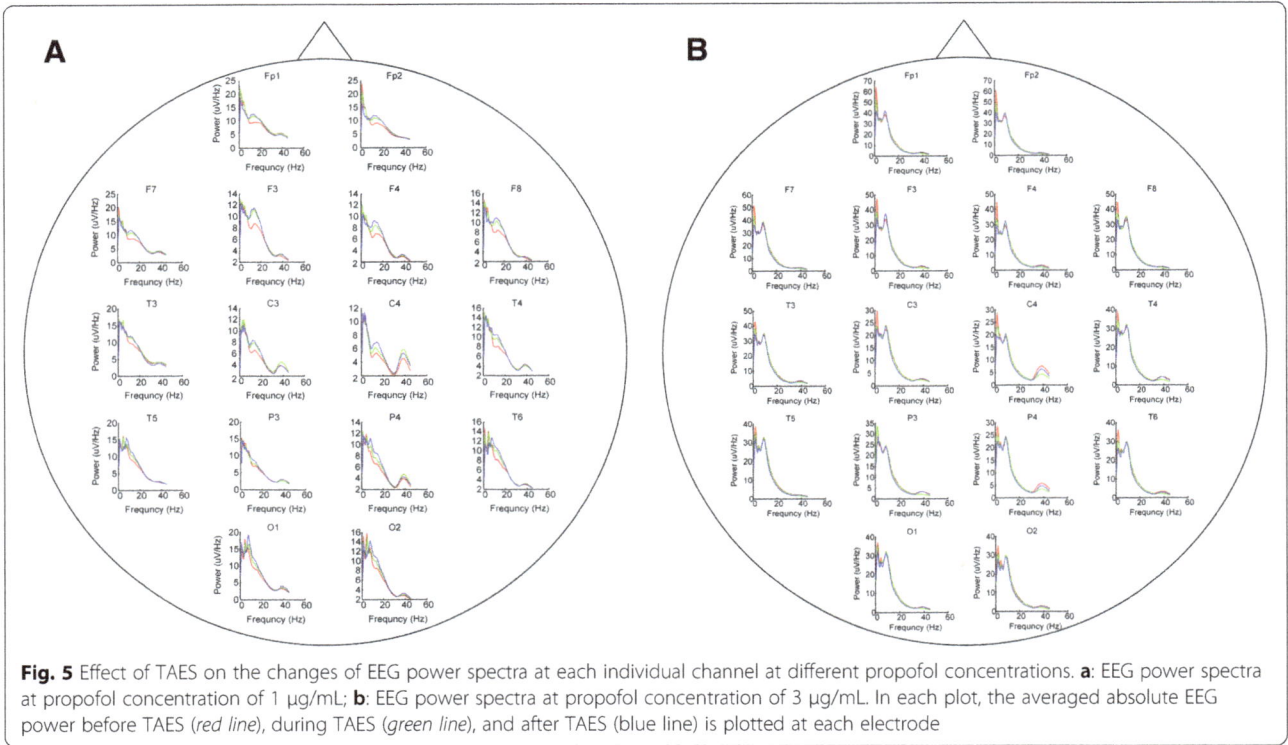

Fig. 5 Effect of TAES on the changes of EEG power spectra at each individual channel at different propofol concentrations. **a**: EEG power spectra at propofol concentration of 1 μg/mL; **b**: EEG power spectra at propofol concentration of 3 μg/mL. In each plot, the averaged absolute EEG power before TAES (*red line*), during TAES (*green line*), and after TAES (blue line) is plotted at each electrode

Discussion

We adopted a self-control design to compare the changes of brain oscillations before and after TAES in patients undergoing pituitary adenoma resection. The individual difference of EEG data was large. The self-control design can minimize the interference of the individual difference to the results. We used a computer-controlled infusion to achieve stable propofol target effect-site concentrations of 1 μg/mL and 3 μg/mL before and after TAES, respectively. Bonhomme et al. reported that the objects become slightly drowsy at 0.5 μg/mL propofol, inarticulate and sluggish at 1.5 μg/mL, and irresponsive at all at 3.5 μg/mL [19]. Purdon et al. identified two states, one where subjects had a nonzero probability of response to auditory stimulated another where subjects were unconscious with a zero probability of response [9]. Then, some researchers defined upper two states as propofol-induced unconsciousness trough-max (TM) and peak-max (PM), respectively [20]. Furthermore, Akeju's team found that the neurophysiological signatures were stably maintained over changing propofol effect-site concentrations: approximately 1 to 2 μg/mL for TM and approximately 3 to 5 μg/mL for

PM [20]. Thus, we defined 1 μg/mL and 3 μg/mL propofol as light and deep sedation respectively in present study. It not only made it easy to investigate the effect of TAES in a stable neurophysiological state, but also reduced the dose of propofol used for the research.

Brain oscillation at low- and high-concentrations of propofol

Compared with baseline, the power of alpha and beta oscillations had a significant increase at 1 μg/mL propofol, and power of delta, theta, alpha, and beta significantly increased at 3 μg/mL propofol. Numerous studies have investigated the effect of propofol on EEG, and propofol might exhibit anesthetic effect by potentiating $GABA_A$ receptors. The effects on macroscopic dynamics were noticeable in the EEG, which contained several stereotyped patterns during maintenance of propofol anesthesia. These patterns were like that powers in (0.5–4 Hz) delta range increase in light anesthetic level [21, 22]; with the increasing concentration, an alpha (~10 Hz) rhythm [23–25] is coherent across frontal cortex; powers in alpha range

Table 1 Channels with significant change ($p < 0.05$) at different frequency bands, induced by TEAS at two propofol concentrations

Propofol concentration	Frequency band				
	Delta	Theta	Alpha	Beta	Gama
1 μg/mL			O1 O2P4	C3 O1 F7 T5 Fp2 F4 C4 P4 O2 F8 T6	
3 μg/mL	T3 C4T6	O1 O2		Fp1F3P3O1F7T3T5FP2F4C4P4O2F8T4T6	

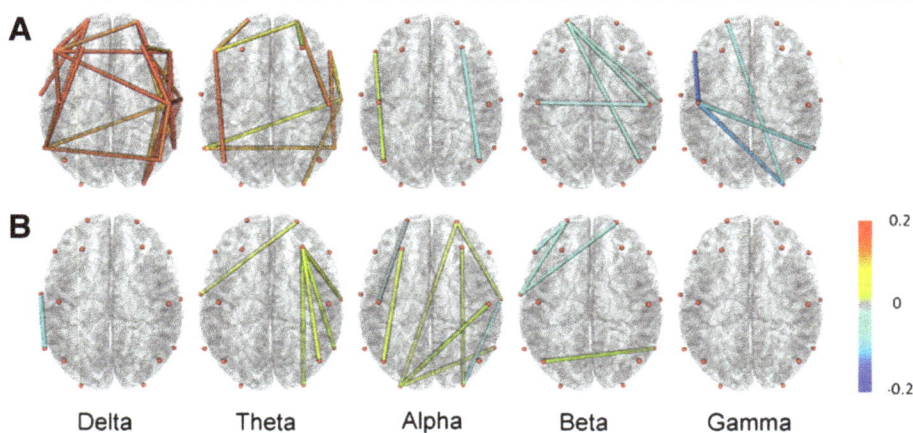

Fig. 6 The effect of TAES on synchronization among EEG channels at different frequency bands at different propofol concentrations. **a**: Synchronization among EEG channels at propofol concentration of 1 μg/mL; **b**: Synchronization among EEG channels at propofol concentration of 3 μg/mL. Red nodes indicate electrodes projected onto the cortex. Lines between nodes indicate a significant change in synchronization between the two channels before and after TAES. The color of lines represents the strength of synchronization. The red color indicates an increase in synchronization, and the blue indictaed a decrease

then became smaller and theta or delta powers become dominant in deeper levels. With further deeper levels, burst suppression, an alternation between bursts of high-voltage activity and phases of flat EEG was lasting for several seconds [26, 27]. Some researchers investigated the change of EEG power at the loss of consciousness and sedation induced by propofol, a significant increase of beta and alpha bands were observed at sedation of propofol, corresponding to 15–25 Hz and 12–15 Hz, respectively. Additionally, they noticed an enhancement in delta, alpha, and theta power were noticed during propofol induced loss of consciousness [22]. Our results were not completely concordant with pervious study. The reason might be the different propofol concentration used that leading to the different level of sedation, or TAES might influence the brain oscillation, since all patients accepted TAES before the increase in popofol concentration.

TAES modulation on brain oscillation in light and deep propofol sedation

The validity of TAES in anesthesia was controversial. Some researchers argued that acupuncture was "only" a placebo procedure based on sensory input. However, we observed significant changes of the ongoing power spectra in different frequency oscillations ranging from delta to beta band except for the gamma band.

It is known that alpha oscillation mainly serves as a top-down controlled inhibitory mechanism. Beta oscillation may be involved in the maintenance of the current sensorimotor or cognitive state, and the extraordinary enhancement of beta oscillation may result in an abnormal persistence of the current situation and a deterioration of flexible behaviors and cognitive controls [28].

Theta oscillation serves as an essential network-level role in hippocampal learning and memory. For example, theta oscillations promote plasticity [29] and support memory processes requiring interregional signal integration [30–32]. Conversely, suppression of the theta rhythm impairs learning and memory [33–35]. Delta-band oscillation is more often seen to be related to deep-sleep states and compromise of neuronal function [36]. The latter findings support the belief that low-frequency oscillations might actually influence in active processing [37]. For our result, the brain oscillations induced by TAES in light and deep propofol sedation were different. The power increase in light propofol sedation following TAES intervention occurred at alpha and beta bands, while reduction of power at delta and beta bands was in deep propofol sedation.

As mentioned before, the alpha power has become a reverse measure of activation [38–40]. The beta oscillation might be related to deterioration of cognitive control. The power increases of alpha and beta bands after TAES in propofol sedation might indicate that TAES could strengthen the sedation effect of propofol. The power of delta and beta oscillation was significantly induced after TAES, especially for beta oscillation at 3 μg/mL propofol. The decrease in beta oscillation occurred at all channels. Elevated endogenous GABA levels could cause the elevation of beta power [41, 42]. Electro acupuncture may induce release of endogenous endomorphins that activate μ opioid receptors in GABA-nergic neurons to suppress the release of GABA [43]. Taken together, it is conceivable that the decreased power of beta oscillations in our results might reflect the inhibition of GABAergic interneurons by TAES.

More importantly, we found an enhancement of synchronization at low frequency and a decline in synchronization at high frequency between different channels after TAES, and at different propofol concentrations. Synchronous rhythms represent a vital mechanism for expressing temporal coordination of neural activity in the brain wide network. Coherent oscillations are generated by many generally neuronal synchrony. It may contribute to well-timed coordination and communication between neural populations simultaneously engaged in a cognitive process. It is well known that slow waves oscillations are the electrophysiological correlate of millions of neurons switching between up and down states. The large slow waves may link to decreases in effective connectivity, which presence of widespread cortical disability between up and down states during early NREM sleep [44, 45]. The high frequency oscillations like beta and gamma may play an important role in integrating the unity of conscious perception [46]. It has been accepted that low-frequency oscillations might be involved in the integration of information across widely spatial distribution of neural assemblies and high-frequency oscillations distributed over a more limited topographic area. In our study, we found that the synchronization of low frequency (delta, theta) oscillation occurred widely across brain areas, while the coherence of high frequency (beta, gamma) occurred within more limited areas. Taken together, we speculated that TAES exerted antinociceptive effect by modulation of the power and coherence between different channels, which disturbed the cortex excitability and effective connectivity.

The deficiency of this article and the future directions of research

There are still some limitations in this view, including limited samples. In the future studies, we will enlarge the sample size to solve this problem. Moreover, there is a washout phase in the self-control design. Although we did not find the conclusive evidence about corporation effect of TAES for 2 min, the post effect of TAES should be taken into consideration when analyze and discuss the EEG changes at 3 μg/mL propofol.

Conclusion

Changes in EEG signature induced by TAES under light or deep sedation were different. TAES might strengthen the effect of propofol during light sedation, whereas it might have an antagonism to propofol in deep sedation. TAES may exert antinociceptive effect by modulating the power and coherence between different channels, which disturbed the cortex excitability and effective connectivity. However, it is difficult for us to simply come

to the conclusion that whether TAES is beneficial or harmful in propofol anesthesia, and a large cohort studies are still needed to further clarify the potential mechanisms of TAES.

Competing interests
The authors have no conflicts of interest to declare.

Authors' contributions
Xing Liu, Qing Lei Teng, and Shang Yan Wang collected data and Xing Liu draft the manuscript, Jing Wang reviewed the data collection, analysis and manuscript, Ying Hua Wang and Jia Qing Yan draw the figures, analyzed data and performed statistics, YW and GBW designed the study, analyzed the data and finalized the manuscript. All authors read and approved the final manuscript.

Acknowledgments
This research was supported by grants from the National Basic Research Program of the Ministry of Science and Technology of China (2013CB531905), the National Natural Science Foundation of China (81230023 and 81221002).

Author details
[1]Department of Anesthesiology, Beijing Sanbo Brain Hospital, Capital Medical University, Beijing 100093, China. [2]Department of Neurobiology, Capital Medical University, Beijing 100069, China. [3]Center for Collaboration and Innovation in Brain and Learning Sciences, Beijing Normal University, Beijing 100875, China. [4]State Key Laboratory of Cognitive Neuroscience and Learning & IDG/Mc Govern Institute for Brain Research, Beijing Normal University, Beijing 100875, China. [5]Institute of Electrical Engineering, Yanshan University, Qinhuangdao 066004, China. [6]Neuroscience Research Institute, Key Lab for Neuroscience, Peking University Health Science Center, Beijing 100191, China.

References
1. Wang J, Weigand L, Lu W, Sylvester J, Semenza GL, Shimoda LA. Hypoxia inducible factor 1 mediates hypoxia-induced TRPC expression and elevated intracellular Ca2+ in pulmonary arterial smooth muscle cells. Circ Res. 2006; 98(12):1528–37.
2. Nayak S, Wenstone R, Jones A, Nolan J, Strong A, Carson J. Surface electrostimulation of acupuncture points for sedation of critically ill patients in the intensive care unit–a pilot study. Acupunct med. 2008;26(1):1–7.
3. Ding YH, Gu CY, Shen LR, Wu LS, Shi Z, Chen YL. [Effects of acupuncture combined general anesthesia on endorphin and hemodynamics of laparoscopic cholecystectomy patients in the perioperative phase]. Zhongguo Zhong Xi Yi Jie He Za Zhi. 2013;33(6):761–5.
4. Wang H, Xie Y, Zhang Q, Xu N, Zhong H, Dong H, et al. Transcutaneous electric acupoint stimulation reduces intra-operative remifentanil consumption and alleviates postoperative side-effects in patients undergoing sinusotomy: a prospective, randomized, placebo-controlled trial. Br J Anaesth. 2014;112(6):1075–82.
5. Wang B, Tang J, White PF, Naruse R, Sloninsky A, Kariger R, et al. Effect of the intensity of transcutaneous acupoint electrical stimulation on the postoperative analgesic requirement. Anesth Analg. 1997;85(2):406–13.
6. Liu X, Li S, Wang B, An L, Ren X, Wu H. Intraoperative and postoperative anaesthetic and analgesic effect of multipoint transcutaneous electrical acupuncture stimulation combined with sufentanil anaesthesia in patients undergoing supratentorial craniotomy. Acupunct Med. 2015;33(4):270–6.
7. Chen Y, Zhang H, Tang Y, Shu J. Impact of bilateral ST36 and PC6 electroacupuncture on the depth of sedation in general anaesthesia. Acupunct Med. 2015;33(2):103–9.

8. Baker GW, Sleigh JW, Smith P. Electroencephalographic indices related to hypnosis and amnesia during propofol anaesthesia for cardioversion. Anaesth Intensive Care. 2000;28(4):386–91.

9. Purdon PL, Pierce ET, Mukamel EA, Prerau MJ, Walsh JL, Wong KF, et al. Electroencephalogram signatures of loss and recovery of consciousness from propofol. Proc Natl Acad Sci U S A. 2013;110(12):E1142–1151.

10. Alkire MT, Hudetz AG, Tononi G. Consciousness and anesthesia. Sci (New York, NY). 2008;322(5903):876–80.

11. Mashour GA. Consciousness unbound: toward a paradigm of general anesthesia. Anesthesiology. 2004;100(2):428–33.

12. Hsu SF, Chen CY, Ke MD, Huang CH, Sun YT, Lin JG. Variations of brain activities of acupuncture to TE5 of left hand in normal subjects. Am J Chin Med. 2011;39(4):673–86.

13. Chen AC, Liu FJ, Wang L, Arendt-Nielsen L. Mode and site of acupuncture modulation in the human brain: 3D (124-ch) EEG power spectrum mapping and source imaging. NeuroImage. 2006;29(4):1080–91.

14. Lewith GT, White PJ, Pariente J. Investigating acupuncture using brain imaging techniques: the current state of play. Evid Based Complement Alternat Med. 2005;2(3):315–9.

15. Marsh B, White M, Morton N, Kenny G. Pharmacokinetic model driven infusion of propofol in children. Br J Anaesth. 1991;67(1):41–8.

16. Wang J, Li D, Li X, Liu FY, Xing GG, Cai J, et al. Phase-amplitude coupling between theta and gamma oscillations during nociception in rat electroencephalography. Neurosci Lett. 2011;499(2):84–7.

17. Wang J, Wang J, Li X, Li D, Li XL, Han JS, et al. Modulation of brain electroencephalography oscillations by electroacupuncture in a rat model of postincisional pain. Evid Based Complement Alternat Med. 2013;2013:160357.

18. Welch PD. The use of fast fourier transform for the estimation of power spectra: a method based on time averaging over short, modified periodograms. IEEE Trans Audio Electroacoust. 1967;15:70–3.

19. Bonhomme V, Fiset P, Meuret P, Backman S, Plourde G, Paus T, et al. Propofol anesthesia and cerebral blood flow changes elicited by vibrotactile stimulation: a positron emission tomography study. J Neurophysiol. 2001; 85(3):1299–308.

20. Akeju O, Pavone KJ, Westover MB, Vazquez R, Prerau MJ, Harrell PG, et al. A comparison of propofol- and Dexmedetomidine-induced electroencephalogram dynamics using spectral and coherence analysis. Anesthesiology. 2014;121(5):978–89.

21. Steriade M, Nunez A, Amzica F. A novel slow (<1 Hz) oscillation of neocortical neurons in vivo: depolarizing and hyperpolarizing components. J Neurosci. 1993;13(8):3252–65.

22. Murphy M, Bruno MA, Riedner BA, Boveroux P, Noirhomme Q, Landsness EC, et al. Propofol anesthesia and sleep: a high-density EEG study. Sleep. 2011;34(3):283–291a.

23. Feshchenko VA, Veselis RA, Reinsel RA. Propofol-induced alpha rhythm. Neuropsychobiology. 2004;50(3):257–66.

24. Supp GG, Siegel M, Hipp JF, Engel AK. Cortical hypersynchrony predicts breakdown of sensory processing during loss of consciousness. Curr Biol. 2011;21(23):1988–93.

25. Cimenser A, Purdon PL, Pierce ET, Walsh JL, Salazar-Gomez AF, Harrell PG, et al. Tracking brain states under general anesthesia by using global coherence analysis. Proc Natl Acad Sci U S A. 2011;108(21):8832–7.

26. Akrawi WP, Drummond JC, Kalkman CJ, Patel PM. A comparison of the electrophysiologic characteristics of EEG burst-suppression as produced by isoflurane, thiopental, etomidate, and propofol. J Neurosurg Anesthesiol. 1996;8(1):40–6.

27. Ching S, Purdon PL, Vijayan S, Kopell NJ, Brown EN. A neurophysiological-metabolic model for burst suppression. Proc Natl Acad Sci U S A. 2012; 109(8):3095–100.

28. Engel AK, Fries P. Beta-band oscillations–signalling the status quo? Curr Opin Neurobiol. 2010;20(2):156–65.

29. Masquelier T, Hugues E, Deco G, Thorpe SJ. Oscillations, phase-of-firing coding, and spike timing-dependent plasticity: an efficient learning scheme. J Neurosci. 2009;29(43):13484–93.

30. Siapas AG, Lubenov EV, Wilson MA. Prefrontal phase locking to hippocampal theta oscillations. Neuron. 2005;46(1):141–51.

31. Paz R, Bauer EP, Pare D. Theta synchronizes the activity of medial prefrontal neurons during learning. Learn Mem. 2008;15(7):524–31.

32. Mizuseki K, Sirota A, Pastalkova E, Buzsaki G. Theta oscillations provide temporal windows for local circuit computation in the entorhinal-hippocampal loop. Neuron. 2009;64(2):267–80.

33. Pan WX, McNaughton N. The medial supramammillary nucleus, spatial learning and the frequency of hippocampal theta activity. Brain Res. 1997; 764(1–2):101–8.

34. Robbe D, Montgomery SM, Thome A, Rueda-Orozco PE, McNaughton BL, Buzsaki G. Cannabinoids reveal importance of spike timing coordination in hippocampal function. Nat Neurosci. 2006;9(12):1526–33.

35. McNaughton N, Ruan M, Woodnorth MA. Restoring theta-like rhythmicity in rats restores initial learning in the Morris water maze. Hippocampus. 2006; 16(12):1102–10.

36. Steriade M. Grouping of brain rhythms in corticothalamic systems. Neuroscience. 2006;137(4):1087–106.

37. Fries P, Schroder JH, Roelfsema PR, Singer W, Engel AK. Oscillatory neuronal synchronization in primary visual cortex as a correlate of stimulus selection. J Neurosci. 2002;22(9):3739–54.

38. Klimesch W, Doppelmayr M, Rohm D, Pollhuber D, Stadler W. Simultaneous desynchronization and synchronization of different alpha responses in the human electroencephalograph: a neglected paradox? Neurosci Lett. 2000; 284(1–2):97–100.

39. Klimesch W, Sauseng P, Hanslmayr S. EEG alpha oscillations: the inhibition-timing hypothesis. Brain Res Rev. 2007;53(1):63–88.

40. Pfurtscheller G, Neuper C, Krausz G. Functional dissociation of lower and upper frequency mu rhythms in relation to voluntary limb movement. Clin Neuropathol. 2000;111(10):1873–9.

41. Hall SD, Stanford IM, Yamawaki N, McAllister CJ, Ronnqvist KC, Woodhall GL, et al. The role of GABAergic modulation in motor function related neuronal network activity. NeuroImage. 2011;56(3):1506–10.

42. Muthukumaraswamy SD, Myers JF, Wilson SJ, Nutt DJ, Lingford-Hughes A, Singh KD, et al. The effects of elevated endogenous GABA levels on movement-related network oscillations. NeuroImage. 2013;66:36–41.

43. Zhang Y, Li A, Lao L, Xin J, Ren K, Berman BM, et al. Rostral ventromedial medulla mu, but not kappa, opioid receptors are involved in electroacupuncture anti-hyperalgesia in an inflammatory pain rat model. Brain Res. 2011;1395:38–45.

44. Massimini M, Ferrarelli F, Huber R, Esser SK, Singh H, Tononi G. Breakdown of cortical effective connectivity during sleep. Science. 2005;309(5744):2228–32.

45. Esser SK, Hill S, Tononi G. Breakdown of effective connectivity during slow wave sleep: investigating the mechanism underlying a cortical gate using large-scale modeling. J Neurophysiol. 2009;102(4):2096–111.

46. Antunes LM, Roughan JV, Flecknell PA. Effects of different propofol infusion rates on EEG activity and AEP responses in rats. J Vet Pharmacol Ther. 2003; 26(5):369–76.

12

Electroacupuncture for tapering off long-term benzodiazepine use

Wing-Fai Yeung[1], Ka-Fai Chung[2*], Zhang-Jin Zhang[3], Wai-Chi Chan[2], Shi-Ping Zhang[4], Roger Man-Kin Ng[5], Connie Lai-Wah Chan[6], Lai-Ming Ho[7], Yee-Man Yu[1] and Li-Xing Lao[3]

Abstract

Background: Conventional approaches for benzodiazepine tapering have their limitations. Anecdotal studies have shown that acupuncture is a potential treatment for facilitating successful benzodiazepine tapering. As of today, there was no randomized controlled trial examining its efficacy and safety. The purpose of the study is to evaluate the efficacy of using electroacupuncture as an adjunct treatment to gradual tapering of benzodiazepine doses in complete benzodiazepine cessation in long-term benzodiazepine users.

Methods/Design: The study protocol of a randomized, assessor- and subject-blinded, controlled trial is presented. One hundred and forty-four patients with histories of using benzodiazepines in ≥50% of days for more than 3 months will be randomly assigned in a 1:1 ratio to receive either electroacupuncture or placebo electroacupuncture combined with gradual benzodiazepine tapering schedule. Both experimental and placebo treatments will be delivered twice per week for 4 weeks. Major assessments will be conducted at baseline, week 6 and week 16 post-randomization. Primary outcome is the cessation rate of benzodiazepine use. Secondary outcomes include the percentage change in the doses of benzodiazepine usage and the severity of withdrawal symptoms experienced based on the Benzodiazepine Withdrawal Symptom Questionnaire, insomnia as measured by the Insomnia Severity Index, and anxiety and depressive symptoms as evaluated by the Hospital Anxiety and Depression Scale. Adverse events will also be measured at each study visit.

Discussion: Results of this study will provide high quality evidence of the efficacy and safety of electroacupuncture as an adjunct treatment for benzodiazepine tapering in long-term users.

Trial registration: ClinicalTrials.gov NCT02475538.

Keywords: Benzodiazepine discontinuation, Withdrawal, Acupuncture, Sham, RCT

Background

Benzodiazepines are commonly prescribed for short-term relief of anxiety and insomnia symptoms. Despite the initial intention, some patients continue taking the drugs and become long-term benzodiazepine users. Cross-sectional studies indicated that 58–84% of benzodiazepine users reported taking the drugs for longer than 6 months [1, 2]. In a population-based survey in Switzerland, nearly one-tenth of 520,000 participants reported at least one benzodiazepine use in the last 6 months and among the benzodiazepine users, 56% were taking the drug for more than 90 days [3]. The potential harms due to long-term benzodiazepine use, including abuse, dependence, overdose, cognitive impairment, household, work and road accidents, and falls, often outweigh its benefits [4–6]. Particularly in the elderly, benzodiazepine use, both short and long term, has been associated with increased risk of daytime drowsiness, accidents and falls, hip fractures and mortality [5]. Studies have shown that a high proportion of long-term benzodiazepine users have attempted to stop or reduce taking the drug; however, many of them have failed due to benzodiazepine withdrawal symptoms [7].

* Correspondence: kfchung@hkucc.hku.hk
[2]Department of Psychiatry, University of Hong Kong, Pokfulam, Hong Kong SAR, China
Full list of author information is available at the end of the article

Benzodiazepine withdrawal symptoms, such as insomnia, anxiety, hand tremor, sweating, muscle pain and irritability are common [8]. A study showed that 43% of 180 participants who were taking diazepam for longer than 8 months experienced withdrawal symptoms on cessation of use [9]. Another study indicated that 35% of 109 patients with panic disorder reported withdrawal symptoms when an 8-week course of alprazolam was stopped [10]. Gradual reduction or in combination with substitutive pharmacotherapy or psychological intervention are conventional approaches for tapering benzodiazepines [11, 12]. According to a meta-analysis including both adults and older adults, the average cessation rate was 42% for gradual benzodiazepine reduction in routine care. There were no significant benefits for gradual reduction in combination with substitutive pharmacotherapy [11]; however, combining gradual reduction with psychological intervention was more effective than gradual reduction alone (OR = 1.82, 95% CI = 1.25–2.67) [11]. Psychological intervention may have helped patients to attain motivation and confidence or have reduced their levels of anxiety and insomnia during benzodiazepine withdrawal [13]. While the existing conventional tapering approaches need further trials to confirm their effectiveness, exploring complementary and alternative therapies is therefore suggested.

Complementary and alternative medicine is a group of diverse medical and healthcare practices that are not presently considered to be a part of conventional medicine. A recent systematic review showed that the 12-month prevalence of complementary and alternative medicine use ranged between 9.8 and 76% [14]. Complementary and alternative medicine therapies can be an alternative treatment to patients than substitutive pharmacotherapy or psychological intervention as treatments of benzodiazepine tapering. Acupuncture is one of the commonly-used complementary and alternative medicine therapies. According to the traditional Chinese medicine theory, fine needles are inserted at special points on the body, called acupoints, to produce therapeutic effects [15]. Electroacupuncture is a special technique of acupuncture. Instead of manual stimulation, electricity is used to stimulate acupoints via inserted acupuncture needles. Previous systematic reviews have shown that acupuncture is efficacious in alleviating anxiety symptoms in subjects with anxiety [16] and in improving sleep quality in subjects with a chief complaint of insomnia [17, 18]. Anecdotal reports have been performed to examine whether acupuncture can augment gradual benzodiazepine tapering in enhancing benzodiazepine cessation rate [19–21]. Ruan et al. showed that the use of hypnotics was reduced from 7.6 times per week to 3.2 times per week after a 2-month course of electroacupuncture in 32 subjects with insomnia and hypnotic dependence [19]. In another study, the cessation rate of hypnotics was over 90% after 10 sessions of manual acupuncture [20]. Another study showed that all subjects could stop using their benzodiazepines for anxiety following a 2-month manual acupuncture treatment and 80% of the subjects attained a Hamilton Anxiety Rating Scale score below 14 [21]. However, these studies adopted a retrospective recall on the use of benzodiazepine, which is vulnerable to recall bias and the reliability is limited. Besides these uncontrolled studies, to the best of our knowledge, there has been no randomized placebo-controlled study on the efficacy and safety of electroacupuncture as an adjunct treatment of gradual benzodiazepine withdrawal in enhancing benzodiazepine cessation rate. We therefore planned to conduct a randomized controlled trial to examine the short- (2-week posttreatment) and medium-term (12-week posttreatment) effects of electroacupuncture in a group of long-term benzodiazepine users in Hong Kong.

Methods

Objective

This study aims to examine the efficacy and safety of electroacupuncture as an adjunct treatment to gradual benzodiazepine withdrawal in enhancing benzodiazepine cessation rate in long-term (at least 3 months) benzodiazepine users. The short-term and medium-term effects of electroacupuncture were defined as within 4 weeks and 4–12 weeks after completion of the electroacupuncture treatment course. We hypothesize that subjects receiving electroacupuncture will have a higher benzodiazepine cessation rate than those receiving non-invasive placebo acupuncture at 2-week posttreatment (short-term, week 6 post-randomization) and 12-week posttreatment (medium-term, week 16 post-randomization).

Trial design

This study is a randomized, parallel-group, assessor- and subject-blinded controlled trial with a 1:1 ratio of group allocation to receive electroacupuncture plus gradual tapering of benzodiazepines or placebo electroacupuncture plus gradual tapering. Design and reporting of the study will follow the CONSORT [22] and STRICTA [23] recommendations.

Ethical approval

The study will be conducted in compliance with local law, Declaration of Helsinki (1989), institutional policies and the Good Clinical Practice (ICH-GCP) guidelines to protect subjects' right and safety. Ethics approval has been obtained from the Institutional Review Board of the University of Hong Kong/Hospital Authority Hong Kong West Cluster (UW 14–554), Research Ethics Committee of Hospital Authority Kowloon Central/Kowloon East Cluster (KC/KE-15-0178/FR-3) and Human Subjects Ethics Subcommittee of the Hong Kong Polytechnic University

(HSEARS20160509002). The trial has been registered at ClinicalTrials.gov (NCT02475538).

Participants

A total of 144 subjects who are long-term benzodiazepine users will be recruited from psychiatric outpatient clinics of three regional hospitals in Hong Kong and an integrative health clinic. We have planned an 18-month recruitment period starting from July 2015.

Inclusion criteria

Subjects will be included if they are: (1) 18 years or above in age including elderly patients; (2) having at least one of the psychiatric diagnoses that are listed in Table 1; (3) taking one or more benzodiazepines, coded as N05BA, N05CD, N05CF, and M03BX07 according to the World Health Organization Anatomical Therapeutic Chemical classification system [24], on more than 50% of days for at least 3 months and during a prospective 2-week period prior to baseline; and (4) willing to taper benzodiazepines as per protocol.

Exclusion criteria

We will exclude participants who have: (1) any increase by 50% or higher in the dosage of antidepressants or anxiolytics in the past 1 year; (2) scored ≥8 in either the depression or anxiety subscale of the Hospital Anxiety and Depression Scale (HADS) [25]; (3) any concurrent psychiatric disorders on the exclusion list (Table 1); (4) any unstable psychiatric conditions or serious physical illnesses which are judged by the investigator to render unsuitable or unsafe to join the study; (5) valvular heart defects or bleeding disorders, taking anticoagulant drugs, or are fitted with any implanted electrical device such as pacemaker, defibrillator, or brain stimulation; (6) acupuncture during the previous 6 months prior to baseline; (7) pregnancy, breastfeeding or childbearing potential but not using adequate contraception; (8) infection or abscess close to the site of selected acupoints and in the investigator's opinion inclusion is unsafe; and (9) significant suicidal risk as rated by the Hamilton Depression Rating Scale (HDRS) [26] item on suicide (a score ≥ 3).

Trial procedure (Fig. 1)

Potential subjects will be invited to attend a face-to-face interview for written consent, psychiatric history, and history of benzodiazepine use. We will request participants to complete a daily record of benzodiazepine use in the 2 weeks prior to baseline. Those who use benzodiazepines for more than 50% of days are eligible for randomization. Participants will be randomly assigned to receive electroacupuncture plus gradual tapering or placebo electroacupuncture plus gradual tapering in a 1:1 ratio. Block randomization will be administrated by an independent administrator using a computer-generated list of random sequence. Group allocation will be kept in sequentially-numbered opaque-sealed envelopes and will be opened by acupuncturists after all baseline assessments have been completed by the research assistant who is blind to treatment allocation.

Intervention

Electroacupuncture combined with gradual tapering.

Subjects will receive electroacupuncture twice per week for 4 consecutive weeks. The frequency and duration

Table 1 Lists of included and excluded psychiatric disorders according to the ICD-10 system

Included

  F32.0 Mild depressive episode;
  F32.1 Moderate depressive episode;
  F32.8 Other depressive episodes;
  F32.9 Depressive episode, unspecified;
  F33.0 Recurrent depressive disorder, current episode mild;
  F33.4 Recurrent depressive disorder, currently in remission;
  F33.1 Recurrent depressive disorder, current episode moderate;
  F33.8 Other recurrent depressive disorders;
  F33.9 Recurrent depressive disorder, unspecified;
  F41.0 Panic disorder;
  F41.1 Generalized anxiety disorder;
  F41.2 Mixed anxiety and depressive disorder;
  F43.2 Adjustment disorders;
  F51.0 Nonorganic insomnia

Excluded

  F31.0 Bipolar affective disorder;
  F42.0 Obsessive-compulsive disorder;
  F43.1 Post-traumatic stress disorder;
  F20.0 Schizophrenia;
  F21–29 other Schizotypal and delusional disorders;
  F55.0 Abuse of non-dependence-producing substances;
  F10–12, F14–19 Abuse of other psychoactive substances

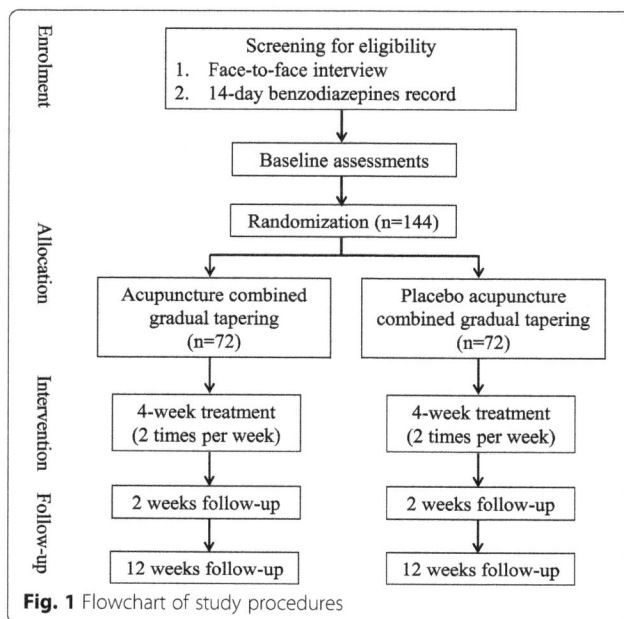

Fig. 1 Flowchart of study procedures

are based on previous systematic reviews [16–18] and experts' opinions. Subjects will be needled at bilateral EX-HN1 (Sishencong), EX-HN22 (Anmian), GB8 (Shuaigu), ST8 (Touwei), EX-HN5 (Taiyang), GB15 (Toulinqi), PC6 (Neiguan), HT7 (Shenmen), SP6 (Sanyinjiao), LV3 (Taichong), unilateral EX-HN3 (Yintang), GV24 (Shenting), and GV20 (Baihui). The location and indication are summarized in Table 2. The total number of needles used in each session will be fixed to 23. The acupoints have been used for treating insomnia and mood disorders [16, 27–29] and modified for the purpose of benzodiazepine tapering according to our expert team.

After sterilizing the skin around the acupoints with 75% alcohol, sterilized disposable needles (Blister Needle, Dong Bang, Korean, 0.25x30mm) will be inserted. "De qi" (a radiating feeling of numbness or distension considered to be indicative of effective needling as reported by the participant) will be achieved if possible. It is an indication of "effective needling" in terms of TCM theory. Four pairs of needles (left and right EX-HN1; GV20-EX-HN3; left GB8- ST8; and right GB8- ST8) will be connected to an electric-stimulator (AWQ 104 L, Hong Kong) for continuous stimulation at constant current and a frequency of 4 Hz. In clinical practice, acupuncturists usually select 1–4 pairs of acupoints to deliver electric stimulation. These four pairs of acupoints were chosen to deliver electric-stimulation because they are the main acupoints that are supposed to have anxiolytic and sedative effects according to the TCM theory. The amplitude of electrical stimulation will be adjusted to a comfortable level. The needles will be left for 30 min and then removed which resembles the duration used in clinical practice.

All the included subjects will be advised to taper their benzodiazepines over 4 weeks according to a protocol as suggested by Rickels et al. [30]. The baseline benzodiazepine dosage in diazepam equivalent will be calculated based on the average daily consumption in the 2 weeks prior to baseline [31]. Subjects will be asked to reduce their daily dose by 25% in the first and second week. For the remaining 50%, we will advise reduction by 12.5% for 3–4 days each time (Fig. 2). Where tablets do not allow precise dose reduction, tablets will be either cut in half or spaced over alternative days as required. After the second, fourth, sixth, and eighth electroacupuncture sessions, the subjects will be asked to complete a Benzodiazepine Withdrawal Symptom Questionnaire [32] to assess their withdrawal symptoms, then a trained research assistant who is blinded to the treatment allocation will use about 10–15 min to evaluate subjects' benzodiazepine withdrawal symptoms and other adverse events, discuss the problems encountered due to benzodiazepine tapering, count the surplus of benzodiazepines due to dose reduction, set the withdrawal schedule for the following weeks, and provide support and encouragement to follow the

withdrawal schedule. If subjects find it too difficult to cope, feel unable to meet the reduction goal, or have at least one item in the Benzodiazepine Withdrawal Symptom Questionnaire [32] rated as severe, we will suggest keeping the dosage unchanged or slowing down the tapering, e.g., the 25% per week tapering in the first 2 weeks can be reduced to 12.5% per week.

Placebo electroacupuncture combined with gradual tapering

The sterilization procedure will be the same as in electroacupuncture group. Placebo needles, designed by Streitberger [33], have a blunt tip that cannot penetrate the skin. The handles of placebo needles will slide over the needle when they are pressed, giving an appearance of penetrating the skin. The placebo needles will be placed 1 in. beside the acupoints in order to avoid acupressure effect. The needles are held by surgical tape or hair pin to imitate the procedure of electroacupuncture. The needles are connected to an electric-stimulator with zero frequency and amplitude. The number, duration and frequency of treatment session will be the same as in the electroacupuncture group.

Electroacupuncture will be performed according to a standard operating procedure (SOP) manual which is developed to standardize the treatment procedure and dialogue between acupuncturists and subjects (Additional file 1).

Fidelity of the intervention

The acupuncturists are registered Chinese medicine practitioners in Hong Kong with a Bachelor degree in Chinese Medicine and at least 5 years' experience in providing needle acupuncture. Their first 10 electroacupuncture treatments will be assessed and guided by the PI (WY) using a standardized checklist to ensure fidelity of the intervention. The PI will also randomly visit to check the acupuncturists' adherence to the research protocol.

Outcome measures (Table 3)
Primary outcome

Primary outcome is the proportion of participants who successfully discontinue benzodiazepines at 2-week posttreatment (week 6) and 12-week posttreatment (week 16). Previous randomized controlled trials of benzodiazepine tapering [10] have used cessation rate as the main outcome measure. The primary end-point is 12-week posttreatment (Fig. 2).

Secondary outcomes

Secondary measures include percentage benzodiazepine dose reduction, Benzodiazepine Withdrawal Symptom Questionnaire (BWSD), Insomnia Severity Index (ISI),

Table 2 Location and indication of acupoints used in the treatment protocol

Acupoints	Location	Indication in Traditional Chinese Medicine
EX-HN1 (Sishencong)	At the vertex of the scalp, four points, 1 *cun* respectively anterior, posterior and lateral to GV 20 (baihui)	Tranquilize and calm the mind, helps in headache, insomnia and forgetfulness
EX-HN22 (Anmian)	Midpoint between SJ 17 and GB 20	Helps in insomnia, palpitations and restlessness
GB8 (Shuaigu)	Head, directly above auricular apex, 1.5 *cun* superior to the hairline	Clear haet and extinguish wind, helps in headache and dizziness
ST8 (Touwei)	On the head 0.5 *cun* directly superior to anterior hairline, at the corner of forehead, 4.5 *cun* lateral to the anterior median line	Clear the head, helps in headache, dizziness and eye pain
EX-HN5 (Taiyang)	At the temple in the depression about one finger-breadth posterior to the midpoint of the lateral end of the eyebrow and the outer canthus	Helps in mental disorders such as headache, insomnia, forgetfulness, epilepsy and eye disorders
GB15 (Toulinqi)	On the head 0.5 *cun* within the anterior hairline, directly superior to the center of the pupil	Calm the mind, helps in headache, dizziness, double vision and tinnitus
PC6 (Neiguan)	On the medial aspect of the forearm between the palmers longus and flexor carpi radials tendons, 2 *cun* proximal to the palmers wrist crease	Calm the heart and mind, helps in palpitations, vexation, insomnia, depression, mania and other heart and mind disorders
HT7 (Shenmen)	Posteromedial aspect of the wrist radial to the flexor carpi ulnaris tendon at the palmer wrist crease	Calm the heart and mind, helps in insomnia, depression, mania, forgetfulness, headache and dizziness
SP6 (Sanyinjiao)	On the tibial aspect of leg posterior to the medial border of the tibia, 3 *cun* superior to the prominence of the medial mallcolus	Helps in insomnia and mania
LV3 (Taichong)	Dorsum of foot, within the depression distal between first and second metatarsal bones.	Calm the liver and extinguish win, helps in depressive psychosis, manic psychosis and insomnia.
EX-HN3 (Yintang)	At the midpoint between the medial ends of the eyebrows	Clear liver heat and improve vision
GV24 (Shenting)	One the head at the anterior median line, 0.5 *cun* superior to the anterior hairline	Subdue yang and calm the mine, helps in depression, mania, insomnia, other mental disorders, headache and dizziness
GV20 (Baihui)	On the head at the anterior median line, 5 *cun* superior to the anterior hairline	Helps in palpitations due to fright, insomnia, forgetfulness and other mental disorders

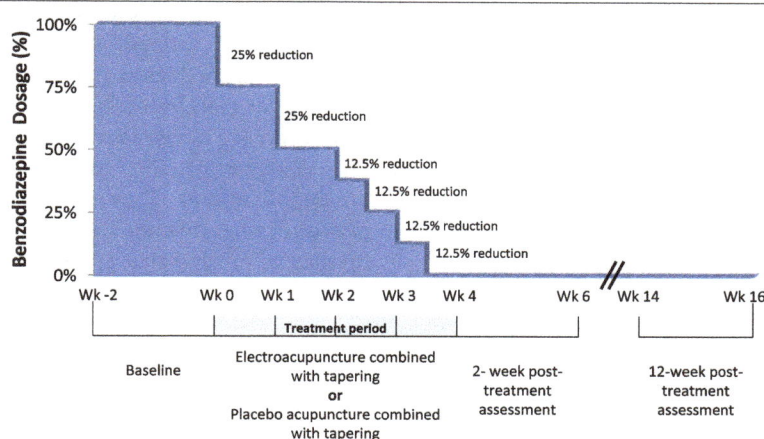

Fig. 2 Benzodiazepine gradual tapering schedule

and HADS. A daily dose of benzodiazepine in diazepam equivalent and percentage reduction as compared to baseline will be derived from a 14-day record form. Previous studies have suggested that prospective usage diary is more accurate than retrospective recall of consumption [34, 35]. The subject will be asked to bring back their un-used medications at each visit for cross-checking with the usage record.

Benzodiazepine withdrawal symptoms will be assessed by the 20-item self-administrated BWSQ [32]. The items include main symptoms experienced during withdrawal from benzodiazepine dependent patients including dizziness, pains in muscle, muscle twitching, and so on [32]. Withdrawal symptoms are rated as "absent", "moderate" or "severe" (0, 1, or 2), yielding a total score ranging between 0 and 40. The original English version has been translated into Chinese for use in this study. The back-translated version has been compared with the original version to ensure it appropriately reflects the original version. Insomnia, one of the most common benzodiazepine withdrawal symptoms, will be further evaluated

by the ISI [36]. The ISI is a 7-item 5-point self-rating Likert scale to indicate subjects' perceived severity of insomnia symptoms. The total score ranges from 0 to 28. The Chinese version of ISI has been demonstrated to have adequate validity and reliability [37]. The HADS [25], a validated and widely-used self-reported questionnaire, will be adopted to measure the severity of depressive and anxiety symptoms. It consists of 14 items; seven of them are on depression and seven on anxiety, which generates the anxiety and depression subscales. Somatic symptoms are not included in the HADS. The validated Chinese version of HADS will be used in the present study [38].

Treatment expectancy
The Credibility of Treatment Rating Scale (CTRS), a 4-item scale, will be used for assessing subjects' confidence and expectation towards treatment [39]. The Chinese version CTRS has been adopted in previous studies [27, 29]. Higher scores indicate greater confidence and expectation towards treatment.

Table 3 Summary of outcome measures and assessment schedule

Measure	Baseline	Intervention				2-week posttreatment	12-week posttreatment
		2nd	4th	6th	8th		
BZ cessation rate[a]	✓					✓	✓
BZ dose reduction, %	✓	✓	✓	✓	✓	✓	✓
BWSQ	✓	✓	✓	✓	✓	✓	✓
ISI	✓		✓			✓	✓
HADS	✓		✓			✓	✓
SDS	✓						
CTRS	✓	✓			✓		
AE monitoring		✓	✓	✓	✓	✓	✓

BZ Benzodiazepine, BWSQ Benzodiazepine Withdrawal Symptom Questionnaire, ISI Insomnia Severity Index, HADS Hospital Anxiety and Depression Scale, SDS Substance Dependence Scale, CTRS Credibility of Treatment Rating Scale, AE adverse events
[a]Primary outcome

Assessment for substance dependence

The Substance Dependence Scale (SDS) measures the severity of dependency towards a particular substance in the last 12 months [40]. The SDS contains five items and the Chinese version has been shown to be reliable and valid [41]. The term "particular substance" in the SDS will be revised to "benzodiazepine" in this study.

Safety concern

Subjects will be provided with sufficient information regarding the potential adverse events of benzodiazepine withdrawal. Benzodiazepine withdrawal symptoms, and electroacupuncture-related adverse events will be assessed at each study visit. Benzodiazepine withdrawal symptoms will be assessed by the BWSQ. A standardized electroacupuncture-related adverse event form [42, 43], consisting of eight items on adverse events around the needle sites, 13 items on systemic adverse events, and three items on serious adverse events, will be used. Severity of each adverse event will be rated as "absent", "mild", "moderate" or "severe" and the causality of adverse event will be reported using a 5-point Likert scale, ranging from "unrelated" to "certain". In addition, worsening of pre-existing medical and psychiatric conditions is counted as adverse events. Subjects with heart rate over 100 beats per minute, systolic blood pressure higher than 140 mmHg, diastolic blood pressure higher than 90 mmHg, and any suicidal risk based on the HDRS suicidality item will be evaluated by the Principal Investigator before continuing in the study. Those with moderate suicidal risk will be excluded from the study and referred to their case doctors as early as possible.

Blinding assessment

As all outcome measures are self-reported, assessments are deemed to be blinded. Success of participant blinding will be measured at the last electroacupuncture session. Subjects will be asked a standard question: "When you volunteered for the trial, you were informed that you would receive traditional acupuncture, or acupuncture-like placebo treatment. Which acupuncture do you think you received?" The standard question is adapted from the paper by Park et al. [44].

Sample size calculation

Sample size calculation is based on benzodiazepine cessation rate, the primary outcome. No previous studies have been conducted on the efficacy of electroacupuncture and placebo electroacupuncture for tapering benzodiazepines; hence the effect size for sample size calculation is estimated according to previous randomized controlled trials using psychological intervention. A median cessation rate of 74% (range = 13–85%) was reported in a previous systematic review on benzodiazepine tapering using psychological intervention [11]. We estimate that electroacupuncture will produce a cessation rate similar to that of psychological intervention (75%) and the cessation rate in placebo control group is about 50%; hence. a 25% difference in cessation rate between groups is assumed [27]. A power of 80% has been regarded as a reasonable protection against Type II error [45]. Based on a 25% between-group difference and a power of 80%, the minimal number of subjects that are required to avoid a Type I error of 0.05 is 108 (54 per group). The final sample size is 144 (72 per group) after allowing a 25% attrition rate at 12-week posttreatment.

Statistical analysis

Data will be double-entered and checked for consistency. Data analysis will be performed with an identification code of group A and group B according to a pre-specified statistical analysis plan. The coding of group allocation will be revealed after the completion of data analysis or in case of reports of serious adverse events associated with electroacupuncture or benzodiazepine withdrawal. Between-group difference will be assessed by two-sample t-test or chi-square test at baseline, week 4 (end of treatment), week 6 (2-week posttreatment), and week 16 (12-week posttreatment). The absolute risk reduction and number of subjects that are needed to be treated to obtain one benzodiazepine withdrawal will be estimated at week 16. Attempts will be made for minimizing missing data among subjects who do not return for assessment or have withdrawn from study by mail and phone reminders. Both per protocol and intention-to-treat analyses will be performed. Multiple imputation technique will be used to handle missing values, assuming data are missing at random (MAR). Ten sets of imputed values will be generated to adjust for variability due to imputation, and so ten completed data sets will be created. These completed data sets will be analyzed separately with standard statistical methods, and the results are combined into a single multiple-imputation result [46]. Sensitivity analysis will be conducted to examine the effect of departures from the assumption of MAR on clinical outcomes. The missing data due to dropout cases may be associated with those who rebound in insomnia or anxiety levels, or those who fail to decrease consumption of benzodiazepine. Pattern mixture models with various possible values of the informative missing parameters will be employed to conduct the sensitivity analysis [47]. For dichotomous outcomes, the informative missing parameter specifies the odds ratio between the outcome and missingness indicator. For continuous outcomes, it specifies the mean difference between the unobserved outcome and observed outcome. By varying the informative missing parameter, it is possible to examine the magnitude of departures from MAR assumption on different outcomes. Stata rctmiss will be used to do the sensitivity analysis [48].

Trial status

Subject recruitment has been started in late July 2015 and is expected to complete in March 2017. Results of the study will be available by the end of 2017. The current study does not include any interim analyses.

Discussion

Benzodiazepine is one of the most frequently prescribed drugs. Although benzodiazepines play an important role in the treatment of anxiety disorders, insomnia, and physical illnesses such as epilepsy, their use has been questioned due to public concerns about adverse effects and liability to lead to physical dependence and abuse. Despite legislative measures to control the prescription of benzodiazepines [49], long-term benzodiazepine use remains common. Gradual reduction of benzodiazepines with or without substitutive pharmacotherapy or psychological intervention have their limitations, the present study will explore using electroacupuncture as an adjunct for benzodiazepine tapering. In this trial, we aimed to examine the specific effects of electroacupuncture such as needle insertion, *deqi* sensation, and electric-stimulation in tapering off benzodiazepine use. Therefore, we used a non-invasive sham as a control. Our next step is to perform a pragmatic trial on the effectiveness of electroacupuncture compared to other standard interventions (e.g. psychological or pharmacological intervention) for tapering benzodiazepines.

To the best our knowledge, we are the first group to perform a randomized placebo-controlled trial using a well-documented screening process and validated scales to examine the efficacy and safety of electroacupuncture for benzodiazepine tapering. Results of this study will enrich our understanding on the use of electroacupuncture for benzodiazepine cessation.

Abbreviations
AE: Adverse events; BWSQ: Benzodiazepine Withdrawal Symptom Questionnaire; CONSORT: Consolidated Standards of Reporting Trials; CTRS: Credibility of Treatment Rating Scale; DSM-IV (SCID): Diagnostic And Statistical Manual Of Mental Disorders, Fourth Edition (Structured Clinical Interview for DSM Disorders); HADS: Hospital Anxiety and Depression Scale; ICD: International Classification of Diseases; ICH-GCP: Good Clinical Practice from International Conference on Harmonisation of Technical Requirements for Registration of Pharmaceuticals for Human Use; ISI: Insomnia Severity Index; SDS: Substance Dependence Scale; SOP: Standard operating procedure; STRICTA: Standards for Reporting Interventions in Clinical Trials of Acupuncture

Acknowledgements
The authors would like to thank all the subjects participating at the current study.

Funding
The study is supported by the Health and Medical Research Fund (HMRF), Food and Health Bureau, Hong Kong SAR (Project no. 12133661).

Authors' contributions
WFY and KFC are responsible for the study design. ZJZ, WCC and XLL provide clinical advice for the treatment design. LMH provides statistical advice. KFC, RMKN and CLWC are the site coordinators and help in monitoring recruitment progress. YMY is responsible for data collection. ZJZ, SPZ, and LL are responsible for monitoring the operation of acupuncture. WFY, KFC and YMY draft the manuscript. WFY, KFC, ZJZ, SPZ, WCC, RMKN, CLWC, LMH, YMY and XLL are responsible for revising the manuscript. All authors have read and approved the manuscript.

Competing interests
The authors declare that they have no competing interests.

Ethics approval and consent to participate
This study has obtained ethics approval from the Institutional Review Board of the University of Hong Kong/Hospital Authority Hong Kong West Cluster (UW 14–554), Research Ethics Committee of Hospital Authority Kowloon Central/Kowloon East Cluster (KC/KE-15-0178/FR-3) and Human Subjects Ethics Sub-committee of the Hong Kong Polytechnic University (HSEARS20160509002). All participants, included in the current study, gave their informed consent prior to their inclusion in the study.

Author details
[1]The Hong Kong Polytechnic University, Hunghom, Kowloon, Hong Kong SAR, China. [2]Department of Psychiatry, University of Hong Kong, Pokfulam, Hong Kong SAR, China. [3]School of Chinese Medicine, University of Hong Kong, Pokfulam, Hong Kong SAR, China. [4]School of Chinese Medicine, Hong Kong Baptist University, Kowloon Tong, Kowloon, Hong Kong SAR, China. [5]Department of Psychiatry, Kowloon Hospital, 147A Argyle Street, Kowloon, Hong Kong SAR, China. [6]Department of Psychiatry, United Christian Hospital, 130 Hip Wo Street, Kwun Tong, Kowloon, Hong Kong SAR, China. [7]School of Public Health, University of Hong Kong, Pokfulam, Hong Kong SAR, China.

References
1. Holden JD, Hughes IM, Tree A. Benzodiazepine prescribing and withdrawal for 3234 patients in 15 general practices. Fam Pract. 1994;11:358–62.
2. Australian Bureau of Statistics. National Health Survey, first results, Australia, 1995. Canberra: Australian Bureau of Statistics; 1996.
3. Petitjean S, Ladewig D, Meier CR, Amrein R, Wiesbeck GA. Benzodiazepine prescribing to the Swiss adult population: results from a national survey of community pharmacies. Int Clin Psychopharmacol. 2007;22:292–8.
4. Kan CC, Breteler MH, Zitman FG. High prevalence of benzodiazepine dependence in out-patient users, based on the DSM-III-R and ICD-10 criteria. Acta Psychiatr Scand. 1997;96:85–93.
5. Lader M, Tylee A, Donoghue J. Withdrawing benzodiazepines in primary care. CNS Drugs. 2009;23:19–34.
6. Verwey B, Eling P, Wientjes H, Zitman FG. Memory impairment in those who attempted suicide by benzodiazepine overdose. J Clin Psychiatry. 2000;61: 456–9.

7.   Chung KF, Cheung RC, Tam JW. Long-term benzodiazepine users-characteristics, views and effectiveness of benzodiazepine reduction information leaflet. Singap Med J. 1999;40:138–43.

8.   Schweizer E, Rickels K. Benzodiazepine dependence and withdrawal: a review of the syndrome and its clinical management. Acta Psychiatr Scand Suppl. 1998;393:95–101.

9.   Rickels K, Case WG, Downing RW, Winokur A. Long-term diazepam therapy and clinical outcome. JAMA. 1983;250:767–71.

10. Pecknold JC. Discontinuation reactions to alprazolam in panic disorder. J Psychiatr Res. 1993;27:155–70.

11. Parr JM, Kavanagh DJ, Cahill L, Mitchell G, McD YR. Effectiveness of current treatment approaches for benzodiazepine discontinuation: a meta-analysis. Addiction. 2009;104:13–24.

12. Gould RL, Coulson MC, Patel N, Highton-Williamson E, Howard RJ. Interventions for reducing benzodiazepine use in older people: meta-analysis of randomised controlled trials. Br J Psychiatry. 2014;204:98–107.

13. Krystal AD. The changing perspective on chronic insomnia management. J Clin Psychiatry. 2004;65:20–5.

14. Harris PE, Cooper KL, Relton C, Thomas KJ. Prevalence of complementary and alternative medicine (CAM) use by the general population: a systematic review and update. Int J Clin Pract. 2012;66:924–39.

15. Kaptchuk TJ. Acupuncture: theory, efficacy, and practice. Ann Intern Med. 2002;136:374–83.

16. Pilkington K, Kirkwood G, Rampes H, Cummings M, Richardson J. Acupuncture for anxiety and anxiety disorders–a systematic literature review. Acupunct Med. 2007;25:1–10.

17. Yeung WF, Chung KF, Leung YK, Zhang SP, Law AC. Traditional needle acupuncture treatment for insomnia: a systematic review of randomized controlled trials. Sleep Med. 2009;10:694–704.

18. Cheuk DK, Yeung WF, Chung KF, Wong V. Acupuncture for insomnia. Cochrane Database Syst Rev. 2012;9:CD005472.

19. Ruan JW, Zheng PY. Therapeutic analysis on the acupuncture for drug-dependence insomnia. Chin J Rehab Med. 2002;17:167–8.

20. Zhang Y, Liu SW, Hou YC. Acupuncture treatment of drug-dependence insomnia. Chin Acupunct Moxibust. 2001;22:85.

21. Qiao YY. Thirty cases of anxiety symptom treated with Shenmen-through-Shaohai point. Chin Acupunct Moxibust. 2002;21:81–2.

22. Moher D, Hopewell S, Schulz KF, Montori V, Gotzsche PC, Devereaux PJ, Elbourne D, Egger M, Altman DG, Consort. CONSORT 2010 explanation and elaboration: updated guidelines for reporting parallel group randomised trials. Int J Surg. 2012;10:28–55.

23. MacPherson H, Altman DG, Hammerschlag R, Li Y, Wu T, White A, Moher D, Group SR. Revised STandards for Reporting Interventions in Clinical Trials of Acupuncture (STRICTA): extending the CONSORT statement. Acupunct Med. 2010;28:83–93.

24. World Health Organisation Collaborating Centre for Drug Statistics Methodology. Guidelines for ATC Classification and DDD Assignment. 5th ed. Oslo, Norway: World Health Organisation; 2002.

25. Zigmond AS, Snaith RP. The hospital anxiety and depression scale. Acta Psychiatr Scand. 1983;67:361–70.

26. Hamilton M. A rating scale for depression. J Neurol Neurosurg Psychiatry. 1960;23:56–62.

27. Chung KF, Yeung WF, Yu YM, Yung KP, Zhang SP, Zhang ZJ, Wong MT, Lee WK, Chan LW. Acupuncture for residual insomnia associated with major depressive disorder: A placebo- and sham-controlled, subject- and assessor-blind, randomized trial. J Clin Psychiatry. 2015;76:e752–60.

28. Yeung WF, Chung KF, Poon MM, Ho FY, Zhang SP, Zhang ZJ, Ziea ET, Wong TV. Prescription of chinese herbal medicine and selection of acupoints in pattern-based traditional chinese medicine treatment for insomnia: a systematic review. Evid Based Complement Alternat Med. 2012;2012:902578.

29. Yeung WF, Chung KF, Tso KC, Zhang SP, Zhang ZJ, Ho LM. Electroacupuncture for residual insomnia associated with major depressive disorder: a randomized controlled trial. Sleep. 2011;34:807–15.

30. Rickels K, Schweizer E, Case WG, Greenblatt DJ. Long-term therapeutic use of benzodiazepines. I. Effects of abrupt discontinuation. Arch Gen Psychiatry. 1990;47:899–907.

31. Zitman FG, Couvée JE. Chronic benzodiazepine use in general practice patients with depression: an evaluation of controlled treatment and taper-off: report on behalf of the Dutch Chronic Benzodiazepine Working Group. Br J Psychiatry. 2001;178:317–24.

32. Tyrer P, Murphy S, Riley P. The benzodiazepine withdrawal symptom questionnaire. J Affect Disord. 1990;19:53–61.

33. Streitberger K, Kleinhenz J. Introducing a placebo needle into acupuncture research. Lancet. 1998;352:364–5.

34. Morin CM, Bastien C, Guay B, Radouco-Thomas M, Leblanc J, Vallières A. Randomized clinical trial of supervised tapering and cognitive behavior therapy to facilitate benzodiazepine discontinuation in older adults with chronic insomnia. Am J Psychiatry. 2004;161:332–42.

35. Voshaar RC, Gorgels WJMJ, Mol AJJ, Van Balkom AJLM, Van de Lisdonk EH, Breteler MHM, van den Hoogen HJ, Zitman FG. Tapering off long-term benzodiazepine use with or without group cognitive-behavioural therapy: three conditioned, randomised controlled trial. Br J Psychiatry. 2003;182:498–504.

36. Bastien CH, Vallières A, Morin CM. Validation of the Insomnia Severity Index as an outcome measure for insomnia research. Sleep Med. 2001;2:297–307.

37. Chung KF, Kan KK, Yeung WF. Assessing insomnia in adolescents: comparison of Insomnia Severity Index, Athens Insomnia Scale and Sleep Quality Index. Sleep Med. 2011;12:463–70.

38. Leung CM, Wing YK, Kwong PK, Lo A, Shum K. Validation of the Chinese-Cantonese version of the hospital anxiety and depression scale and comparison with the Hamilton Rating Scale of Depression. Acta Psychiatr Scand. 1999;100:456–61.

39. Vincent C. Credibility assessment in trials of acupuncture. Complement Med Res. 1990;4:8–11.

40. Gossop M, Darke S, Griffiths P, Hando J, Powis B, Hall W, Strang J. The Severity of Dependence Scale (SDS): psychometric properties of the SDS in English and Australian samples of heroin, cocaine and amphetamine users. Addiction. 1995;90:607–14.

41. Chen VC, Chen H, Lin TY, Chou HH, Lai TJ, Ferri CP, Gossop M. Severity of heroin dependence in Taiwan: Reliability and validity of the Chinese version of the Severity of Dependence Scale (SDS[Ch]). Addict Behav. 2008;33:1590–3.

42. Chung KF, Yeung WF, Kwok CW, Yu YM. Risk factors associated with adverse events of acupuncture: a prospective study. Acupunct Med. 2014;32:455–62.

43. Chung KF, Yeung WF, Yu YM, Kwok CW, Zhang SP, Zhang ZJ. Adverse Events Related to Acupuncture: Development and Testing of a Rating Scale. Clin J Pain. 2015;31:922–8.

44. Park J, White AR, James MA, Hemsley AG, Hohnson P, Chambers J, Ernst E. Acupuncture for subacute stroke rehabilitation. A sham-controlled, subject- and assessor-blind, randomized trial. Arch Intern Med. 2005;165:2026–31.

45. Portney LG, Watkins MP. Foundations of clinical research: applications to practice. 3rd ed. Upper Saddle River, N.J: Pearson/Prentice Hall; 2009.

46. Little RJA, Rubin DB. Statistical Analysis with Missing Data. 2nd ed. Hoboken, NJ: Wiley; 2002.

47. Little RJA. Pattern-Mixture Models for Multivariate Incomplete Data. J Am Stat Assoc. 1993;88:125–34.

48. rctmiss – analyse a RCT allowing for informatively missing outcome data. http://www.mrc-bsu.cam.ac.uk/software/stata-software. Accessed 27 Mar 2017.

49. Chung KF. Benzodiazepine prescribing trend after its inclusion as a dangerous drug under the Hong Kong Dangerous Drugs Ordinance. Hong Kong Med J. 1997;3:16–20.

13

Self-administered acupressure for symptom management among Chinese family caregivers with caregiver stress

Agnes Tiwari[1], Lixing Lao[2], Amy Xiao-Min Wang[3], Denise Shuk Ting Cheung[1]* ⓘ, Mike Ka Pui So[4],
Doris Sau Fung Yu[5], Terry Yat Sang Lum[6], Helina Yin King Yuk Fung[7], Jerry Wing Fai Yeung[2]
and Zhang-Jin Zhang[2]

Abstract

Background: Caregiving can be stressful, potentially creating physical and psychological strain. Substantial evidence has shown that family caregivers suffer from significant health problems arising from the demands of caregiving. Although there are programs supporting caregivers, there is little evidence regarding their effectiveness. Acupressure is an ancient Chinese healing method designed to restore the flow of Qi (vital energy) by applying external pressure to acupoints. A randomized, wait-list controlled trial was developed to evaluate the effectiveness of a self-administered acupressure intervention on caregiver stress (primary objective) and stress-related symptoms of fatigue, insomnia, depression, and health-related quality of life (secondary objectives) in Chinese caregivers of older family members.

Methods: Two hundred Chinese participants, aged ≥ 21 years, who are the primary caregivers of an older family member and screen positive for caregiver stress and symptoms of fatigue/insomnia/depression will be recruited from a community setting in Hong Kong. Subjects will be randomized to receive either an immediate treatment condition (self-administered acupressure intervention) or a wait-list control condition. The self-administered acupressure intervention will include (i) an individual learning and practice session twice a week for 2 weeks, (ii) a home follow-up visit once a week for 2 weeks, and (iii) 15-min self-practice twice a day for 6 weeks. The wait-list control group will receive the same acupressure training after the intervention group has completed the intervention. We hypothesize that Chinese family caregivers in the intervention group will have lower levels of caregiver stress, fatigue, insomnia, depression, and higher health-related quality of life after completion of the intervention than participants in the wait-list control group.

Discussion: This study will provide evidence for the effectiveness of self-administered acupressure in reducing stress and improving symptoms of fatigue, insomnia, depression, and health-related quality of life in Chinese family caregivers. The findings will inform the design of interventions to relieve negative health effects of caregiving. Furthermore, the results can raise community awareness and serve as a basis for policymaking, planning, and allocation of resources regarding empowerment of family caregivers for self-care.

Trial registration: Current Controlled Trials NCT02526446. Registered August 10, 2015.

Keywords: Acupressure, Self-administered acupressure, Family caregivers, Caregiver stress, Fatigue, Insomnia, Depression, Health-related quality of life, Intervention, Chinese, Randomized controlled trial (RCT)

* Correspondence: denisech@hku.hk
[1]School of Nursing, Li Ka Shing Faculty of Medicine, The University of Hong Kong, 4/F, William M.W. Mong Block, 21 Sassoon Road, Pokfulam, Hong Kong
Full list of author information is available at the end of the article

Background

It is estimated that 1.5 billion people, representing 16 % of the world's population, will be aged 65 years or older by 2050 [1]. With increasing population age, noncommunicable diseases increase in prevalence, including chronic disease and disability. This leads to an increased demand for care, and the primary caregiver role often falls on family members [2]. In this study, the primary caregiver of an older family member is defined as one who provides unpaid care to the care recipient for no less than 14 h per week, and the care recipients are older family members (aged ≥ 65 years) irrespective of their health problems/disabilities.

While caring for an older family member can be rewarding for some, evidence shows that family caregivers are at risk of emotional, mental, and physical health problems arising from the complexity and strains of caregiving [2–5]. Caregiver stress, defined as "the burden or strain that caregivers face when caring for a person with a chronic disease," is prevalent and associated with stress-related symptoms, notably fatigue, insomnia, and depression [3]. Fatigue is often the initial and most difficult problem resulting from the stressful caregiving process, and leads to sleep disturbance, anxiety, and depression [6]. It is estimated that more than one-third of family caregivers suffer from poor health [7].

Not only does caregiver stress put family caregivers at risk for poor health outcomes, it may also affect their quality of life [8] and hinder their ability to provide care, with negative consequences for their care recipients [9]. The adverse impact of caregiver stress on the health and safety of both caregivers and care recipients can lead to increased social and healthcare costs [2]. Despite the recognition that stress-related health symptoms among family caregivers is a public health priority [1], there is little evidence about the effectiveness of symptom management for these caregivers.

We aim to study Chinese family caregivers because China comprises 19 % of the world's population and is expected to have an older population of 25 % by 2030 [10]. Furthermore, with 90 % of older Chinese living at home [11], much of the caregiving responsibilities are likely to fall on their family members. Although the Confucian value of filial piety may buffer the demands of caregiving, Chinese family caregivers are not exempt from caregiver stress [12]. Therefore, these caregivers, similar to their Western counterparts, are in need of effective, achievable, and acceptable interventions to help them manage caregiver stress.

Acupressure and symptom management

Acupressure, defined as the application of pressure on acupoints using the hands, fingers, or thumbs [13–15], is a non-invasive technique based on the meridian theory of Traditional Chinese medicine (TCM). TCM theory holds that meridians, which are channels in a network of energy pathways throughout the body, regulate the flow of Qi (vital energy) and the unbalanced flow of Qi results in disease [16]. By applying pressure to acupoints (trigger or active points) on the surface of the skin, acupressure stimulates the meridians, resulting in the opening of the channels and balancing of energy, thus restoring health [14, 16]. Because acupressure uses the application of pressure to acupoints without penetrating the skin, it is noninvasive and painless [17, 18]. The use of acupressure for positive symptom management in healthy people and patients by trained practitioners has been reported [17–22].

In addition to the administration of acupressure by trained practitioners, self-administered acupressure has also been used for symptom management. Self-administered acupressure is acupressure performed by the recipients themselves after undergoing appropriate training. This technique has a number of advantages including flexibility, low cost, and empowerment [18]. Studies have reported on the clinical application of self-administered acupressure [14, 23]. In addition, systematic reviews of the effect of self-administered acupressure for symptom management have been conducted. These reviews included perceived stress, insomnia, and sleep disturbances, and the studies found positive effects and safety. However, attention was also drawn to the need for well-designed randomized controlled trials [13, 18].

Self-administered acupressure is likely to suit the family caregivers because their caregiver responsibilities often leave them with little time and flexibility to seek their own treatment. Once they have mastered the technique of self-administered acupressure, they can choose when and where to conduct the intervention to suit their caregiver activities and their own needs.

In the present study protocol, we detail a self-administered acupressure intervention protocol for Chinese family caregivers with caregiver stress based on our previous study on: (i) a similar model of self-administered acupressure previously tested in women with osteoarthritic knee pain that was shown to be feasible and safe [14]; (ii) factors aggravating or buffering caregiver stress among Chinese family caregivers [12]; (iii) a case management approach to improve the health outcomes of Chinese family caregivers of dementia patients [24]; and (iv) the scientific basis of symptom management [25]. In light of the needs of these caregivers and the little evidence on the effectiveness of self-administered acupressure in symptom management, a specifically designed self-administered acupressure intervention for Chinese family caregivers will be implemented and evaluated in this study.

Aims and hypotheses

The primary aim of this randomized, wait-list controlled trial is to evaluate the effectiveness of a self-administered acupressure intervention on caregiver stress among Chinese caregivers of older family members. The secondary aim is to evaluate the effectiveness of the self-administered acupressure intervention on the Chinese family caregivers' stress-related symptoms of fatigue, insomnia, and depression and their health-related quality of life.

We hypothesize that, on completion of a self-administered acupressure intervention, and as compared with the wait-list control group, Chinese family caregivers in the intervention group will have:

(i) lower levels of caregiver stress, as measured by the Caregiver Burden Inventory;
(ii) lower scores of fatigue symptoms, as measured by the Piper Fatigue Scale;
(iii) lower scores of insomnia symptoms, as measured by the Pittsburgh Sleep Quality Index;
(iv) lower scores of depression symptoms, as measured by the Patient Health Questionnaire; and
(v) higher scores of health-related quality of life, as measured by the SF-12 Health Survey.

Methods/Design

This is a randomized, wait-list controlled trial. There will be two groups: an intervention group and a wait-list control group. The participants randomly assigned to the intervention group will receive an immediate treatment condition (the self-administered acupressure intervention), while those assigned to the wait-list control group will receive a wait-list control condition (the same self-administered acupressure intervention but after the intervention group has completed the treatment condition). The design allows all participants to receive the intervention eventually but at the same time also controls the confounding variables that could cause spurious causality.

Participants

A total of 200 participants will be recruited for the study. Chinese family caregivers will be eligible to participate if they meet all of the following criteria:

1. Chinese men or women, 21 years of age or older, able to communicate in Cantonese or Putonghua. Justifications: an ability to command the Chinese language (Cantonese or Putonghua) is essential because the acupressure protocol is written and conducted in Chinese. Furthermore, the intervention requires participants to have the self-discipline for compliance, hence the decision to select more mature participants of age ≥ 21 years.
2. Primary caregiver of an older family member aged ≥ 65 years. Justifications: the literature has shown that caring for an older family member is a key source of

caregiver stress, hence our decision to adopt a more inclusive approach to target older family members who are the care recipients, irrespective of their health problems/disabilities. We recognize that the older care recipients likely have different health problems/disabilities, which may affect their dependency on the caregivers and the level of caregiver stress. Therefore, we will take into account the care recipients' health problems/disabilities in the data analysis.

3. Providing unpaid care to the care recipient at no less than 14 h per week. Justification: this criterion will exclude paid or occasional caretakers whose needs and caregiver stress, if any, are likely to be different from that studied in this project.
4. Primarily responsible for making day-to-day decisions and providing assistance to the care recipient in tasks relating to activities of daily living (e.g., bathing, dressing, and toileting) and/or instrumental activities of daily living (e.g., housework, grocery shopping, preparing meals, and managing medications). Justification: this criterion will exclude those who are not the primary caregivers.
5. Screened positive for caregiver stress (a summed score of ≥ 25 as measured by the Caregiver Burden Inventory), with symptoms of fatigue (a mean score of ≥ 4 as measured by the Piper Fatigue Scale), insomnia (a global score of > 5 as measured by the Pittsburgh Sleep Quality Index), or depression (a total score of ≥ 10 as measured by the Patient Health Questionnaire). Justifications: caregivers with caregiver stress are the participants targeted while fatigue, insomnia, and depression are the outcome measures in the proposed study.

Chinese family caregivers will be excluded if they have:

1. Cognitive impairment (a Mini Mental State Examination score of ≤ 23). Justification: cognitive impairment will interfere with their comprehension of the intervention.
2. Major chronic illness (e.g., cancer) or are currently taking medication (e.g., opiates) that may prevent them from performing the intervention. Justification: they may have difficulty completing the intervention.
3. Participated in interventional studies involving acupressure or acupuncture previously. Justification: their prior experience may affect their response to the proposed intervention.

Sample size

The power calculation is based on the test for significant difference between the mean pre-post differences of the caregiver stress scores in the intervention and control groups. Because no study has used self-administered acupressure as an intervention to reduce caregiver stress, we determined our study sample size based on the findings of a previous study measuring caregiver burden of those caring for community-residing patients with Alzheimer's disease [24]. This study reported the mean and standard deviation of the CBI score to be 47.54 and 17.61, respectively. Assuming a moderate correlation ($p = 0.7$) between the pre and post intervention CBI scores, we approximate the pooled standard deviation of a two-sample t-test as $17.61\sqrt{2(1-p)} = 13.64$. Taking a clinical difference of $d = 6$, which is considered a 10–15 % improvement owing to intervention (using the mean 47.54 as a reference) and a Type I error rate of 5 %, $n = 83$ was determined to have a power greater than 80 %. Assuming an attrition rate of 15 %, the target sample size is at least 98 per group. We rounded up the number of participants to 100 in each group, which makes a total of 200 participants.

Setting

The proposed trial will be conducted in a nongovernment organization (NGO) in Hong Kong. The NGO has more than 40 outreach centers covering three densely populated districts with an older population of around 14 %. This is comparable to the average older population of 13.5 % in Hong Kong [26]. The NGO has been providing caregiver support and older services in the districts for several decades.

Recruitment

A flyer with a brief description of the present project and an invitation to participate will be displayed in the host NGO center and its outreach sites. An advertisement will also be placed in the NGO's newsletters. Additionally, promotional sessions will be conducted during the activities for family caregivers organized by the NGO. Potential participants who express an interest will be referred by the center staff to our research team. The research assistant responsible for recruitment will contact the individual and provide information about the project together with the rights as a research subject and the voluntary nature of the participation. If the person agrees to participate, a written consent form will be signed. After obtaining informed consent, an assessment of eligibility will be made according to the inclusion and exclusion criteria as described above. Those assessed to be not eligible will be thanked for their interest and no further contact will be made. Those who meet the inclusion criteria will be enrolled in the study.

Randomization and blinding

Eligible participants will be randomly assigned to either the intervention group ($n = 100$) or the wait-list control group ($n = 100$) using a computerized blocked randomization scheme operated by the study programmer (SP) who is not involved in the recruitment. A series of random numbers will be generated to determine the group assignment of the participants. The group assignment results will be kept in separate, sealed, opaque envelopes. The entire randomization process will be securely conducted by the SP and the group assignment of participants will be centrally controlled. Neither the research assistant conducting the recruitment, nor the participant will know the group assignment until the envelope is opened.

Questionnaires will be completed by each of the participants and numerically coded to ensure that the group allocation of the participant is not revealed. The numerical codes and the names of the participants will be stored separately and securely in the central office. Researchers conducting data collection and analysis will be blinded to the group allocation of the participants.

Intervention

The intervention, 28 h in total, extends over an 8-weeks period and includes: (i) individual learning and practice (1st–2nd wk): a one-time 1-h introduction and ice-breaking exercise at the start of the first session to be followed by a 1-h training session on self-administered acupressure provided by certified trainers in the participant's home twice a week for 2 consecutive weeks (total, 5 h); (ii) home follow-up (3rd–4th wk): a 1-h home visit by certified trainers to reinforce learning and self-practice once a week for 2 consecutive weeks (total, 2 h); and (iii) self-practice (3rd–8th wk): self-administered acupressure by the participant at home, to be undertaken not less than one h after a meal, for 15 min twice a day for 6 weeks following the completion of the 2-weeks training session (total, 21 h).

For each of the 1-h training sessions during the first 2 weeks, a brief introduction to the basic theories of TCM and acupressure therapy will be provided (15 min). The introduction will be followed by a demonstration of self-administered acupressure by the trainers (15 min). Self-administered acupressure will then be practiced, until proficient, by the participant under the guidance of the trainers (30 min). The trainers, made up of a senior year TCM student and a senior year nursing student, will be trained and certified by a licensed TCM practitioner from the researchers' School of Chinese Medicine.

For monitoring of compliance, during the 5th through 8th weeks of the intervention, once a week, phone calls will be made by the same team of trainers to remind the participant to perform the self-administered acupressure with feedback for any questions or expressed concerns. Any medical incidents (e.g., visits to hospital or doctor for caregiver health problems) will be documented. Each participant will use an "acupressure" diary to record the frequency, duration, and time of the acupressure conducted each day, and the record will be checked by the trainer during the telephone calls.

Training materials will be provided to each participant. The self-administered acupressure protocol (Table 1), a poster illustrating the acupoints, and stickers used to label each acupoint will be provided to the participant at the first training session. Acupoint selection will be demonstrated step-by-step by the trainers, and the participants will be asked to find the selected acupoints by themselves under the guidance of the trainers. Once they have mastered the location of the selected acupoints, the participants will be guided, with assistance from the trainers as required, to perform the self-administered acupressure as described in the protocol. An audio-recorded step-by step procedure of the self-administered acupressure will be provided to the participants for reinforcement of learning. The audio recording, protocol, posters, and stickers are designed to enhance accuracy and compliance during home practice.

Instruments

The following study instruments (with the exception of the Demographic Questionnaire) will be administered at four time points: (a) pre-intervention (T0, baseline), i.e., on entry to study after randomization but before intervention; (b) post-training (T1, end of 2nd week), i.e., on completion of the 2-weeks individual learning and practice; (c) post-intervention (T2, end of 8th wk), i.e., on completion of the 8-weeks self-administered acupressure intervention; and (d) follow-up (T3, end of 12th wk), i.e., 4 weeks after the completion of the intervention.

(a) The Chinese version of the Caregiver Burden Inventory (C-CBI, 24 items) [27] will be used to (i) initially screen potential participants for caregiver stress, and (ii) assess levels of caregiver stress at different time points in the study. The C-CBI has been validated for the Chinese population and demonstrated satisfactory internal consistency (Cronbach's alpha 0.9) [27]. Each item is assessed using a 5-point Likert scale ranging from 0 (never) to 4 (nearly always). For the initial screening, participants with a summed score of ≥ 25 will be identified as experiencing caregiver stress and recruited into the study.

(b) The Chinese version of the Piper Fatigue Scale (C-PFS, 22 items) will be used to (i) initially screen potential participants for the symptom of fatigue, and (ii) assess the levels of fatigue experienced by the participant at different time points in the study. The C-PFS has been validated with good reliability (Cronbach's alpha 0.93) [28]. Each item is assessed using a numeric scale of "0" to "10" with higher scores representing more fatigue. For the initial screening, participants with a mean score of ≥ 4 will be identified as experiencing fatigue and recruited into the study.

(c) The Chinese version of the Pittsburgh Sleep Quality Index (C-PSQI, 19 items) will be used to (i) initially screen potential participants for the symptom of insomnia, and (ii) assess the levels of insomnia experienced by the participant at different time points of the study. The C-PSQI has been validated with good reliability (Cronbach's alpha 0.86) [29]. Insomnia (sleep disturbances in subjective sleep quality, sleep latency, sleep duration, habitual sleep efficiency, sleep disturbances, use of sleeping medication, and daytime dysfunction) will be assessed on a 4-point Likert scale ranging from 0 (no difficulty) to 3 (severe difficulty). For the initial screening, participants with a global (summed) score of > 5 will be classified as experiencing insomnia and recruited into the study.

(d) The Chinese version of the Patient Health Questionnaire (C-PHQ, nine items) will be used to (i) initially screen potential participants for the symptom of depression, and (ii) assess the levels of depression experienced by the participant at different time points of the study. The C-PHQ is one of the most popular self-administered screening tools for the symptom of depression that has been validated in the Hong Kong Chinese population [30]. Each item is scored from 0 (not at all) to 3 (nearly every day), with a total score ranging from 0 to 27. Cutoff values of 5, 10, 15, and 20 have been widely used to define mild, moderate, moderately severe, and severe depressive symptoms. For the initial screening, participants with a total score of ≥ 10 will be identified as experiencing the symptom of depression and recruited into the study.

(e) The Chinese version of the SF-12 version 2 Health Survey (C-SF-12v2, 12 items) has demonstrated validity and equivalence for Chinese populations [31] and will be used to assess health-related quality of life. The 12 items are grouped under the mental component summary and physical component summary. The survey is scored by recoding the items, computing the raw scale scores, and transforming the scores to a range from 0 to 100 according to the standard scoring algorithm. Higher scores indicate a better health status.

(f) Health economics assessment (HEA) will be assessed to determine the cost minimization [32] related to the intervention, with items on: (i) number of physician visits, (ii) use of prescription drugs, and (iii) incidence of inpatient hospitalization.

Table 1 Standard protocol- self-administered acupressure for symptom management

Sequence/acupoint	Location		Function	How-to-do	Frequency (Times/duration)
1.Baihui (GV20, 百會)	On the vertex of the head at the sagittal midline of the scalp at the midpoint of the line connecting the apexes of both ears		Treatment of various mental disorders, in particular insomnia, depression, anxiety, headache and decreased memory	Using 4 finger pads gently tap the area of this acupoint on the scalp	60/1 min
2.Fenchi (GB20, 風池)	On the nape, in a depression between the upper portion of the sternocleidomastoid muscle and the trapezius		A commonly used point for acupressure to treat headache, neck and shoulder pain and stiffness. Also beneficial in relieving convulsion, agitation, insomnia and stress-related symptoms	Using two thumbs press on the points bilaterally while the other four fingers should hold the back of the head naturally	60/1 min
6.Hegu (LI4, 合谷)	On the dorsum of the hand, between the 1st and 2nd metacarpal bones, in the middle of the 2nd metacarpal bone on the radial side		Expels Wind and releases the exterior, tonifies qi and strengthens immunity; used to manage every type of pain and psychogenic tense	Using thumb pad firmly massage the surrounding area of this acupoint on the dorsum of the hand unilaterally	30/1 min for each side

Table 1 Standard protocol- self-administered acupressure for symptom management *(Continued)*

Acupoint	Location	Image	Function	Technique	Reps/Time
4.Shenshu (UB 23, 腎俞)	On the low back at 1.5 cun lateral to the posterior midline at the level of the 2nd lumbar vertebral spine		Well known For all kidney related issues which affect the brain, bone, hair, teeth and/or hearing. Useful for deficiency conditions: exhaustion, weakness, chronic fatigue, good point for the elderly as Kidney Jing is naturally depleted	Using the fists gently tap the lumbar area of this acupoint at the low back bilaterally	60/1.5mins
5.Zhongwan (CV12, 中脘)	On the **upper abdomen** and on the anterior midline, 4 cun above the centre of the umbilicus.		Innervated by the spinal nerves originating from the same segments of the spinal cord that sends visceral nerve fiber innervating the stomach. Can improve digestive function and relieve abdominal distention/pain, constipation and insomnia	Using finger pads in clockwise circle gently massage the upper abdomen area, 4 cun above the umbilicus	200/2mins
6.Qihai (CV6, 氣海) GuanyYuan (CV4, 關元)	On the **lower abdomen** on the anterior midline at 1.5 cun and 3 cun below the centre of the umbilicus, respectively.		Often applied together in acupressure to tonify Qi because Essential Qi (元氣) is housed and circulated in these two points. Beneficial for constipation, retention of urination, frequent nocturia and indigestion. Modulate the limbic-medial prefrontal network related to cognitive function	Using finger pads in clockwise circle gently massage the lower abdomen area, 3 cun below the umbilicus	200/2mins

Table 1 Standard protocol- self-administered acupressure for symptom management (*Continued*)

7.Zusanli (ST36, 足三里)	On the anterior lateral side of the leg at 3 cun below the knee joint, one middle finger breadth from the anterior crest of the tibia.		Broad therapeutic effects, from gastro, intestinal and endocrinal diseases to neuropsychiatric disorders. Stimulation at Zu-San-Li evokes the robust response in limbic-paralimbic-neocortical network involved in autonomic, pain, mood and cognitive function	Using thumb pad firmly massage the area bilaterally on the anterior lateral side of the leg, 3 cun below the knee joint	60/1.5mins for each side
8.Yongquan (KD1,涌泉)	On sole, in a depression with foot in plantar flexion, at the junction of the anterior 1/3 and posterior 2/3 of line connecting base of the 2nd and 3rd toes with the heel		Useful for headaches, hypertension, low back pain, insomnia, palpitations, anxiety, poor memory, mania, hot flashes, night sweats, and loss of consciousness or yang collapse	Using 4 finger pads firmly massage the area bilaterally on each sole, in depression with foot in plantar flexion	100/2.5mins for each side

Consent to publish the images in the table has been obtained from the patients featured

(g) A demographic questionnaire (DQ) will be used to collect information on age, education level, marital status, number and age of children, employment status, financial hardship, number of care recipients, total number of hours of caregiving per week (for the older adult care recipient and children, if appropriate), length of caring (years/months of caregiving), assistance received from other family members (including number of people providing care), paid/occasional caregivers, receipt of comprehensive social security assistance, need for financial support, and number of years living in Hong Kong. Information will also be collected regarding the care recipient's health and dependency including age, health problems, disabilities, and degree of dependency on the caregiver.

Procedures

Upon study entry, participants in both groups will be asked to complete the Chinese version of the questionnaires (T0, baseline assessment), including C-CBI for caregiver stress, C-PFS for fatigue, C-PSQI for insomnia, C-PHQ for depression, C-SF-12v2 for quality of life, HEA for cost minimization, and DQ for participant profile. The participants assigned to the intervention group will then receive the intervention as described. When the intervention group reaches post-training, post-intervention, and follow-up time points (T1, T2, and T3, respectively), participants in both groups will complete C-CBI, C-PFS, C-PSQI, C-PHQ, C-SF-12v2, and HEA. After the completion of data collection at T3, participants in the wait-list control group will then receive the self-administered acupressure training. The immediate treatment received by the intervention group, the wait-list control condition received by the control group, and the data collection points are shown in Fig. 1.

Data analysis

The primary outcome is caregiver stress and the secondary outcomes are symptoms of fatigue, insomnia, depression, and health-related quality of life.

The effectiveness of the self-administered acupressure intervention on caregiver stress, symptoms of fatigue, insomnia and depression, and health-related quality of life will be assessed. To do this, the scores of the C-CBI, C-PFS, C-PSQI, C-PHQ-9, SF-12v2, and HEA collected at four different time points will be analyzed for changes from baseline (T0) to the post-intervention (T2) and from the post-intervention (T2) to the follow-up (T3).

For the primary analysis, the levels of caregiver stress on completion of the intervention (T2) between the intervention and wait-list control groups will be assessed by a regression analysis with adjustment of baseline values and accounting for any possible effect of the demographics. Residuals will be checked to ensure adequacy of the method. In addition, changes in caregiver stress from baseline (T0) to follow-up (T3) will be assessed by paired t-tests. The intention-to-treat principle will be adopted and all study subjects will be included in the analysis with missing values replaced by the last observed values or imputed by regression substitution.

For secondary analysis, the scores of the C-PFS, C-PSQI, C-PHQ, C-SF-12v2, and HEA will be compared for differences between the intervention and wait-list control groups by a linear mixed effects model with the baseline value of the scale and the intervention group as fixed factors and the intercept as a random factor. Moreover, effects of the demographics, care recipients' health problems/disability, and dependency on the outcomes will be explored by considering them as fixed factors in the linear mixed effects model. Changes in mean scores from baseline will also be assessed by a linear mixed effects model with the use of linear contrasts. Multivariate analysis will also be conducted to simultaneously study changes in clusters of mean scores.

Baseline characteristics (T0) between the intervention and wait-list control groups will be assessed by chi-square test and Mann–Whitney U test for categorical and continuous data, respectively.

Statistical significance is defined as $p < 0.05$ with a two-sided test. All statistical analyses will be conducted with Statistical Package for the Social Sciences (SPSS) program.

Ethics, consent and permissions

This study protocol was approved by the Institutional Review Board of the University of Hong Kong/Hospital Authority Hong Kong West Cluster (HKU/HA HKW IRB: UW 15–367) on June 26, 2015. The study will be conducted according to the Declaration of Helsinki. Participation in the study is entirely voluntary. An information sheet is provided and a written consent is required from all participants. If participants choose to withdraw from this study, they may do so at any time with no questions asked.

Discussion

This study protocol describes the implementation and evaluation of a self-administered acupressure intervention for Chinese family caregivers with caregiver stress. This will be the first randomized controlled trial to test the effectiveness of self-administered acupressure in reducing the stress of caregivers and improving their stress-related symptoms of fatigue, insomnia, depression, and health-related quality of life.

The emotional and physical strain of caregiving and its adverse impact on family caregivers' health and well-being is recognized as a serious public health problem [3, 33, 34]. Although a variety of pharmacological and

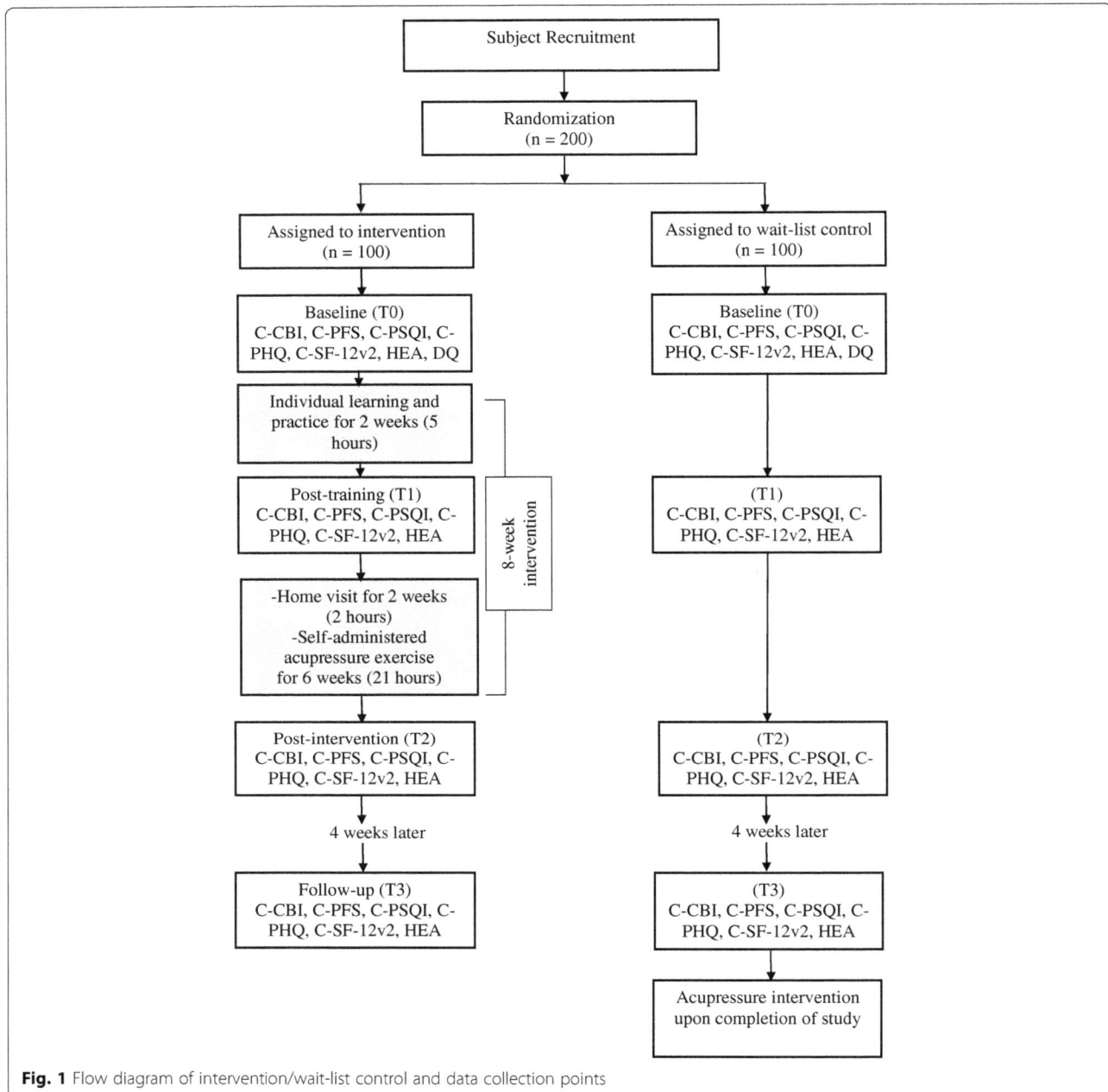

Fig. 1 Flow diagram of intervention/wait-list control and data collection points

psychosocial interventions have been developed to alleviate caregiver stress, the therapeutic benefits are modest [35–37]. Therefore, there is a need to find interventions that are not only effective but also acceptable to caregivers. Providing interventions to these caregivers is challenging; not only may their motivation be hampered by the stress of never-ending caregiving responsibilities, but their needs often have to take second place after those of their care recipients. If proven effective, the self-administered acupressure intervention would open up an attainable avenue for family caregivers to release their caregiving stress in a safe, feasible, and affordable manner.

By reducing the burden of caregiver stress, it is intended that the self-administered acupressure intervention will not only alleviate health declines, but also lower health and social care costs for these caregivers and their care recipients. Furthermore, the realization of what they can achieve in promoting health and well-being through self-administered intervention may also empower the caregivers to make optimal lifestyle choices.

This study has the potential of informing health and social care providers about the design and implementation of interventions to buffer the adverse effects of caregiver stress. In addition, the trial findings will also provide the much-needed evidence to apprise policy-makers of the need for socioeconomic policies to more effectively empower family caregivers to take care of themselves and their care recipients.

Abbreviations

C-CBI: Chinese version of the Caregiver Burden Inventory; C-PFS: Chinese version of the Piper Fatigue Scale; C-PHQ: Chinese version of the Patient Health Questionnaire; C-PSQI: Chinese version of the Pittsburgh Sleep Quality Index; C-SF-12v2: Chinese version of the SF-12 version 2 Health Survey; DQ: Demographic questionnaire; HEA: Health economics assessment; NGO: Nongovernment organization; RCT: Randomized controlled trial; SP: Study programmer; SPSS: Statistical Package for the Social Sciences; TCM: Traditional Chinese medicine

Acknowledgements

The authors acknowledge the staff of HKSKH Lady MacLehose Centre for their advice on the implementation of the intervention.

Funding

This study is funded by the Health and Medical Research Fund, Food and Health Bureau of the Hong Kong SAR Government (Project Number 13143191).

Authors' contributions

Conceptualization and design of the study: AT, LL, AXMW, MKPS, DSFY, TYSL, HYKYF, ZJZ, and JWFY. Preparation of the manuscript: AT, AXMW, DSTC, and MKPS. Reviewing of the manuscript: AT, LL, AXMW, DSTC, MKPS, DSFY, TYSL, HYKYF, ZJZ, and JWFY. All authors read and approved the final manuscript.

Competing interests

The authors declare that they have no competing interests.

Author details

[1]School of Nursing, Li Ka Shing Faculty of Medicine, The University of Hong Kong, 4/F, William M.W. Mong Block, 21 Sassoon Road, Pokfulam, Hong Kong. [2]School of Chinese Medicine, Li Ka Shing Faculty of Medicine, The University of Hong Kong, 10 Sassoon Road, Pokfulam, Hong Kong. [3]Department of Social Sciences, The University of Hong Kong, 11/F, The Jockey Club Tower, Centennial Campus, The University of Hong Kong, Pokfulam Road, Hong Kong, Hong Kong. [4]Department of Information Systems, Business Statistics and Operations Management, Hong Kong University of Science and Technology, Clear Water Bay, Kowloon, Hong Kong. [5]The Nethersole School of Nursing, The Chinese University of Hong Kong, 6/F, Esther Lee Building, The Chinese University of Hong Kong, Shatin, N.T., Hong Kong. [6]Department of Social Work and Social Administration, The University of Hong Kong, Room 534, Jockey Club Tower, The Centennial Campus, The University of Hong Kong, Pokfulam, Hong Kong. [7]HKSKH Lady MacLehose Centre, No.22, Wo Yi Hop Road, Kwai Chung, New Territories, Hong Kong.

References

1. National Institute on Aging (NIA), National Institutes of Health (NIH). Global Health and Aging. https://www.nia.nih.gov/research/publication/global-health-and-aging/overview. Accessed 24 Oct 2016.
2. Family Caregiver Alliance. Impact of Caregiving on Caregiver Mental and Emotional Health. https://www.caregiver.org/caregiver-health. Accessed 24 Oct 2016.
3. Adelman RD, Tmanova LL, Delgado D, Dion S, Lachs MS. Caregiver burden: a clinical review. JAMA. 2014;311(10):1052–9.
4. Schulz R, Sherwood PR. Physical and mental health effects of family caregiving. Am J Nurs. 2008;108(9 Suppl):23–7.
5. Smith L, Onwumere J, Craig T, McManus S, Bebbington P, Kuipers E. Mental and physical illness in caregivers: results from an English national survey sample. Br J Psychiatry. 2014;205(3):197–203.
6. Choi J, Tate JA, Hoffman LA, Schulz R, Ren D, Donahoe MP, Given BA, Sherwood PR. Fatigue in family caregivers of adult intensive care unit survivors. J Pain Symptom Manage. 2014;48(3):353–63.
7. Chiu YC, Lee YN, Wang PC, Chang TH, Li CL, Hsu WC, Lee SH. Family caregivers' sleep disturbance and its associations with multilevel stressors when caring for patients with dementia. Aging Ment Health. 2014;18(1):92–101.
8. Andrieu S, Rive B, Guilhaume C, Kurz X, Scuvee-Moreau J, Grand A, Dresse A. New assessment of dependency in demented patients: impact on the quality of life in informal caregivers. Psychiatry Clin Neurosci. 2007;61(3):234–42.
9. Jessup NM, Bakas T, McLennon SM, Weaver MT. Are there gender, racial or relationship differences in caregiver task difficulty, depressive symptoms and life changes among stroke family caregivers? Brain Inj. 2015;29(1):17–24.
10. Sant SV. China's rapidly aging population strains resources. In: Voice of America. 2015. http://www.voanews.com/content/china-rapidly-aging-population-strains-resources/2817406.html. Accessed 1 Mar 2016.
11. Hua X. China to increase elderly bed numbers. In: China daily. 2016. http://www.chinadaily.com.cn/china/2016-01-25/content_23241315.htm. Accessed 1 Mar 2016.
12. Chow C, Tiwari AF. Experience of family caregivers of community-dwelling stroke survivors and risk of elder abuse: a qualitative study. J Adult Protection. 2014;16(5):276–93.
13. Yeung WF, Chung KF, Poon MM, Ho FY, Zhang SP, Zhang ZJ, Ziea ET, Wong VT. Acupressure, reflexology, and auricular acupressure for insomnia: a systematic review of randomized controlled trials. Sleep Med. 2012;13(8):971–84.
14. Zhang Y, Shen CL, Peck K, Brismee JM, Doctolero S, Lo DF, Lim Y, Lao L. Training self-administered acupressure exercise among postmenopausal women with osteoarthritic knee pain: a feasibility study and lessons learned. Evid-Based Complement Alternat Med. 2012;2012:570431.
15. Zhang ZJ, Chen HY, Yip KC, Ng R, Wong VT. The effectiveness and safety of acupuncture therapy in depressive disorders: systematic review and meta-analysis. J Affect Disord. 2010;124(1–2):9–21.
16. Zhang J, Zhao B, Lao LX, editors. Acupuncture and Moxibustion (International Standard Library of Chinese Medicine). Beijing China: People's Medical Publishing House; 2014.
17. Lee EJ, Frazier SK. The efficacy of acupressure for symptom management: a systematic review. J Pain Symptom Manage. 2011;42(4):589–603.
18. Song HJ, Seo HJ, Lee H, Son H, Choi SM, Lee S. Effect of self-acupressure for symptom management: a systematic review. Complement Ther Med. 2015; 23(1):68–78.
19. Harris RE, Jeter J, Chan P, Higgins P, Kong FM, Fazel R, Bramson C, Gillespie B. Using acupressure to modify alertness in the classroom: a single-blinded, randomized, cross-over trial. J Altern Complement Med (New York, N Y). 2005; 11(4):673–9.
20. Hmwe NT, Subramanian P, Tan LP, Chong WK. The effects of acupressure on depression, anxiety and stress in patients with hemodialysis: a randomized controlled trial. Int J Nurs Stud. 2015;52(2):509–18.
21. Nordio M, Romanelli F. Efficacy of wrists overnight compression (HT 7 point) on insomniacs: possible role of melatonin? Minerva Med. 2008;99(6):539–47.
22. Tsay SL, Cho YC, Chen ML. Acupressure and transcutaneous electrical acupoint stimulation in improving fatigue, sleep quality and depression in hemodialysis patients. Am J Chin Med. 2004;32(3):407–16.
23. Molassiotis A, Sylt P, Diggins H. The management of cancer-related fatigue after chemotherapy with acupuncture and acupressure: a randomised controlled trial. Complement Ther Med. 2007;15(4):228–37.
24. Yu H, Wang X, He R, Liang R, Zhou L. Measuring the caregiver burden of caring for community-residing people with Alzheimer's disease. PLoS One. 2015;10(7):e0132168.
25. Wang XM, Walitt B, Saligan L, Tiwari AF, Cheung CW, Zhang ZJ. Chemobrain: a critical review and causal hypothesis of link between cytokines and epigenetic reprogramming associated with chemotherapy. Cytokine. 2015;72(1):86–96.
26. Social Analysis and Research Section (2), Census and Statistics Department, HKSAR. Population and Household Statistics Analysed by District Council District 2013. http://www.statistics.gov.hk/pub/B11303012013AN13B0100.pdf. Accessed 1 Mar 2016.
27. Chou KR, Jiann-Chyun L, Chu H. The reliability and validity of the Chinese version of the caregiver burden inventory. Nurs Res. 2002;51(5):324–31.
28. Cho YC, Tsay SL. The effect of acupressure with massage on fatigue and depression in patients with end-stage renal disease. J Nurs Res. 2004;12(1):51–9.

29. Tsay SL, Chen ML. Acupressure and quality of sleep in patients with end-stage renal disease–a randomized controlled trial. Int J Nurs Stud. 2003;40(1):1–7.
30. Chen S, Chiu H, Xu B, Ma Y, Jin T, Wu M, Conwell Y. Reliability and validity of the PHQ-9 for screening late-life depression in Chinese primary care. Int J Geriatr Psychiatry. 2010;25(11):1127–33.
31. Lam ET, Lam CL, Fong DY, Huang WW. Is the SF-12 version 2 Health Survey a valid and equivalent substitute for the SF-36 version 2 Health Survey for the Chinese. J Eval Clin Pract. 2013;19(1):200–8.
32. Araujo CD, Veiga DF, Hochman B, Abla LE, Novo NF, Ferreira LM. Health economics and health preference concepts to orthopedics practitioners. Acta Ortopédica Brasileira. 2014;22:102–5.
33. McLennon SM, Bakas T, Jessup NM, Habermann B, Weaver MT. Task difficulty and life changes among stroke family caregivers: relationship to depressive symptoms. Arch Phys Med Rehabil. 2014;95(12):2484–90.
34. Mosher CE, Bakas T, Champion VL. Physical health, mental health, and life changes among family caregivers of patients with lung cancer. Oncol Nurs Forum. 2013;40(1):53–61.
35. Gitlin LN, Belle SH, Burgio LD, Czaja SJ, Mahoney D, Gallagher-Thompson D, Burns R, Hauck WW, Zhang S, Schulz R, et al. Effect of multicomponent interventions on caregiver burden and depression: The REACH multisite initiative at 6-month follow-up. Psychol Aging. 2003;18(3):361–74.
36. Schulz R, Martire LM. Family caregiving of persons with dementia: prevalence, health effects, and support strategies. Am J Geriatr Psychiatry. 2004;12(3):240–9.
37. Van't Leven N, Prick AE, Groenewoud JG, Roelofs PD, de Lange J, Pot AM. Dyadic interventions for community-dwelling people with dementia and their family caregivers: a systematic review. Int Psychogeriatr. 2013;25(10):1581–603.

The electroacupuncture-induced analgesic effect mediated by 5-HT$_1$, 5-HT$_3$ receptor and muscarinic cholinergic receptors in rat model of collagenase-induced osteoarthritis

Byung-Kwan Seo[†], Won-Suk Sung[†], Yeon-Cheol Park and Yong-Hyeon Baek[*]

Abstract

Background: Osteoarthritis (OA) is an degenerative disease characterized by chronic joint pain. Complementary and alternative treatment such as acupuncture have been utilized to alleviate pain. The objective of this study was to investigate the analgesic mechanisms of electroacupuncture (EA) in the collagenase-induced osteoarthritis (CIOA) rat model.

Methods: Four weeks after inducing CIOA by injecting collagenase solution into the left knee of 5-week-old male Sprague-Dawley rats, 2 Hz and 100 Hz EA on Zusanli (ST 36) was performed. The analgesic effect of EA was evaluated by the tail flick latency (TFL) and paw pressure threshold (PPT) tests. To investigate the analgesic mechanism, serotonergic and muscarinic cholinergic receptor agonists and antagonists were injected 20 min prior to EA and the resultant changes were evaluated by the TFL and PPT tests.

Results: EA on Zusanli (ST 36) demonstrated an analgesic effect in the CIOA rat model. The 2 Hz EA treatment showed a significantly greater analgesic effect than the 100 Hz treatment. The analgesic effect of 2 Hz EA was not strengthened by 5-HT1, 5-HT2, 5-HT3, and muscarinic cholinergic receptor agonist pretreatment, was blocked by 5-HT1, 5-HT3, and muscarinic cholinergic receptor antagonist pretreatment, but not blocked by 5-HT2 receptor antagonist pretreatment.

Conclusions: In the CIOA rat model, EA on Zusanli (ST 36) exhibited analgesic effects, and 2 Hz EA resulted in a significantly greater analgesic effect than 100 Hz EA. The analgesic effect of 2 Hz EA was reduced by pretreatment of 5-HT1 receptor, 5-HT3 receptor and muscarinic cholinergic receptor antagonists.

Keywords: Collagenase-induced osteoarthritis, Electroacupuncture, Analgesic effect, Analgesic mechanism, Serotonergic receptor, Cholinergic receptor

Background

Osteoarthritis (OA) is one of the most prevalent chronic joint disease at present. It is characterized by loss of articular cartilage, osteophyte formation, subchondral bone change, and synovitis [1]. OA has varying effects on the individual and on society. OA patients, especially elderly patients, experience symptoms every day, resulting in a lower quality of life. From a societal perspective, the increasing financial costs of treatment and management of OA are a challenging problem. The healthcare costs associated with OA in the USA exceed $60 billion annually and can increase up to $185.5 billion [2], demonstrating the importance of more effective OA treatments. To date, as complementary and alternative options for various treatment modalities including medications, patient education, exercise and physical therapy, non-pharmacological alternative modailities such as acupuncture and electroacupuncture (EA) have been administered [3, 4].

Acupuncture has been widely used to alleviate many types of pain, particularly chronic pain [5]. Human and

* Correspondence: byhacu@khu.ac.kr
[†]Equal contributors
Department of Clinical Korean Medicine, Graduate School, Kyung Hee University, 26, Kyungheedae-ro, Dongdaemun-gu, Seoul 02447, Korea

animal study models have shown that acupuncture-induced analgesia is mediated through various neurotransmitters, modulators, and related factors including β-endorphin, enkephalin, endomorphin, and dynorphin [6].

The analgesic effects of EA have also been established through many studies. Researchers have conducted clinical trials and animal model studies on neuropathic pain and collagen-induced arthritis and demonstrated the descending modulation of nociceptive processing [7–11]. The analgesic effects and its adrenergic or opioidergic mechanisms of EA in CIOA in vivo study was reported [12, 13], but the serotonergic and cholinergic roles in EA analgesia have not been fully clarified. Current study was designed to investigate which receptors agonists and antagonists were involved in the analgesic effect of EA in CIOA in vivo model.

Methods
Animals
Five-week-old male Sprague-Dawley rats weighing 200 mg were obtained from Samtaco (Osan, Korea) and housed under controlled temperature (22 ± 1°C), humidity (55 ± 5 %), and 1:1 light-dark cycle (light from 6 AM to 6 PM). All animals had free access to food and water. All experiments were approved and conducted under the guidelines of the International Association for the Study of Pain and the Institutional Animal Care and Use Committee of Kyung Hee University [14].

Induction of collagenase-induced osteoarthritis
After one week of adaptation to the laboratory conditions, intra-articular collagenase injection was performed; 0.05 ml of 4 mg/ml collagenase solution (Clostridium histolyticum, type II; enzyme activity 425 U/mg) was injected into the left knee of all rats. Four days after the first injection, a booster injection was administered. The gross articular manifestations were assessed and histopathological and serological analyses were performed according to previous CIOA studies [12, 13]. Briefly, the severity of stiffness was scored on a scale of 0–4 in the affected articulation as a reflection of edema and movement impairment. Two independent examiners assessed gross articular manifestations in a blind manner. At the end of the fourth week, the rats were sacrificed for histopathological analysis. Six parameters, i.e., including loss of the superficial layer, erosion of cartilage, fibrillation and/or fissures, disorganization of chondrocytes, loss of chondrocytes, and cluster formation, were evaluated for the histological analysis. Serum from each subject was prepared for the measurement of COX-1, COX-2, PGE2 activity (data not shown).

Behavioral test
After four weeks of induction of CIOA and adaptation in the laboratory room conditions, tail flick latency

(TFL) and paw pressure threshold (PPT) tests were performed at baseline, 10, 20, 30, 45, 60, and 90 min after initiation of EA.

To evaluate the analgesic effect on the thermal stimuli, the TFL test was performed using the tail flick unit (Ugo Basile Model 7360, Comrio, Italy) [15]. The rat was fixed in a 5.3 cm diameter × 15 cm length holder and the proximal third portion of six parts of the tail was laid on the 50-W infrared light bulb. The time lapse between the onset of irradiation and the flick of the tail was measured on the unit. The mean time was calculated after three continuous measurements and expressed in seconds. TFL test was performed at baseline, 10, 20, 30, 45, 60, and 90 min after initiation of EA. The time of irradiation was limited at 20 s and the portion of the tail exposed to the light bulb was shifted to prevent thermal injury. The change of TFL was calculated as a percentage of change of tail flick latency. The increase in the degree of TFL change represents the analgesic effect on the thermal stimuli.

$$\text{The degree of TFL change (\%)} = \frac{\text{post.EA TFL} - \text{baseline TFL}}{\text{baseline TFL}} \times 100$$

For evaluation of the analgesic effect on the mechanical stimuli, a PPT test was performed [16]. Rats were gently held in the cap and the algesiometer device (modified Randall-Selitto test; Ugo Basile, Comerio, Italy) was applied to the dorsal surface of the hind paw. The mechanical device increased the pressure by gram units until the rat withdrew its paw. The mean pressure was calculated after three consecutive measurements and expressed in grams. With 10-s intervals, the PPT test was performed at baseline, 10, 20, 30, 45, 60, and 90 min after initiation of EA. The upper limit of pressure was 250g to prevent tissue damage. The increase in the mean pressure represents the analgesic effect on the mechanical stimuli.

Electroacupuncture treatment
After four weeks of induction of CIOA and adaptation to the laboratory condition, EA was performed into Zusanli (ST36), located laterally from tibial tuberosity and caudally below knee joint on the anterior tibialis muscle. The Zusanli acupoint is generally used to alleviate pain in clinical trials and animal studies [10–13, 17]. Two disposable sterile stainless needles (0.25 mm diameter × 40 mm length) were inserted into Zusanli (ST 36) and another point 5 mm away from the selected point. The acupuncture needle was inserted to the depth of 5 mm and stimulated with a train pulse (0.3 ms, 0.07 mA) for 30 min by an electrical stimulator (Nihon Kohden). At first, EA was performed at 2 Hz and 100 Hz to compare analgesic

effects at different frequencies. The frequency that showed a better analgesic effect was selected when conducting experiments on the analgesic mechanism of EA.

Pretreatment with agonists and antagonists

To investigate the analgesic mechanism, the 5-HT1 receptor agonist 8-OH-DPAT (8 ODT) and antagonist spiroxatrine (SPROX), the 5-HT2 receptor agonist DOI (DOI) and antagonist ketanserin (KTSRN), the 5-HT3 receptor agonist m-chlorophenyl-biguanide (mCLBG) and antagonist ondansetron (ODSTN), and the muscarinic cholinergic receptor agonist neostigmine (NSTM) and antagonist atropine (ATRP) were dissolved in sterile 10 % DMSO (dimethyl sulfoxide) and intraperitoneally injected 20 min before EA.

Statistical analysis

All results were expressed in mean ± standard error of mean. In nonparametric procedures, statistically significant differences ($p < 0.05$) were determined by Friedman's rank test followed by Dunnett's post-hoc test within a group, Mann–Whitney U test between two groups, and Kruskal–Wallis ANOVA followed by Dunnett's post-hoc test among groups.

Results

The analgesic effect of EA and comparison according to latency (2, 100 Hz)

The effects of EA at 2 Hz and 100 Hz in the CIOA rat model are shown in Fig. 1. The degree of TFL change increased during 10–60 min and peaked at 30 min after initiation of EA. Both EA treatment groups showed statistically significant differences compared with the no treatment group ($n = 10$). The 2 Hz EA treatment group ($n = 10$) showed a significantly greater TFL change than the 100 Hz EA treatment group ($n = 10$) (Fig. 1a). PPT also increased during 10–60 min and peaked at 30 min after initiation of EA. Both EA treatment groups showed significant differences compared with the no treatment group ($n = 10$). Between the two EA treatment groups, the 2 Hz EA treatment group ($n = 10$) showed a

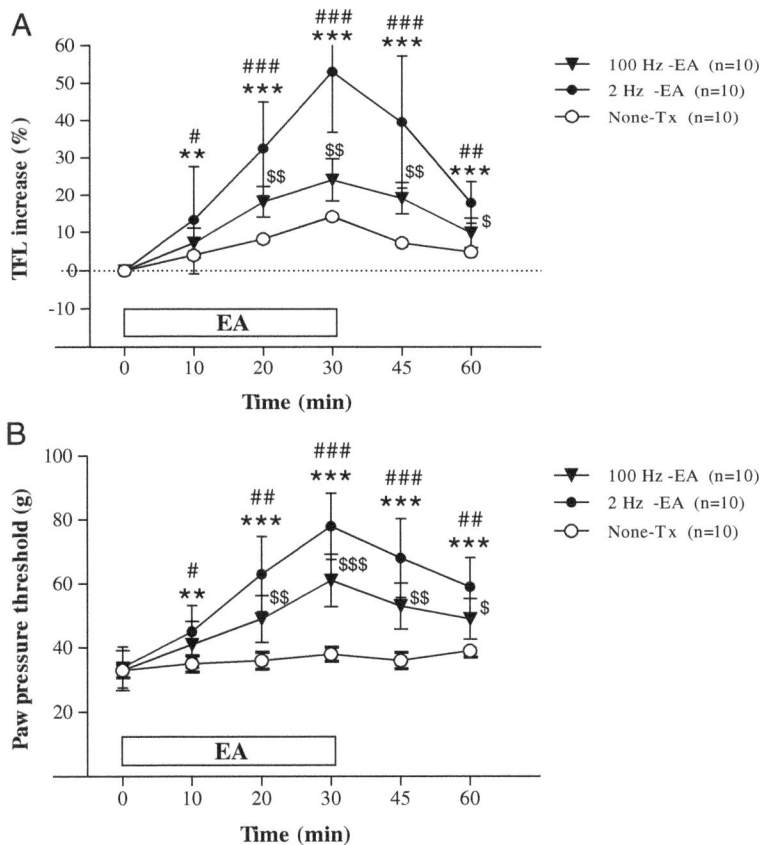

Fig. 1 The effects of EA at 2 Hz and 100 Hz in the CIOA rat model assessed by TFL (a) and PPT (b). 2 Hz EA treatment group (2 Hz-EA, $n = 10$), 100 Hz EA treatment group (100 Hz-EA, $n = 10$) and no treatment group (None-Tx, $n = 10$). $p < 0.05$, $$p < 0.01$, $$$ $p < 0.001$: compared with None-Tx; **$p < 0.01$, ***$p < 0.001$: compared with None-Tx; #$p < 0.05$, ##$p < 0.01$, ###$p < 0.001$: compared with 100 Hz-EA

significantly higher PPT than the 100 Hz EA treatment group (n = 10) (Fig. 1b).

The 5-HT1 receptor Involvement of EA-induced analgesia

The effects of the 5-HT1 receptor agonist 8-ODT and antagonist SPROX on the analgesia induced by 2 Hz EA in the CIOA rat model are shown in Fig. 2. In the TFL test, there were no significant differences between the EA + 8 ODT group (n = 10) and the EA + DMSO group (n = 10). However, TFL increases induced by ST36 EA were significantly suppressed by SPROX pretreatment (n=10) 10–90 min after initiation of EA (Fig. 2a). In the PPT test, there were no significant differences between the EA + 8 ODT group (n = 10) and the EA + DMSO group (n = 10). However, PPT increases induced by ST36 EA were significantly suppressed by SPROX pretreatment (n=10) 10–90 min after initiation of EA (Fig. 2b).

The 5-HT2 receptor Involvement of EA-induced analgesia

The effects of the 5-HT2 receptor agonist DOI and antagonist KTSRN on the analgesia induced by 2 Hz EA in the CIOA rat model are shown in Fig. 3. In the TFL test, there were no significant differences between the EA + DOI group (n = 10), the EA + KTSRN group, and the EA + DMSO group (n = 10) (Fig. 3a). In the PPT test, there were also no significant differences between the EA + DOI group (n = 10), the EA + KTSRN group, and the EA + DMSO group (n = 10) (Fig. 3b).

The 5-HT3 receptor Involvement of EA-induced analgesia

The effects of the 5-HT3 receptor agonist mCLBG and antagonist ODSTN on the analgesia induced by 2 Hz EA in the CIOA rat model are shown in Fig. 4. In the TFL test, there were no significant differences between the EA + mCLBG group (n = 10) and the EA + DMSO group (n = 10) except 30 min after initiation of EA.

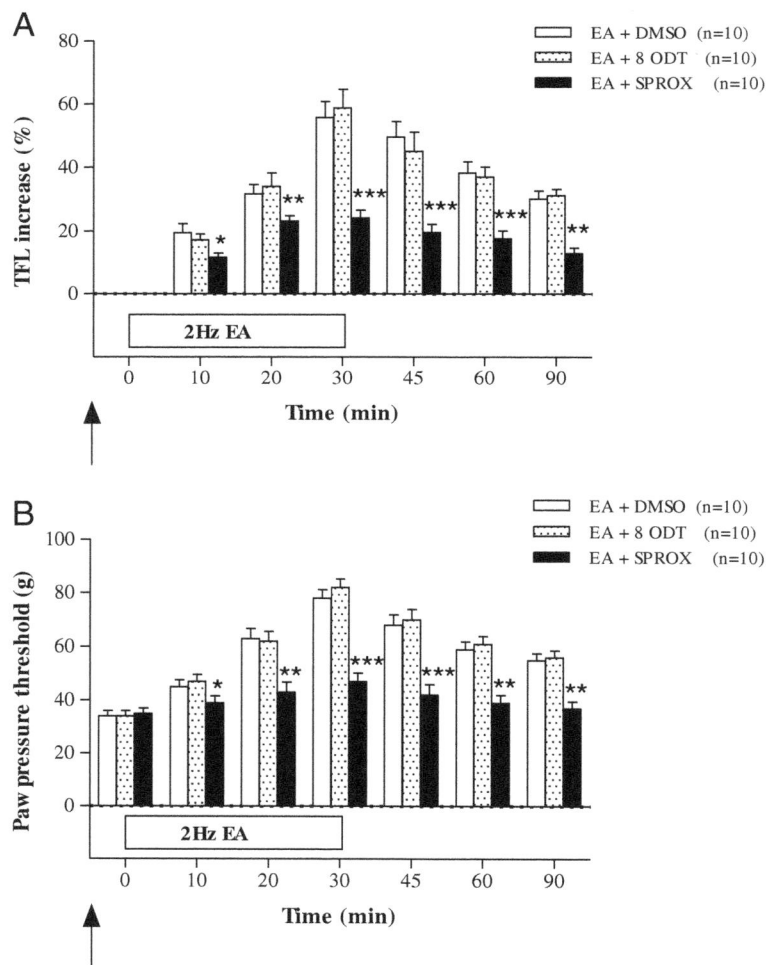

Fig. 2 The effects of pretreatment of 5-HT1 receptor agonist (8-OH-DPAT, EA+8 ODT, n = 10) and antagonist (spiroxatrine, EA+SPROX, n = 10) in the CIOA rat treated by 2 Hz EA (EA+DMSO, n = 10) assessed by TFL (**a**) and PPT (**b**). Pretreatment with DMSO, 8 ODT, and SPROX was performed 20 min before 2 Hz EA. *p < 0.05, **p < 0.01, ***p < 0.001: compared with EA+DMSO

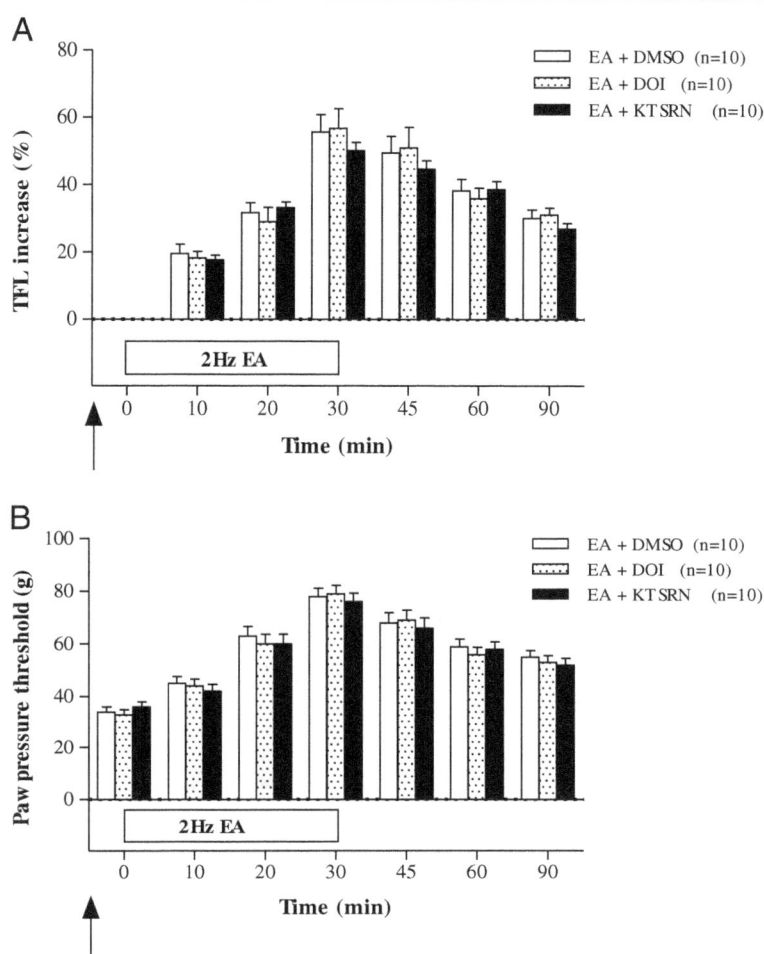

Fig. 3 The effects of pretreatment of 5-HT2 receptor agonist (DOI, EA+DOI, $n = 10$) and antagonist (ketanserin, EA+KTSRN, $n = 10$) in the CIOA rat treated by 2 Hz EA (EA+DMSO, $n = 10$) assessed by TFL (**a**) and PPT (**b**). Pretreatment with DMSO, DOI, and KTSRN was performed 20 min before 2 Hz EA

However, TFL increases induced by ST36 EA were significantly suppressed by ODSTN pretreatment ($n=10$) 20–90 min after initiation of EA (Fig. 4a). In the PPT test, there were no significant differences between the EA + mCLBG group ($n = 10$) and the EA + DMSO group ($n = 10$) except 30 min after initiation of EA. However, PPT increases induced by ST36 EA were significantly suppressed by ODSTN pretreatment ($n=10$) 20–90 min after initiation of EA (Fig. 4b).

The muscarinic cholinergic receptor Involvement of EA-induced analgesia

The effects of the muscarinic cholinergic receptor agonist NSTM and antagonist ATRP on the analgesia induced by 2 Hz EA in the CIOA rat model are shown in Fig. 5. In the TFL test, there were no significant differences between the EA + NSTM group ($n = 10$) and the

EA + DMSO group ($n = 10$). However, TFL increases induced by ST36 EA were significantly suppressed by ATRP pretreatment ($n = 10$) 10–90 min after initiation of EA (Fig. 5a). In the PPT test, there were no significant differences between the EA + NSTM group ($n=10$) and the EA + DMSO group ($n=10$). However, PPT increases induced by ST36 EA were suppressed by ATRP pretreatment ($n=10$) 10–90 min after initiation of EA (Fig. 5b).

The involvement of each receptor agonists and antagonists in EA-induced analgesia

The effects of each receptor agonist and antagonist on the analgesia in the CIOA rat model are shown in Fig. 6. In both the TFL and PPT test, there were no significant differences between each receptor agonist and antagonist group except the None-Tx + mCLBG group at 30 min after measurement (Fig. 6).

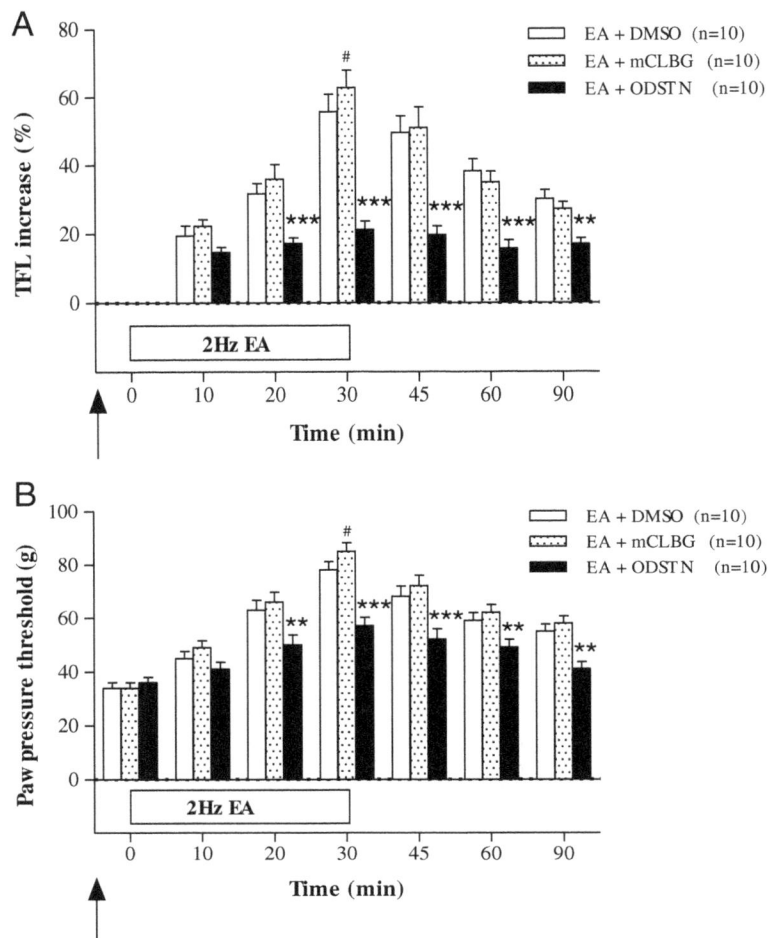

Fig. 4 The effects of pretreatment of 5-HT3 receptor agonist (m-chlorophenyl-biguanide, EA+mCLBG, $n = 10$) and antagonist (ondansetron, EA+ODSTN, $n = 10$) in the CIOA rat treated by 2 Hz EA (EA+DMSO, $n = 10$) assessed by TFL (**a**) and PPT (**b**). Pretreatment with DMSO, mCLBG, and ODSTN was performed 20 min before 2 Hz EA. #$p < 0.05$, **$p < 0.01$, ***$p < 0.001$: compared with EA+DMSO

Discussion

OA is the most common degenerative joint disorder characterized by the progressive erosion of articular cartilage. The aching pain may worsen with use, and can be accompanied by morning stiffness, crepitus contributes to limited articular function and deteriorated quality of life [18]. The pathogenesis of OA is not entirely established, but is likely related to inflammatory cytokines that mediate cartilage destruction [19].

The current standard care for OA focuses on alleviating pain and managing symptoms. For the pharmacological treatment options, non-steroidal anti-inflammatory drugs (NSAIDs) have been considered as the primary therapy for OA [20]. Despite their universal administration for pain relief in osteoarthritis patients, the long term use of NSAIDs is controversial due to the gastrointestinal disorders and cardiovascular events related to their safety profile [21, 22]. The demands of osteoarthritis patients for non-pharmacologic therapies, especially acupuncture,

have increased due to failure to alleviate pain and improve articular function.

EA has been used to treat a diverse range of painful conditions. Previous research has suggested a relationship between pain modulatory mechanisms and acupuncture analgesia, focusing on the role of transmitters and modulators [23]. The EA analgesia is initiated by needles triggering stimulation of afferent nerves and related with systemic activation of a variety of bioactive chemicals through peripheral, spinal and supraspinal mechanisms [24]. Research on EA analgesia induction and recovery profiles has demonstrated the possible involvement of humoral factors [25]. Several studies have been performed to prove the analgesic effect and mechanism of EA in various animal models, considering EA stimulation parameters such as frequency, intensity, and wave form [9–11]. However, there are limited studies on EA in CIOA model.

Various methods, including surgical procedures and intra-articular injections, can be used to induce OA.

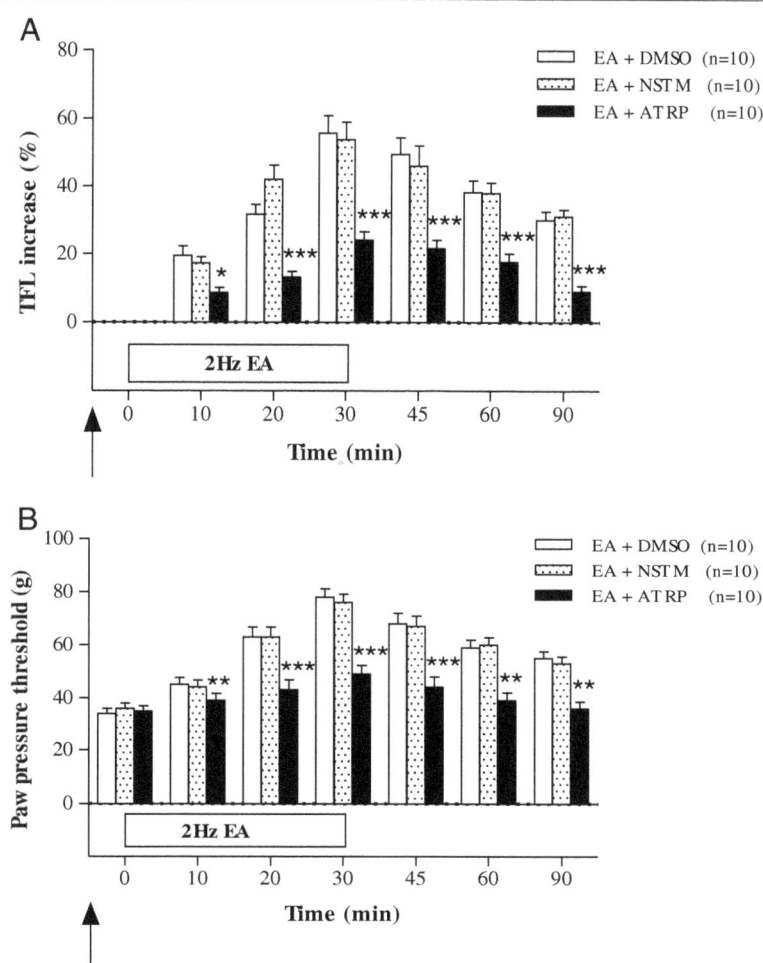

Fig. 5 The effects of pretreatment of muscarinic cholinergic receptor agonist (neostigmine, EA+NSTM, $n = 10$) and antagonist (atropine, EA+ATRP, $n = 10$) in the CIOA rat treated by 2 Hz EA (EA+DMSO, $n = 10$) assessed by TFL (**a**) and PPT (**b**). DMSO, NSTM, and ATRP were pretreated 20 min before 2 Hz EA. *$p < 0.05$, **$p < 0.01$, ***$p < 0.001$: compared with EA+DMSO

Intra-articular injection with chemical substances can be more conveniently performed in many studies because surgical procedures are complicated and take a longer period of time to induce degeneration [26]. When selecting a chemical substance, some studies have used papain but its use is limited by both its unclear mechanism of action and large dose requirement (4–12 mg) [27]. In contrast, a previous study demonstrated that CIOA was characterized by severe degenerative cartilage lesions, sclerosis of the subchondral bone below the cartilage erosions, osteophyte formation, and consequent deformity [28]. Other research showed that in the progression of OA, a larger amount of collagenase was detected [29] and cytokines stimulated the production of collagenase as a proteolytic enzyme [30]. In this regard, collagenase was considered to be appropriate to induce OA in rats that would be similar to the clinical manifestations in human version of OA.

In order to determine the proper time to conduct experiments with the CIOA model, the gross articular manifestations and histopathological and serological features were evaluated. In accordance with the results of previous studies, most of the osteoarthritic clinical and histopathological features were observed from 4 weeks after first collagenase injection. These features included altered pain-related behaviors, gross articular manifestations, cartilage-destructive features and serological biomarker activities [12, 13].

TFL and PPT tests are commonly used to evaluate the degree of nociception through the change of animal behavior. TFL is focused on the thermal stimuli and PPT is focused on the mechanical stimuli. Pain in OA is associated with thermal and mechanical hyperalgesia and affected by local mechanical and thermal factors [31]. TFL and PPT tests are appropriate to evaluate analgesic effects on thermal and mechanical stimuli in the CIOA, in

A

B

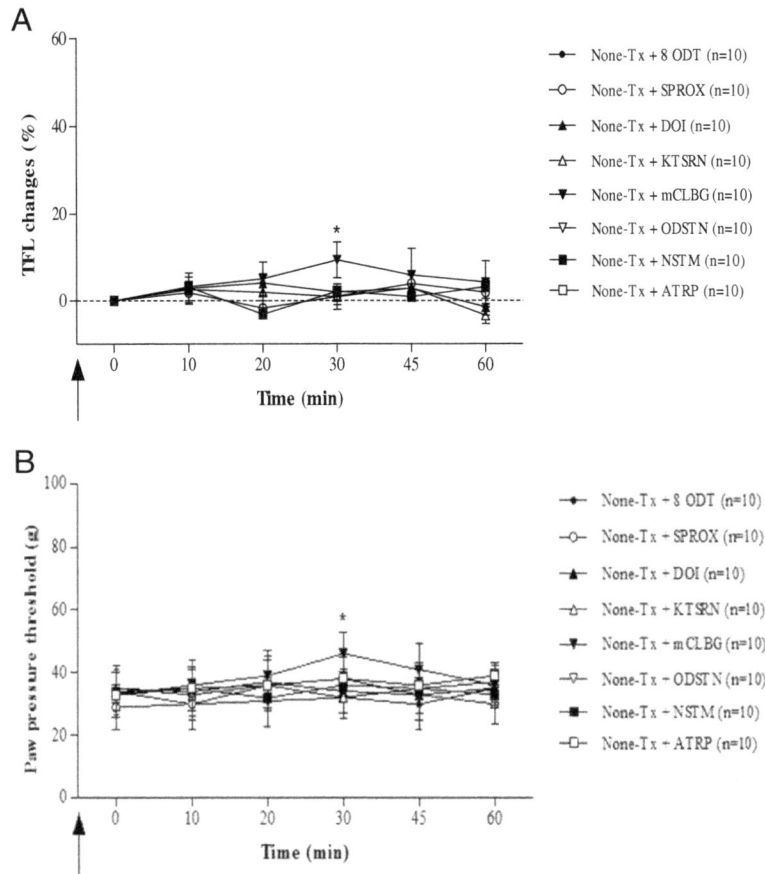

Fig. 6 The effects of each receptor agonists and antagonists on the pain threshold in CIOA rat model assessed by TFL (**a**) and PPT (**b**). *$p < 0.05$: compared with each group

accordance with other painful condition experiments [32]. However, there are few existing studies that have conducted TFL and PPT at the same time and showed positive results in the CIOA.

The acupoint Zusanli (ST 36) is traditionally used to reduce pain. Previous studies showed that EA on Zusanli (ST 36) led to analgesia using the tail flick method and c-Fos expression in the brain [33], and its effect was related to peripheral nerve receptors and biomarkers like β-endorphin and cortisol [34, 35].

Our results demonstrated that both 2 Hz and 100 Hz EA showed analgesic effect, evidenced in the TFL and PPT tests. The 2 Hz EA more effectively relieved thermal and mechanical hyperalgesia than the 100 Hz EA, in accordance with the results of previous studies. It has been shown that low-frequency EA is more effective for nociceptive pain whereas high-frequency EA is more effective for neurogenic pain [36]. Recent studies also showed that 2 Hz EA provides better and longer-lasting analgesic effects on mechanical allodynia [37, 38]. These results suggest

that low-frequency EA is appropriate for the treatment of OA related pain.

In order to investigate the analgesic mechanism of EA, we conducted experiments with serotonergic and muscarinic cholinergic receptor agonists and antagonists. With respect to the serotonergic mechanism, our study showed that the analgesic effect of 2 Hz EA was not strengthened by the 5-HT1, 5-HT2, and 5-HT3 receptor agonists. In experiments with antagonists, the analgesic effect of 2 Hz EA was blocked by the 5-HT1 and 5-HT3 receptor antagonists, but not blocked by the 5-HT2 receptor antagonist. These results suggest that the 5-HT1 and 5-HT3 receptors partially mediate the analgesia induced by 2 Hz EA in the CIOA rat model. Ryu et al. [10] conducted experiments on the analgesic effects and mechanism of 2 Hz EA in the collagen-induced arthritis (CIA) model using 5-HT1A, 5-HT1B, and 5-HT4 receptor antagonists, and demonstrated that the analgesic effect of EA was blocked by 5-HT1A, 5-HT1B, and 5-HT4 receptor antagonists. Baek et al. [39] conducted experiments on the analgesic effects and mechanism of 2 Hz

The electroacupuncture-induced analgesic effect mediated by 5-HT1, 5-HT3 receptor and muscarinic...

139

EA in a CIA model using 5-HT1A, 5-HT2, and 5-HT3 receptor agonists and antagonists, and demonstrated that the analgesic effect of EA was blocked by the 5-HT1A and 5-HT3 receptor antagonists, but not blocked by the 5-HT2 receptor antagonist. Chang et al. [40] demonstrated that 5-HT1A and 5-HT3 receptor antagonist blocked EA analgesia at three different frequencies (2, 10, and 100 Hz) and Kim et al. [41] suggested that 5-HT1A and 5-HT3 receptors had important roles in mediating the relieving effect 2 Hz EA on cold allodynia. In this regard, 2 Hz EA induces an analgesic effect through 5-HT1 and 5-HT3 receptors.

With respect to the cholinergic mechanism, our study showed that the analgesic effect of 2 Hz EA was not strengthened by the muscarinic cholinergic receptor agonist and blocked by muscarinic cholinergic receptor antagonist. These results suggest that the muscarinic cholinergic receptor partially mediates the analgesia induced by 2 Hz EA in the CIOA rat model. Baek et al. [39] also conducted experiments on the analgesic effects and mechanism of 2 Hz EA in the CIA model using a muscarinic cholinergic receptor agonist and antagonist, and demonstrated that the analgesic effect of EA was blocked by the muscarinic cholinergic receptor antagonist. Park et al. [42] studied the effects of 2 Hz EA on cold and warm allodynia in a neuropathic rat model using several muscarinic receptor antagonists and demonstrated that spinal muscarinic receptors, especially M1 subtype, mediate the EA antiallodynia. In this regard, 2 Hz EA induces analgesic effect through muscarinic cholinergic receptor.

Conflicting study results have been reported in the role of the serotonergic agonists and antagonists themselves in pain modulatioin. McCleane et al. [43] suggested that ondansetron could have an analgesic effect in neuropathic pain in a double-blind study and Ali Z et al. [44] showed that ondansetron reduced nociceptive response in behavioral and electrophysiological studies. Houde RW [45] showed the analgesic effectiveness of narcotic agonists and antagonists. Takagi et al. [46] examined the effects of several serotonin (5-HT) antagonists on 2 Hz EA analgesia in tooth pulp stimulation rat models and suggested that 5-HT1, except 5-HT1A; 5-HT2, except 5-HT2A; and 5-HT3 receptors are positively related to EA-induced analgesia.

The present study demonstrated that 5-HT antagonists ODSN intraperitoneal pretreatment suppressed the ST-36 2Hz EA-induced analgesia but there was no significant TFL and PPT changes when EA was not administered. It appears that 5-HT3 agonist mCLBG intraperitoneal pretreatment increased pain thresholds assessed by TFL and PPT not only in absence of EA treatment and also in ST-36 2Hz EA. Ali Z et al. [44] demonstrated that intrathecal administration of mCLBG increased the responsiveness of dorsal

horn neurons to noxious stimulation. Sasaki et al. [47] reported that intrathecal 5-HT3 receptor agonist, 2-methyl-5-HT mediates antinociception to chemical stimuli.

In summary of the results of our research and previous studies, we speculate that the pain threshold-modulatory effects of serotonergic agonists and antagonits could depend on differences among the agonists, antagonists, time of agonists and antagonits pretreatment, administrative maneuver (intraperitoneal or intrathecal), and the type of pain models.

Considering limited knowledge on the therapeutical active components of EA and the physiological reactions followed by EA, restricted conclusive implication whether 2 Hz EA induced analgesia was mediated by serotonergic and cholinergic receptor mechanisms could be made. Because current study did not perform a comparison with the effect of non-acupoint EA, further studies are needed to investigate the acupoint specific effects of ST36 EA using various EA stimulation parameters including frequency.

Conclusion
In summary, these observation suggest that 5-HT1, 5-HT3 and muscarinic cholinergic receptors partially mediate the analgesic effects of EA in CIOA. These results suggests that EA could be a potential option for the relieving osteoarthritic pain.

Abbreviations
8 ODT, 8-OH-DPAT; ATRP, atropine; CIA, collagen-induced arthritis; CIOA, collagenase-induced osteoarthritis; DMSO, dimethyl sulfoxide; DOI, 5-HT2 receptor agonist DOI; EA, electroacupuncture; KTSRN, ketanserin; mCLBG, m-chlorophenyl-biguanide; NSAIDs, Non-steroidal anti-inflammatory drugs; NSTM, neostigmine; OA, osteoarthritis; ODSTN, ondansetron; PPT, paw pressure threshold; SPROX, spiroxatrine; TFL, tail flick latency

Acknowledgements
None.

Funding
This research was supported by the Basic Science Research Program, through the National Research Foundation of Korea (NRF) funded by the Ministry of Education, Science and Technology (NRF-2013R1A1A2010049) and the Traditional Korean Medicine R&D program funded by the Ministry of Health & Welfare through the Korea Health Industry Development Institute (KHIDI) (HI15C0117).

Authors' contributions
BKS and WSS collected and analyzed data and wrote the manuscript. YCP analyzed data and revised the manuscript. YHB designed the study, supervised experimental procedures and drafted the manuscript. All authors have read, revised and approved the final manuscript.

Authors' information
Department of Acupuncture & Moxibustion, College of Korean Medicine, Kyung Hee University, 26, Kyungheedae-ro, Dongdaemun-gu, Seoul, 02447, Korea.

140 The Acuarehandbook

Competing interests
The authors declare that they have no competing interests.

References

1. Dieppe PA, Lohmander LS. Pathogenesis and management of pain in osteo arthritis. Lancet. 2005;365(9463):965–73.
2. Kotlarz H, Gunnarsson CL, Fang H, Rizzo JA. Insurer and out-of-pocket costs of osteoarthritis in the US: evidence from national survey data. Arthritis Rheum. 2009;60(12):3546–53.
3. Sarzi-Puttini P, Cimmino MA, Scarpa R, Caporali R, Parazzini F, Zaninelli A, Atzeni F, Canesi B. Osteoarthritis: an overview of the disease and its treatment strategies. Semin Arthritis Rheum. 2005;35:1–10.
4. Kwon YD, Pittler MH, Ernst E. Acupuncture for peripheral joint osteoarthritis: a systematic review and meta-analysis. Rheumatology. 2006;45(11):1331–7.
5. Zhao ZQ. Neural mechanism underlying acupuncture analgesia. Prog Neurobiol. 2008;85(4):355–75.
6. Lin JG, Chen WL. Acupuncture analgesia: a review of its mechanisms of actions. Am J Chin Med. 2008;36(4):635–45.
7. Sangdee C, Teekachunhatean S, Sananpanich K, Sugandhavesa N, Chiew-Chantanakit S, Pojchamarnwiputh S, Jayasvasti S. Electroacupuncture versus diclofenac in symptomatic treatment of osteoarthritis of the knee: a randomized controlled trial. BMC Complement Altern Med. 2002;2:3.
8. Jubb RW, Tukmachi ES, Jones PW, Dempsey E, Waterhouse L, Brailsford S. A blinded randomised trial of acupuncture (manual and electroacupuncture) compared with a non-penetrating sham for the symptoms of osteoarthritis of the knee. Acupunct Med. 2008;26(2):69–78.
9. Ko J, Na DS, Lee YH, Shin SY, Kim JH, Hwang BG, Min BI, Park DS. cDNA microarray analysis of the differential gene expression in the neuropathic pain and electroacupuncture treatment models. J Biochem Mol Biol. 2002;35(4):420.
10. Ryu SR, Baek YH, Park DS. The Analgesic Effect and Its Mechanism of electroacupuncture in the type II collagen-induced arthritis rats : mediation by serotonergic receptors. J Korean Acupunct Moxibustion Soc. 2006;23(3):77–90.
11. Kim EJ, Baek YH, Kang SK. The analgesic effect and its opioidergic mechanism of electroacupuncture on inflammatory pain in the type II collagen-induced arthritis rats. J Korean Acupunct Moxibustion Soc. 2006; 23(4):149–62.
12. Seo BK, Park DS, Baek YH. The analgesic effect and the mechanism of electroacupuncture on thermal hyperalgesia in the rat model of collagenase-induced arthritis: mediation by adrenergic receptors. J Korean Acupunct Moxibustion Soc. 2011;28(2):57–67.
13. Seo BK, Park DS, Baek YH. The analgesic effect of electroacupuncture on inflammatory pain in the rat model of collagenase-induced arthritis: mediation by opioidergic receptors. Rhematol Int. 2013;33(5):1177–83.
14. Zimmermann M. Ethical guidelines for invetigations of experimental pain in conscious animals. Pain. 1983;16(2):109–10.
15. Grossman ML, Basbaum AI, Fields HL. Afferent and efferent connections of the rat tail flick reflex (a model used to analyze pain control mechanisms). J Comp Neurol. 1982;206(1):9–16.
16. Wang Y, Hackel D, Peng F, Rittner HL. Long-term antinociception by electroacupuncture is mediated via peripheral opioid receptors in free-moving rats with inflammatory hyperalgesia. Eur J Pain. 2013; 17(10):1447–57.
17. Selfe TK, Taylor AG. Acupuncture and osteoarthritis of the knee: a review of randomized, controlled trials. Fam Community Health. 2008;31(3):247–54.
18. Neogi T. The epidemiology and impact of pain in osteoarthritis. Osteoarthritis Cartilage. 2013;21(9):1145–53.
19. Rainbow R, Ren W, Zeng L. Inflammation and joint tissue interactions in OA: implications for potential therapeutic approaches. Arthritis. 2012;741582. doi: 10.1155/2012/741582
20. Ausiello JC, Stafford RS. Trends in medication use for osteoarthritis treatment. J Rheumatol. 2002;29(5):999–1005.
21. Tegeder I, Geisslinger G. Cardiovascular risk with cyclooxygenase inhibitors: general problem with substance specific differences? Naunyn Schmiedebergs Arch Pharmacol. 2006;373:1–17.
22. Hollander D. Gastrointestinal complications of nonsteroidal antiinflammatory drugs: prophylactic and therapeutic strategies. Am J Med. 1994;96:274–81.
23. Han JS, Terenius L. Neurochemical basis of acupuncture analgesia. Annu Rev Pharmacol Toxicol. 1982;22:193–220.

24. Zhang R, Lao L, Ren K, Berman BM. Mechamisms of acupuncture-electoacupuncture on persistent pain. Anesthesiolgy. 2014;120(2):482–503.
25. Ulett GA, Han S, Han JS. Electroacupuncture: mechanisms and clinical application. Biol Psychiatry. 1998;44(2):129–38.
26. Kikuchi T, Sakuta T, Yamaguchi T. Intra-articular injection of collagenase induces experimental osteoarthritis in mature rabbits. Osteoarthritis Cartilage. 1998;6(3):177–86.
27. Farkas T, Bihari-Varga M, Biro T. Thermoanalytical and histological study of intra-articular papain-induced degradation and repair of rabbit cartilage. II. Mature animals. Ann Rheum Dis. 1976;35(1):23–6.
28. van der Kraan PM, Vitters EL, van Beuningen HM, van de Putte LB, van den Berg WB. Degenerative knee joint lesions in mice after a single intra-articular collagenase injection. A new model of OA. J Exp Pathol. 1990;71(1):19–31.
29. Ehrlich MG, Armstrong AL, Treadwell BV, Mankin HJ. The role of proteases in the pathogenesis of OA. J Rheumatol. 1987;14:30–2.
30. Gowen M, Wood DD, Ihrie EJ, Meats JE, Russell RG. Stimulation by human interleukin 1 of cartilage breakdown and production of collagenase and proteoglycanase by human chondrocytes but not by human osteoblasts in vitro. Biochim Biophys Acta. 1984;797(2):186–93.
31. Farrell M, Gibson S, Mcmeeken J, Helme R. Pain and hyperalgesia in osteoarthritis of the hands. J Rheumatol. 2000;27(2):441–7.
32. Maciel LY, da Cruz KM, de Araujo AM, Silva ZM, Badauê-Passos D Jr, Santana-Filho VJ, Desantana JM. Electroacupuncture reduces hyperalgesia after injections of acidic saline in rats. Evid Based Complement Alternat Med. 2014:485043. doi: 10.1155/2014/485043
33. de Medeiros MA, Canteras NS, Suchecki D, Mello LE. Analgesia and c-Fos expression in the periaqueductal gray induced by EA at the Zusanli point in rats. Brain Res. 2003;973(2):196–204.
34. Yu XJ, Zhan R, Huang H, Ding GH. Analysis on the difference of afferent mechanism of analgesic signals from manual acupuncture and electroacupuncture of "Zusanli" (ST 36). Zhen Ci Yan Jiu. 2008;33(5):310–5.
35. Ahsin S, Saleem S, Bhatti AM, Iles RK, Aslam M. Clinical and endocrinological changes after electro-acupuncture treatment in patients with osteoarthritis of the knee. Pain. 2009;147(1–3):60–6.
36. Lundeburg TE, Stener-Victorin E. Is there a physiological basis for the use of acupuncture in pain? Int Congress Series. 2002;1238:3–10.
37. Huang C, Wang Y, Han JS, Wan Y. Characteristics of EA-induced analgesia in mice: variation with strain, frequency, intensity and opioid involvement. Brain Res. 2002;945(1):20–5.
38. Kim JH, Min BI, Na HS, Park DS. Relieving effects of EA on mechanical allodynia in neuropathic pain model of inferior caudal trunk injury in rat: mediation by spinal opioid receptors. Brain Res. 2004;998(2):230–6.
39. Baek YH, Choi DY, Yang HI, Park DS. Analgesic effect of EA on inflammatory pain in the rat model of collagen-induced arthritis: mediation by cholinergic and serotonergic receptors. Brain Res. 2005;1057(1–2):181–5.
40. Chang FC, Tsai HY, Yu MC, Yi PL, Lin JG. The central serotonergic system mediates the analgesic effect of EA on Zusanli (ST36) acupoints. J Biomed Sci. 2004;11(2):179–85.
41. Kim SK, Park JH, Bae SJ, Kim JH, Hwang BG, Min BI, Park DS, Na HS. Effects of EA on cold allodynia in a rat model of neuropathic pain: mediation by spinal adrenergic and serotonergic receptors. Exp Neurol. 2005;195(2):430–6.
42. Park JH, Kim SK, Kim HN, Sun B, Koo S, Choi SM, Bae H, Min BI. Spinal cholinergic mechanism of the relieving effects of EA on cold and warm allodynia in a rat model of neuropathic pain. J Physiol Sci. 2009;59(4):291–8.
43. Mccleane GJ, Suzuki R, Dickenson AH. Does a single intravenous injection of the 5HT3 receptor antagonist ondansetron have an analgesic effect in neuropathic pain? A double-blinded, placebo-controlled cross-over study. Anesth Analg. 2003;97(5):1474–8.
44. Ali Z, Wu G, Kozlov A, Barasi S. The role of 5HT3 in nociceptive processing in the rat spinal cord: results from behavioural and electrophysiological studies. Neurosci Lett. 1996;208(3):203–7.
45. Houde RW. Analgesic effectiveness of the narcotic agonist-antagonists. Br J Clin Pharmacol. 1979;7 Suppl 3:297S–308S.
46. Takagi J, Yonehara N. Serotonin receptor subtypes involved in modulation of electrical acupuncture. Jpn J Pharmacol. 1998;78(4):511–4.
47. Sasaki M, Ishizaki K, Obata H, Goto F. Effects of 5-HT2 and 5-HT3 receptors on the modulation of nociceptive transmission in rat spinal cord according to the formalin test. Eur J Pharmacol. 2001;424(1):45–52.

15

Efficacy of acupuncture for chronic prostatitis/chronic pelvic pain syndromes: study protocol for a randomized, sham acupuncture-controlled trial

Zongshi Qin[1,2], Zhiwei Zang[3], Jiani Wu[1], Jing Zhou[1,2] and Zhishun Liu[1]*

Abstract

Background: Chronic prostatitis/chronic pelvic pain syndrome (CP/CPPS) affects many adult men worldwide. The currently available therapies offer little or no proven benefit for CP/CPPS. We designed this study to assess the efficacy of acupuncture therapy for the treatment of CP/CPPS.

Methods: This study is designed as a randomized, sham acupuncture-controlled trial. We will compare patients with CP/CPPS in an acupuncture group and a sham acupuncture group. Sixty-eight patients will be randomly allocated to receive acupuncture or sham acupuncture. The treatments will consist of 30-min sessions, three times weekly, for 8 weeks. The primary outcome measure is change in the weekly mean National Institutes of Health Chronic Prostatitis Symptom Index (NIH-CPSI) total score from baseline through the 8-week treatment period. Secondary measures include the NIH-CPSI subscale scores, the total International Prostate Symptom Score (IPSS), patients' response rate, and patient satisfaction after treatment. We will also assess changes in the NIH-CPSI total score from baseline at the 20th and 32nd week of follow-up.

Discussion: This is a randomized, sham-controlled trial of acupuncture treatment for CP/CPPS. The results of this trial will provide more evidence on whether acupuncture is efficacious for treating CP/CPPS.

Trial registration: Clinical Trials.gov NCT02588274

Keywords: Chronic prostatitis/chronic pelvic pain syndrome, Acupuncture, Efficacy, Randomized controlled trial

Background

Chronic prostatitis/chronic pelvic pain syndrome (CP/CPPS) is a common prostatic syndrome with a worldwide prevalence of 2 % to 10 % in adult men [1–3]. Based on a survey in China, the prevalence of CP/CPPS-like symptoms among Chinese men is 4.5 % [4]. CP/CPPS can present with a wide range of clinical manifestations; the main symptoms include urogenital pain, lower urinary tract symptoms, psychological issues and sexual dysfunction [5]. Compared with other urological conditions, the aetiologic factors of CP/CPPS are unclear, and its pathophysiological mechanisms are still poorly understood. It is hypothesized that inflammation or abnormal activity of the pelvic nerve and muscle play important roles in this disease [6]. According to the consensus guidelines, there is still no standard treatment for CP/CPPS; as a result, individualized therapy and symptom-based treatment approaches are recommended [5]. The interventions for CP/CPPS include medication (alpha-adrenergic antagonists, antibiotics, pain pharmacotherapies, 5-alpha-reductase inhibitors, and phytotherapy), physiotherapy (biofeedback, acupuncture) and surgical intervention [7–10]. Drugs such as alpha-adrenergic antagonists and antibiotics have been considered the initial treatment options for CP/CPPS, but in most cases, the administration of a single drug does not relieve multiple symptoms [5]. Hence, other approaches to prevent and ameliorate CP/CPPS symptoms are considered essential. Acupuncture may be a

* Correspondence: liuzhishun@aliyun.com
[1]Department of Acupuncture, Guang'anmen Hospital, China Academy of Chinese Medical Sciences, Beijing 100053, China
Full list of author information is available at the end of the article

currently underestimated option for CP/CPPS treatment. Based on prior research by Lee et al., acupuncture may relieve the pain-related symptoms of CP/CPPS [11]. Thus far, although several well-designed randomized controlled trials (RCTs) related to acupuncture for the treatment of CP/CPPS have been published [12–15], the recommendations for CP/CPPS in current guidelines remain at level 5 (the lowest level) [5]. Therefore, we designed this trial to further assess the efficacy of acupuncture for treating CP/CPPS.

Methods/design
Aim
The aim of this study is to evaluate the efficacy of acupuncture in CP/CPPS patients.

Design
This study is a multi-centre, sham-controlled, randomized trial of acupuncture for the treatment of CP/CPPS that will be conducted in the Guang'anmen Hospital of China Academy of Chinese Medical Sciences and Yantai Hospital of Traditional Chinese Medicine from November 2015 to May 2017. All of the patients will be asked to sign an informed consent form prior to randomization. Blinded evaluators and statisticians will manage all data. We developed this protocol according to the Standard Protocol Items: Recommendations for Interventional Trials (SPIRIT) checklist [16]. This trial protocol has been approved by the Research Ethical Committee of Guang'anmen Hospital of China Academy of Chinese Medical Sciences and Yantai Hospital of Traditional Chinese Medicine, and it has been registered under the identifier NCT02588274 at ClinicalTrials.gov in the USA. Figure 1 provides a study flow chart.

Participants
Sixty-eight patients will be recruited from the Guang'anmen Hospital of Chinese Academy of Chinese Medical Sciences and Yantai Hospital of Traditional Chinese Medicine.

Inclusion criteria
Patients must meet the diagnostic criteria from the NIH CP/CPPS consensus [17], including the following:

1. History of pain perceived in the prostate region and absence of other lower urinary tract pathology for a minimum of three of the past 6 months. In addition, any associated lower urinary tract symptoms, sexual function, and psychological factors should be addressed. Physical examinations, urine analyses, and urine cultures will be performed for all subjects.
2. Age 18 to 50 years

3. NIH Chronic Prostatitis Symptom Index (NIH-CPSI) total score ≥ 15 (scale 0–43, with 0 meaning no symptoms).

Exclusion criteria

1. Other urologic diseases, such as acute prostatitis, bacterial prostatitis, benign prostatic hyperplasia (BPH), prostate cancer, urinary tuberculosis, and urinary tract infection. (The 2-glass test will be performed in patients with urinary tract symptoms using their voided bladder 2 (VB2) and VB3, which can provide fairly accurate results and is easy to perform [18].)
2. Serious or acute diseases involving the heart, liver, kidney or blood.
3. Patients receiving acupuncture or medication (including alpha blockers or pain killers) in the week prior to the baseline assessment.

Recruitment procedures
We will recruit the participants using advertisements in newspapers, on television, and on the Internet. Prospective participants will obtain a good understanding of the trial by reading the advertisement, which will include a brief introduction of the population needed, the contact information of the researchers, and details of the acupuncture intervention and of the comparison (all participants will be informed that there are two acupuncture groups, i.e., a traditional acupuncture group and a sham acupuncture group, in which blunt needles are used to stimulate the acupoint skin, and that they have a 50 % chance of being allocated into either of the two groups). If the patient is eligible and interested in the trial, they will be invited to consult with the study doctors; after the doctors have provided a diagnosis, the patients will be recruited. All of the participants will be required to sign an informed consent form before the trial that will include an introduction of CP/CPPS, the inclusion and exclusion criteria of the trial, and an introduction to the interventions. In addition, participants have the right to withdraw from the trial at any time.

Randomization
After the participants have completed a baseline evaluation and met the selection criteria, one research assistant, uninvolved with the treatment and data collection, will be responsible for randomly grouping the participants. The acupuncturists will be blinded to the process of randomized assignment. The random sequence will be generated by the Institute of Clinical Pharmacology affiliated to Guang'anmen Hospital of China Academy of Chinese Medical Sciences. Randomization numbers using a block of four will be sealed in a scheduled

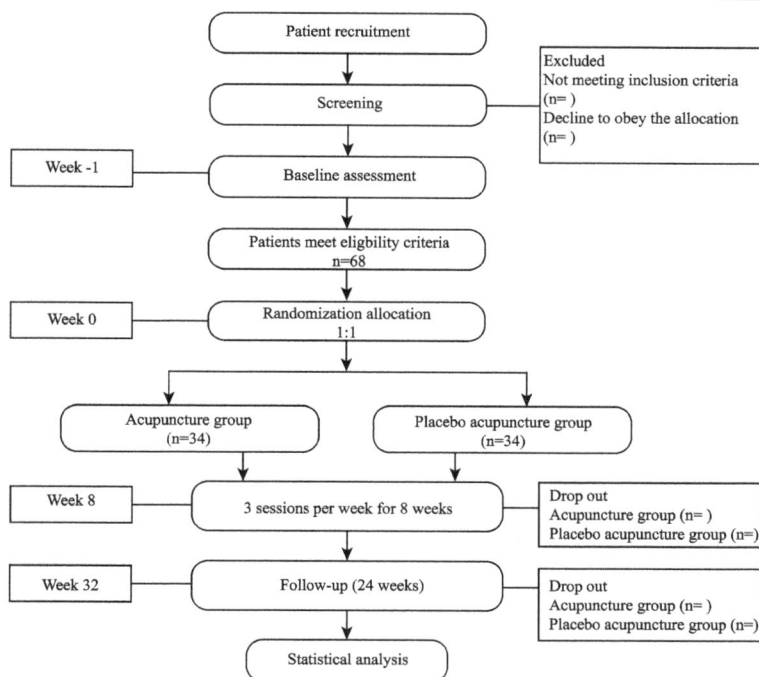

Fig. 1 Flow chart

computer-generated opaque randomization envelope. To ensure that randomization is successfully implemented, the patient's sequence number will be written outside of the envelope, and a paper-written group name will be inside the envelope. All envelopes will be numbered sequentially. The envelopes will be delivered according to the patients' screening sequence numbers. Finally, the acupuncturist will be informed of the random numbers and the group assignment by telephone or e-mail.

Interventions and comparison
Treatment group
According to records in the ancient Traditional Chinese Medicine work *Huangdi Neijing*, acupuncture points belonging to bladder meridian (BL) have a noticeable effect on urinary disease. Furthermore, spleen meridian (SP), kidney meridian (KI), and liver meridian (LR) intersect at Sanyinjiao (SP 6), one of the most frequently used acupuncture points for urogenital disease [19, 20]. In addition, the treatment was based on the theory of neuroanatomy [10, 21, 22] and consensus among acupuncture experts in Guang'anmen Hospital. Therefore, we chose the following acupuncture points: Zhongliao (BL 33), Shenshu (BL 23), Huiyang (BL 35), and Sanyinjiao (SP 6) (Table 1). After the patients are relaxed and in a prone position, acupuncturists will use 75 % alcohol pads to sterilize the skin around the acupuncture points and then insert steel needles (Huatuo, Suzhou, China 0.3 mm*40 mm/0.3 mm*75 mm) into the acupuncture

points. For bilateral Zhongliao (BL 33), the needle will be inserted approximately 50–60 mm with a 45-degree angle. For Huiyang (BL 35), the needle will be inserted approximately 50–60 mm. For Shenshu (BL 23) and Sanyinjiao (SP 6), the needles will be inserted vertically to a depth of 25–30 mm. Acupuncturists will twirl at BL23, BL35 and SP 6 to achieve and enhance the sensation of aches, heaviness or numbness in the area surrounding the inserted needle (known as de qi), and the manipulations will be performed a total of three times during 1 session (every 10 min). For bilateral BL 33, which are located in the 3rd posterior sacral foramina, needles will be inserted without lifting or rotating based on the characteristics of the points. There are 24 treatment sessions after baseline that occur three times a week, and the participants will receive a 30-min treatment each session.

Control group
The control group will receive sham acupuncture at the same acupuncture points as the treatment group. The sham needle with a blunt tip used in the control group is similar to the Streitberger needle (Fig. 2 provides a diagram to illustrate the sham acupuncture applied in this trial) [23]. Acupuncturists will gently lift, thrust, and twist the sham needles to simulate the treatment procedure, thus blinding the patients to the intervention. Each acupuncture point will undergo the same twirling motion as the acupuncture group. The duration and

Table 1 Measurements at different time points

Measurements	baseline	1 week	2 weeks	3 weeks	4 weeks	5 weeks	6 weeks	7 weeks	8 weeks	20 weeks	32 weeks
NIH-CPSI total score	×	×	×	×	×	×	×	×	×	×	×
NIH-CPSI subscales score	×				×				×	×	×
IPSS total score	×				×				×	×	×
Global response assessment	×				×				×	×	×
Degree of expectation	×										
Satisfaction									×	×	×

NIH-CPSI The National Institutes of Health Chronic Prostatitis Symptom Index, *IPSS* International Prostate Symptom Score

frequency of the sessions will be the same as in the acupuncture group. To ensure blinding, the investigators will make appointments with each participant on alternate days to prevent crosstalk between groups. To test the success of the blinding, the participants will be asked to answer the following question after the 4th week treatment: "Do you think you received traditional acupuncture (A) or sham acupuncture (blunt needles used to stimulate the acupoint skin) (B)?" The participants can answer "A", "B" or "unclear" (these two interventions will be demonstrated before the treatment, and all participants will have a good understanding of both interventions). Any medication usage should be recorded, including the name of the medicine, the dosage and the session. We will compare the proportion of subjects using medicine and the mean days of medication use between the groups.

Outcome measures
Primary outcome measures
The primary outcome of this study is the change in the NIH-CPSI total score, which will be measured from baseline to the 8th week. After we have collected data for

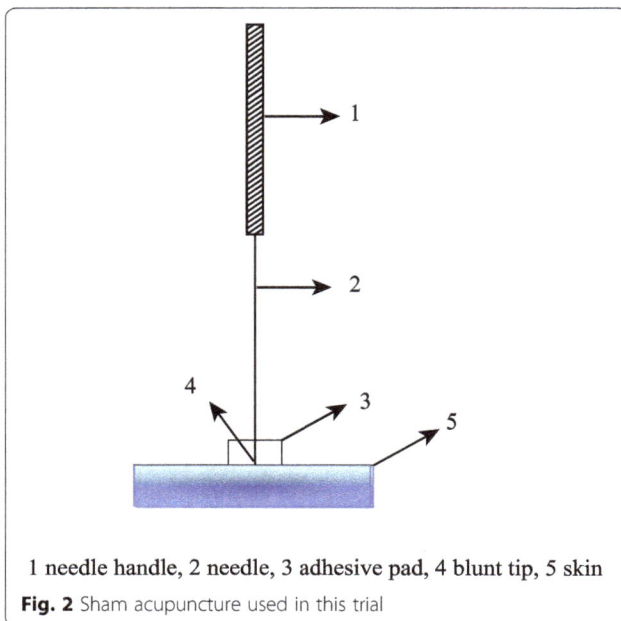

1 needle handle, 2 needle, 3 adhesive pad, 4 blunt tip, 5 skin

Fig. 2 Sham acupuncture used in this trial

8 weeks, the average score from each week will be calculated.

The NIH-CPSI is a validated, self-reported questionnaire that is widely used to assess CP/CPPS patients [24, 25]. It contains 13 items that are scored in three discrete domains: pain, urinary symptoms and impact on quality of life. A score of 0 indicates that the condition described in the question never occurs.

The secondary outcome measures include the following (for the first three secondary outcomes, we will measure the change from baseline):

1. NIH-CPSI total score at the 20th and 32nd week.
2. NIH-CPSI subscale scores at the 4th, 8th, 20th, and 32nd week.
3. IPSS total score at the 4th, 8th, 20th, and 32nd week. The International Prostate Symptom Score (IPSS) is another valid, reliable and sensitive measure for patients with lower urinary tract symptoms (LUTS). The IPSS has been translated into several languages, including Chinese, and it is widely used in clinical practice and research to determine the severity of LUTS, including incomplete bladder emptying, frequency of urination, intermittency, urgency, weak urine stream, straining and nocturia [26, 27]. Each of the questions is rated from 0 (not at all) to 5 (almost always), and according to the total symptom score, the severity of LUTS can be graded as mild (0–7), moderate (8–19) or severe (20–35).
4. Global response assessment at the 4th, 8th, 20th, and 32nd week. Patients who have at least a 50 % decrease compared to baseline in total NIH-CPSI score will be considered "responders". We will compare the response rate between the two groups.
5. Expectations that acupuncture might help CP/CPPS at baseline. This scale includes four brief questions to investigate whether patients are confident that acupuncture treatment will help their CP/CPPS.
6. The degree of satisfaction for patients undergoing acupuncture treatment will be measured at the 8th, 20th, and 32nd week.

Table 1 shows the time to visit and the data collection measurements at different time points.

Safety assessment

Adverse events (AEs) related to acupuncture treatment will be appropriately assessed and recorded by the observers throughout the trial, for instance, pain, haematomas, or nausea. AEs will be managed by acupuncturists and related clinical specialists within 24 h. The principal investigator (Z. Liu) will make the final decision to terminate the trial if severe AEs arise.

Data collection and quality control

Because nonstandard input of clinical data can contribute to the bias of results, two investigators (to assess the effect of treatment) will independently collect the data using case report forms and then input the data into a computer; this process will ensure the safety and reliability of the data. To confirm the quality of the trial, all acupuncturists will be required to have an official license and more than two years of clinical experience.

Sample size calculation and statistical analysis

The calculation of sample size was based on the primary outcome of change in NIH-CPSI total score from baseline to the 8th week of treatment (mean of 8 weeks of data). According to previous literature [12], after 10 weeks of sham acupuncture treatment, NIH-CPSI scores decreased by 6.2, with a standard deviation of 10.3. We estimated that for a 13.3-point difference in the NIH-CPSI score with a standard deviation of 4.5, and based on our clinical experience and data from previous research, the decrease in the NIH-CPSI total score should be more than 6 points (i.e., the minimal clinically important difference, MCID) [28]. Therefore, we will need to recruit 34 patients per group from Guang'anmen Hospital of Chinese Academy of Chinese Medical Sciences and Yantai Hospital of Traditional Chinese Medicine to obtain 90 % power and a significance level of 5 % while allowing for a 20 % dropout rate.

The data will be analysed using SPSS software Ver.19.0 (IBM SPSS Statistics, IBM Corp, Somers, New York), and the data analysis will be based on the intention-to-treat (ITT) principle regarding baseline characteristics. If there are significantly more dropouts in the control group than in the treatment group, we will conduct a secondary analysis of subjects who have completed the treatment according to the protocol. The outcomes for evaluating changes between the groups will be based on the outcome of the NIH-CPSI at different time points. The significance levels will be two-sided and reported at a 5 % level. For continuous measurement data, the mean, standard deviation, median and interquartile range will be represented. If the data are normally distributed, analysis of covariance will be used because the centres and baseline variables in this study are covariates that are not manipulated by the researchers but may still have an effect on the efficacy of acupuncture. If the distribution is not normal, we will use generalized estimating equations, if needed, to account for the cumulative acupuncture frequency and to observe whether increasing treatment sessions results in increased efficacy for patients. Linear regression will be used to explore whether the patients' expectations have an impact on treatment. For categorical data, a CMH (Cochran-Mantel-Haenszel) test will be used, and the data will be represented as case and percentages. Missing data will be assumed to be missing randomly and will be imputed using multiple imputation.

Table 2 summarizes the details of the analysis methods for the primary and secondary outcomes.

Discussion

Acupuncture has been used to treat urinary diseases in China for centuries, and many RCTs have been focused on this illness [29–33]. Several RCTs to date have shown that acupuncture or electro-acupuncture is effective for CP/CPPS [12–14]; however, according to a systematic review and the consensus guidelines, positive evidence for acupuncture-based therapy in CP/CPPS remains poor [17, 34]. The lack of evidence is mainly attributable to the methodological limitations of prior studies, such as inappropriate trial designs, inadequate control groups, lack of follow-up, and lack of suitable outcome measures. Some well-designed trials have indicated that the effect of invasive sham acupuncture may be comparable to that of real acupuncture or standard drug therapy [35, 36]. These results might call into question whether the "invasive sham acupuncture" is a reasonable control for CP/CPPS or whether it is actually a type of shallow acupuncture intervention. Several researchers have also argued about whether invasive sham procedures can be incorporated by acupuncture trials [37, 38]. We are also curious about this question, and we designed the sham acupuncture to use a blunt-tip needle on acupoints without penetration. According to the findings of our prior crossover study, this non-insertion-type needle is a valid sham control for acupuncture research and can achieve good subject blinding effects with a similar appearance to traditional acupuncture [39]. Given a sufficiently thin needle and the manipulation used (lifting, thrusting or rotating), even blunt tips can make participants feel the sensation of piercing. Most of the participants were hardly able to distinguish this device from real acupuncture in the previous trial [39]. In addition, in the current trial, we will use BL 23, BL 33, BL 35 and SP 6 as the selected acupoints instead of conception vessel 1 (CV 1) and CV 4. According to our previous clinical

Table 2 Analysis methods for outcomes

Outcomes	Time frame	Statistics
Primary outcome		
NIH-CPSI total score and change from baseline	baseline, week 1-8	Covariance analysis or generalized estimating equations
Secondary outcomes		
NIH-CPSI subscales score	Baseline, week 4,8,20,32	Covariance analysis or generalized estimating equations
NIH-CPSI total score in follow-up	week 20,32	Covariance analysis or generalized estimating equations
IPSS total score and change from baseline	baseline, week 4,8,20,32	Covariance analysis or generalized estimating equations
Global response assessment improvement	week 4,8,20,32	CMH test or nonparametric test
Degree of expectation	baseline	linear regress
Degree of satisfaction	week 8,20,32	CMH test or nonparametric test

experiences and studies related to BPH, acupuncture on BL 23, BL 33, and BL 35 could significantly improve the condition of patients with LUTS [40]. Furthermore, the selected acupoints mentioned above are located on the participant's lower back and distal lower extremity; therefore, the participants will barely be able to see the treatment procedure and puncture wounds from their prone position. Thus, we anticipate that the acupoints chosen in this trial might increase the possibility of patient-blinding.

In this trial, we aim to clarify the efficacy and safety of acupuncture for treating CP/CPPS. We will calculate the mean NIH-CPSI scores over 8 weeks, and these scores will indicate the weekly efficacy of acupuncture during the 8 weeks of treatment; additionally, the mean value may provide more sufficient evidence for determining whether acupuncture is efficacious for treating CPPS. Furthermore, we will add an expectations scale to explore whether the patients' expectations have a potential impact on the outcomes of acupuncture treatment. Nevertheless, this study has several limitations, including the small sample size and the unblinded acupuncturists. Due to the use of a sham acupuncture control, a relatively high rate of dropouts might be observed in the control group. Additionally, there is a risk that the blinding method may be unsuccessful in control participants, as the blunt tip needle will not leave puncture holes. Finally, a few participants might be recruited mistakenly due to the overlapping symptoms of CP/CPPS and BPH [41]. Nonetheless, the outcome assessors and patients will be blinded to decrease the potential for bias [42]. We hope that the results of this trial can provide both an evidence-based treatment option for patients suffering from CP/CPPS and an enhanced level of evidence on which to base guideline recommendations.

Abbreviations
AEs: Adverse events; BL: Bladder meridian; BPH: Benign prostatic hyperplasia; CMH: Cochran-Mantel-Haenszel; CP/CPPS: Chronic prostatitis/chronic pelvic pain syndrome; CV: Conception vessel; IPSS: International Prostate Symptom Score; ITT: Intention-to-treat; KI: Kidney meridian; LR: Liver meridian;

LUTS: Lower urinary tract symptoms; NIH-CPSI: National Institutes of Health Chronic Prostatitis Symptom Index; RCTs: Randomized controlled trials; SP: Spleen meridian; SPIRIT: Standard Protocol Items: Recommendations for Interventional Trials; VB: Voided bladder

Acknowledgements
Not applicable.

Funding
None.

Availability of data and materials
Not applicable.

Authors' contribution
ZQ: conception, design, and manuscript writing. ZL: conception, design, and manuscript revising. ZZ: recruitment and treatment of participants during the procedure. JW: recruitment and treatment of participants during the procedure. JZ: data collection and analysis. All authors approved the publication of this protocol.

Competing interests
The authors declare that they have no competing interests.

Author details
[1]Department of Acupuncture, Guang'anmen Hospital, China Academy of Chinese Medical Sciences, Beijing 100053, China. [2]Beijing University of Chinese Medicine, Beijing 100029, China. [3]Department of Acupuncture, Yantai Hospital of Traditional Chinese Medicine, Yantai 265200, China.

References
1.   Krieger JN, Riley DE, Cheah PY, Liong ML, Yuen KH. Epidemiology of prostatitis: new evidence for a world-wide problem. World J Urol. 2003;21: 70–4.
2.   Nickel JC, Downey J, Hunter D, Clark J. Prevalence of prostatitis-like symptoms in a population based study using the National Institutes of Health chronic prostatitis symptom index. J Urol. 2001;165:842–5.
3.   Clemens JQ, Meenan RT, O'Keeffe-Rosetti MC, Gao SY, Brown SO, Calhoun EA. Prevalence of prostatitis-like symptoms in a managed care population. J Urol. 2006;176:593–6.

4. Liang CA, Li HJ, Wang ZP, Xing JP, Hu WL, Zhang TF, et al. The prevalence of prostatitis-like symptoms in China. J Urol. 2009;182:558–63.
5. Rees J, Abrahams M, Doble A, Cooper A. Diagnosis and treatment of chronic bacterial prostatitis and chronic prostatitis/chronic pelvic pain syndrome: a consensus guideline. BJU Int. 2015;116:509–25.
6. Schaeffer AJ. Etiology and management of chronic pelvic pain syndrome in men. Urology. 2004;63 Suppl 1:75–84.
7. Yang Q, Wei Q, Li H, Yang Y, Zhang S, Dong Q. The effect of alpha-adrenergic antagonists in chronic prostatitis/chronic pelvic pain syndrome: a meta-analysis of randomized controlled trials. J Androl. 2006;27:847–52.
8. Anothaisintawee T, Attia J, Nickel JC, Thammakraisorn S, Numthavaj P, McEvoy M, et al. Management of chronic prostatitis/chronic pelvic pain syndrome: a systematic review and network meta-analysis. JAMA. 2011;305:78–86.
9. Nickel JC, Baranowski AP, Pontari M, Berger RE, Tripp DA. Management of men diagnosed with chronic prostatitis/chronic pelvic pain syndrome who have failed traditional management. Rev Urol. 2007;9:63–72.
10. Anderson RU, Wise D, Sawyer T, Chan C. Integration of myo-fascial trigger point release and paradoxical relaxation training treatment of chronic pelvic pain in men. J Urol. 2005;174:155–60.
11. Lee SH, Lee BC. Use of acupuncture as a treatment method for chronic prostatitis/chronic pelvic pain syndromes. Curr Urol Rep. 2011;12:288–96.
12. Lee SW, Liong ML, Yuen KH, Krieger JN. Acupuncture versus sham acupuncture for chronic prostatitis/chronic pelvic pain. Am J Med. 2008;121:79.e1–7.
13. Lee SH, Lee BC. Electroacupuncture relieves pain in men with chronic prostatitis/chronic pelvic pain syndrome: three-arm randomized trial. Urology. 2009;73:1036–41.
14. Sahin S, Bicer M, Eren GA, Tas S, Tugcu V, Tasci AI, et al. Acupuncture relieves symptoms in chronic prostatitis/chronic pelvic pain syndrome: a randomized, sham-controlled trial. Prostate Cancer Prostatic Dis. 2015;18:249–54.
15. Küçük EV, Suçeken FY, Bindayı A, Boylu U, Onol FF, Gümüş E. Effectiveness of acupuncture on chronic prostatitis-chronic pelvic pain syndrome category IIIB patients: a prospective, randomized, nonblinded, clinical trial. Urology. 2015;85:636–40.
16. Chan AW, Tetzlaff JM, Altman DG, Laupacis A, Gøtzsche PC, Krleža-Jerić K, et al. SPIRIT 2013 Explanation and Elaboration: Guidance for protocols of clinical trials. BMJ. 2013;346:e7586.
17. Krieger JN, Hyberg L, Nickel JC. NIH consensus definition and classification of prostatitis. JAMA. 1999;282:236–7.
18. Nickel JC, Shoskes D, Wang Y, Alexander RB, Fowler Jr JE, Zeitlin S, et al. How does the pre-massage and post massage 2-glass test compare to the Meares-Stamey 4-glass test in men with chronic prostatitis/chronic pelvic pain syndrome? J Urol. 2006;176:119–24.
19. Xie H. Huangdi Neijing. Publishing House of Ancient Chinese Medical books. 2001.
20. Yuan SY, Qin Z, Liu DS, Yin WQ, Zhang ZL, Li SG. Acupuncture for chronic pelvic pain syndromes (CPPS) and its effect on cytokines in prostatic fluid. Zhongguo Zhen Jiu. 2011;31:11–4.
21. Siegel S, Paszkiewicz E, Kirkpatrick C, Hinkel B, Oleson K. Sacral nerve stimulateon in patients with chronic intractable pelvic pain. J Urol. 2001;166:1742–5.
22. Chen R, Nickel JC. Acupuncture ameliorates symptoms in men with chronic prostatitis/chronic pelvic pain syndrome. Urology. 2003;61:1156–9.
23. Streitberger K, Kleinhenz J. Introducing a placebo needle into acupuncture research. Lancet. 1998;352:364–5.
24. Hong K, Xu QQ, Jiang H, Wang XF, Zhu JC. Chronic Prostatitis Symptom Index of Chinese. Zhonghua Nan Ke Xue. 2002;8:38–41.
25. Litwin MS. A review of the development and validation of the national institutes of health chronic prostatitis symptom index. Urology. 2002;60:14–8.
26. Edmond PH, Cindy LK, Weng YC. Validation of the international prostate symptom score in Chinese males and females with lower urinary tract. Health Qual Life Outcomes. 2014;12:1–9.
27. Szeto PS. Applilcation of the Chinese version of the international prostate symptom score for the management of lower urinary tract symptoms in a primary health care setting. Hong Kong Med J. 2008;14:458–64.
28. Alexander RB, Propert KJ, Schaeffer AJ, Landis JR, Nickel JC, O'Leary MP, et al. Ciprofloxacin or tamsulosin in men with chronic prostatitis/chronic pelvic pain syndrome: a randomized, double-blind trial. Ann Intern Med. 2004;141:581–9.
29. He TY, Xu YL. Clinical observation on acupuncture at "san yin points" plus "yin san points" for treatment of chronic prostatitis. World J Clin Acupunct Moxibust. 2007;23:12–3.
30. Hu BC, Wang S, Zhou ZK, Cai YY. Point-through-point acupuncture for treatment of chronic non-bacterial prostatitis. Cap Med. 2005;21:8–9.
31. Jin XH, Ji LX. Clinical study on acupuncture for the treatment of chronic non-bacterial prostatitis and prostatodynia. Chin Naturopath. 2008;5:9.
32. Chen ZS. Observation of therapeutic effect on chronic non-bacterial prostatitis treated with warm needling moxibustion. World J Acupunct Moxibust. 2009;19:19–29.
33. Li C, Wang HS. Clinical study of acupuncture for the treatment of chronic prostatitis. Beijing J Tradit Chin Med. 2006;25:680–1.
34. Posadzki P, Zhang J, Lee MS, Ernst E. Acupuncture for chronic nonbacterial prostatitis/chronic pelvic pain syndrome: a systematic review. J Androl. 2012;33:15–21.
35. Linde K, Streng A, Jürgens S, Hoppe A, Brinkhaus B, Witt C, et al. Acupuncture for patients with migraine: a randomized controlled trial. JAMA. 2005;293:2118–25.
36. Diener HC, Kronfeld K, Boewing G, Lungenhausen M, Maier C, Molsberger A, et al. Efficacy of acupuncture for the prophylaxis of migraine: a multicenter randomized controlled clinical trial. Lancet Neurol. 2006;5:310–6.
37. Birch S. A review and analysis of placebo treatments, placebo effects and placebo controls in trials of medical procedures when sham is not inert. J Altern Complement Med. 2006;12:303–10.
38. Vickers AJ. Placebo controls in randomized trials of acupuncture. Eval Health Profess. 2002;25:421–35.
39. Liu B, Xu H, Ma R, Mo Q, Yan S, Liu Z. Effect of blinding with a new pragmatic placebo needle: a randomized controlled crossover study. Medicine. 2014;93:e 200.
40. Wang Y, Liu B, Yu J, Wu J, Wang J, Liu Z. Electroacupuncture for moderate and severe benign prostatic hyperplasia: a randomized controlled trial. PLoS ONE. 2013;8:e59449.
41. Nickel JC. The overlapping lower urinary tract symptoms of benign prostatic hyperplasia and prostatitis. Curr Opin Urol. 2006;16:5–10.
42. Altman DG, Dore CJ. Randomisation and baseline comparisons in clinical trials. Lancet. 1990;335:149–53.

16

An investigation of the use of acupuncture in stroke patients in Taiwan

Shu-Wen Weng[1,2†], Ta-Liang Chen[3,4,5], Chun-Chieh Yeh[6,7], Chien-Chang Liao[1,3,4,5†], Hsin-Long Lane[8], Jaung-Geng Lin[1,9†] and Chun-Chuan Shih[8,10*†]

Abstract

Background: Acupuncture is considered a complementary and alternative medicine in many countries. The purpose of this study was to report the pattern of acupuncture use and associated factors in patients with stroke.

Methods: We used claims data from Taiwan's National Health Insurance Research Database and identified 285001 new-onset stroke patients in 2000–2008 from 23 million people allover Taiwan. The use of acupuncture treatment after stroke within one year was identified. We compared sociodemographics, coexisting medical conditions, and stroke characteristics between stroke patients who did and did not receive acupuncture treatment.

Results: The use of acupuncture in stroke patients increased from 2000 to 2008. Female gender, younger age, white-collar employee status, higher income, and residence in areas with more traditional Chinese medicine (TCM) physicians were factors associated with acupuncture use in stroke patients. Ischemic stroke (odds ratio [OR] 1.21, 95 % confidence interval [CI] 1.15–1.28), having no renal dialysis (OR 2.76, 95 % CI 2.45–3.13), receiving rehabilitation (OR 3.20, 95 % CI 3.13–3.27) and longer hospitalization (OR 1.23, 95 % CI 1.19–1.27) were also associated with acupuncture use. Stroke patients using rehabilitation services were more likely to have more acupuncture visits and a higher expenditure on acupuncture compared with stroke patients who did not receive rehabilitation services.

Conclusions: The application of acupuncture in stroke patients is well accepted and increasing in Taiwan. The use of acupuncture in stroke patients is associated with sociodemographic factors and clinical characteristics.

Keywords: Acupuncture, Complementary and alternative medicine, Stroke, Traditional Chinese medicine, Use

Abbreviations: CAM, Complementary and alternative medicine; CI, Confidence interval; ICD-9-CM, International classification of diseases, 9th revision, clinical modification; OR, Odds ratio; TCM, Traditional Chinese medicine

Background

With the increasing use of complementary and alternative medicine (CAM) worldwide [1], the 1-year prevalence of CAM use in the United States and United Kingdom were found to be as high as 33.2 % and 26.3 %, respectively [2, 3]. The estimated out-of-pocket cost for CAM was $33.9 billion in the USA in 2007 [4].

Acupuncture is considered a subtype of traditional Chinese medicine (TCM) [5], which has been used for at least 2000 years in China, and it has gained attention in the United States since 1971. Currently, it is widely used in many countries [1, 5]. A cross-sectional survey showed that at least 1.5 % of adults had used acupuncture in the past 12 months in the United States in 2007 [6].

Stroke remains the leading cause of adult disabilities worldwide, with an estimated direct medical cost of $20.6 billion in the United States in 2010 [7]. The 1-year cost of stroke ranges from $7,342 to $146,149 per patient in several countries [8]. Pneumonia, urinary tract

---

* Correspondence: hwathai@seed.net.tw
Dr. Chien-Chang Liao has equal contribution with the first author; Prof. Jaung-Geng Lin has equal contribution with the corresponding author.
[†]Equal contributors
[8]School of Chinese Medicine for Post-Baccalaureate, College of Medicine, I-Shou University, Kaohsiung City 824, Taiwan
Full list of author information is available at the end of the article

infection, pain, dysphagia, depression, and recurrent stroke are common complications after stroke [9–11].

Acupuncture has been accepted in stroke rehabilitation in many countries, and the treatment is relatively safe and effective in improving post-stroke chronic symptoms, such as disability, shoulder pain, and dysphagia [5, 12–15]. In the United States, acupuncture was used more frequently in stroke compared with non-stroke patients [16]. A previous study also showed the high use of TCM among stroke patients in Taiwan [17]. However, limited information is available on the pattern of use of acupuncture in stroke patients.

Using the National Health Insurance Research Database, we conducted a nationwide, population-based cohort study to evaluate the pattern of acupuncture use in stroke patients. Another purpose of this study was to report the factors associated with acupuncture use among adult stroke patients.

Methods
Source of data
Since 1996, all medical claims of insured beneficiaries have been documented in the National Health Insurance Research Database, which was established by Taiwan's National Health Research Institute. Information available for this study included gender, birth date, disease codes, health care rendered, medicines prescribed, diagnoses at admission and discharge, and medical institutions and physicians providing services. This study employed the All Stroke Database, which consisted of all prevalent and incident stroke patients across Taiwan between 2000 and 2008 [17–19].

Ethical statement
Insurance reimbursement claims used in this study were obtained from Taiwan's National Health Insurance Research Database, which is available for academic access. This study was conducted in accordance with the Helsinki Declaration. To protect personal privacy, the electronic database was decoded with patient identifications scrambled for further public access for research. Although the National Health Research Institute regulations do not require informed consent due to the use of decoded and scrambled patient identification, this study was approved by Taiwan's National Health Research Institute (NHIRD-100-122) and the Institutional Review Board of E-DA Hospital, Kaohsiung, Taiwan (2014012) [17–19].

Study design and population
We identified 285001 newly diagnosed, hospitalized stroke patients aged ≥20 years between 2000 and 2008 as our eligible study subjects from 23 million people allover Taiwan. Those with a previous stroke according to a physician's diagnosis were excluded until 1996. To confirm that all stroke patients in our study were incident cases, only new-onset stroke cases were included. The outcome of this study was the prevalence of acupuncture use in people with a new diagnosis of stroke in the first year. This study compared sociodemographic factors, coexisting medical conditions, and stroke characteristics between stroke patients who used and did not use acupuncture.

Criteria and definition
We defined stroke according to the International Classification of Diseases, 9th Revision, Clinical Modification (ICD-9-CM 430–438). Coexisting medical conditions included diabetes mellitus (ICD-9-CM 250), hypertension (ICD-9-CM 401–405), hyperlipidemia (ICD-9-CM 272.0–272.4), and myocardial infarction (ICD-9-CM 410 and 412). According to the administration codes (D8, D9) from reimbursement claims, regular renal dialysis (including hemodialysis and/or peritoneal dialysis) was also considered a coexisting medical condition among stroke patients in this study. We classified the frequency of acupuncture visits into quartiles. Stroke patients in the highest quartile of acupuncture visits were defined as high acupuncture users. Medical expenditures on acupuncture were also classified into quartiles. Stroke patients who were in the highest quartile of acupuncture expenditure were considered high acupuncture expenditure patients.

As Taiwan has 359 townships and city districts, we calculated the population density (persons/km^2) of each of these administrative units. Based on the population density, these units were stratified into tertiles to designate areas of low, moderate, and high urbanization. We calculated the density of traditional Chinese physicians (traditional Chinese physicians/10,000 persons) based on the number of traditional Chinese physicians per 10,000 residents in each administrative unit. The first, second, and third tertiles were considered areas with low, moderate, and high physician densities, respectively. Based on the Ministry of Health and Welfare criteria, low income status was defined as qualification for waived medical co-payments.

Statistical analysis
To observe the trend of acupuncture use, the annual prevalence of stroke patients using acupuncture treatment was calculated from 2000 to 2008. We used chi-square tests to compare the difference in sociodemographics, coexisting medical conditions, and characteristics of hospitalization between stroke patients who did and did not use acupuncture. Univariate and multivariate logistic regression analyses were performed to calculate crude and adjusted odds ratios (ORs) and 95 % confidence intervals

(CIs) that measured the relationships between acupuncture use and associated characteristics in stroke patients. These characteristics included sex, age, income status, occupation, urbanization, density of traditional Chinese physicians in the area, disease history, use of rehabilitation, type of stroke, and in-hospital characteristics. All analyses were performed using Statistical Analysis Software version 9.1 (SAS Institute Inc., Cary, North Carolina, USA). A two-sided probability value of <0.05 was considered statistically significant.

Results

The prevalence of acupuncture use among stroke patients increased from 12 % in 2000 to 17 % in 2008 ($p < 0.0001$) (Fig. 1). A higher incidence of acupuncture use was found in men, younger patients, higher income people, white-collar employees, residents living in highly urbanized areas, and areas with more TCM physicians.

The multivariate logistic regression analysis yielded the ORs of factors associated with acupuncture use in stroke patients (Tables 1 and 2), including female gender (OR 1.04, 95 % CI 1.01–1.06), age 30–39 years (OR 4.05, 95 % CI 3.77–4.36), very high income status (OR 1.55, 95 % CI 1.47–1.65), white-collar employee status (OR 1.16, 95 % CI 1.12–1.20), residence in highly urbanized areas (OR 1.44, 95 % CI 1.37–1.52), residence in areas with more TCM physicians (OR 1.43, 95 % CI 1.39–1.48), and use of other types of rehabilitation (OR 3.20, 95 % CI 3.13–3.27). Acupuncture users also experienced greater incidences of hypertension (OR 1.18, 95 % CI 1.15–1.21) and hyperlipidemia (OR 1.30, 95 % CI 1.26–1.35) but lower incidences of myocardial infarction (OR 1.18, 95 % CI 1.09–1.28) and renal dialysis (OR 2.76, 95 % CI 2.45–3.13). Ischemic stroke (OR 1.21, 95 % CI 1.15–1.28) and longer hospitalization (OR 1.23, 95 % CI 1.19–1.27) were also associated with acupuncture use.

The average number of acupuncture visits in stroke patients was higher in males than in females (6.5 ± 7.8 vs. 6.4 ± 7.7, $p < 0.001$) (Tables 3 and 4). Stroke patients

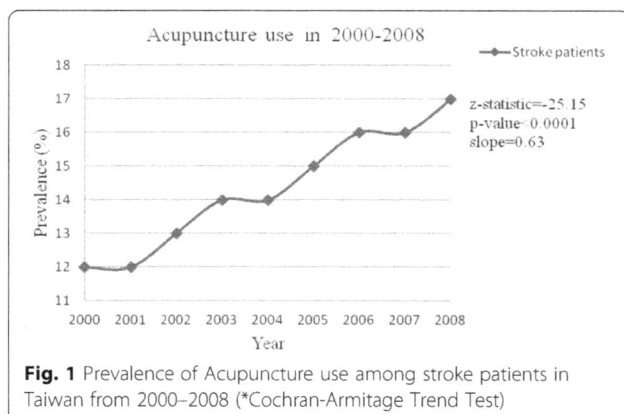

Fig. 1 Prevalence of Acupuncture use among stroke patients in Taiwan from 2000–2008 (*Cochran-Armitage Trend Test)

who had a low income, were white-collar employees, lived in highly urbanized areas and areas with more traditional Chinese physicians, used rehabilitation services, suffered from hemorrhagic stroke or ischemia, or had a longer hospitalization made more acupuncture visits. Patients who had more acupuncture treatment visits also had a higher expenditure on acupuncture.

Discussion

Our study found that the prevalence of acupuncture use among stroke patients significantly increased from 2000 to 2008 in Taiwan, and the sociodemographic characteristics were highly correlated with recent acupuncture use. In contrast to the previous report that was based on a cross-sectional sample [17], this study included all of Taiwan's stroke patients and evaluated the patterns of acupuncture use.

The incidence of acupuncture use in the general population has been reported in the United States as 4.1 % in 2002 and 6.8 % in 2007 [6, 20]. The increasing use of acupuncture was investigated in the western countries [6, 20]. However, Chinese herbal medicine is not common in western countries. In Taiwan, Chinese herbal medicine and acupuncture were covered in the traditional Chinese medicine which is commonly used. Frequent use of acupuncture treatment was found in people with chronic diseases, such as osteoarthritis [21], cancer [22], and stroke [16]. The use of CAM is a trend, and it is not surprising that our study found that the use of acupuncture in stroke patients increased from 12 % in 2000 to 17 % in 2008. Demographic factors, such as age and sex, are associated with the patient's choice of acupuncture [20, 23]. Compared with men, women were more likely to use acupuncture in this study. Several surveys also showed similar findings, namely, women had a higher use of TCM than men [17, 24]. Younger stroke patients were more likely to use acupuncture than older patients in this study. The association between young or middle age and acupuncture use was investigated in previous studies [17, 20, 23, 24]. The finding of better functional outcomes in younger stroke patients is not unexpected, as they had more home support and motivation [25]. A previous study suggested that young people seek more effective ways to improve their well-being and health and to relieve disease symptoms [26]. It is reasonable that younger stroke patients had a higher tendency to use acupuncture and to have a higher acupuncture expenditure than older patients in this study.

The increasing use of TCM is somewhat related to the growth of the number of TCM physicians in Taiwan [17]. A previous investigation reported that the density of TCM increased from 1.39 physicians per 10,000 residents in 1996 to 1.78 physicians per 10,000 residents in 2001 [27]. Our results also showed that the prevalence

Table 1 Comparison of sociodemographic characteristics between stroke patients with and without acupuncture treatment in 2000–2008

	Acupuncture use				p-value	OR	(95 % CI)*
	No (N = 242213)		Yes (N = 42788)				
Sex	n	(%)	n	(%)	<0.0001		
Women	101,397	(85.5)	17,225	(14.5)		1.04	(1.01–1.06)
Men	140,816	(84.6)	25,563	(15.4)		1.00	(reference)
Age, years					<0.0001		
20–29	1819	(83.1)	369	(16.9)		3.44	(3.04–3.89)
30–39	5680	(78.9)	1517	(21.1)		4.05	(3.77–4.36)
40–49	20,319	(79.3)	5298	(20.7)		3.79	(3.60–4.00)
50–59	39,190	(79.6)	10,054	(20.4)		3.56	(3.39–3.73)
60–69	58,684	(82.6)	12,374	(17.4)		3.05	(2.91–3.18)
70–79	74,891	(87.8)	10,424	(12.2)		2.04	(1.95–2.13)
≥ 80	41,630	(93.8)	2752	(6.2)		1.00	(reference)
Mean ± SD	67.4 ± 13.3		62.5 ± 12.5		<0.0001		
Income					<0.0001		
Very low	13,611	(86.1)	2203	(13.9)		1.00	(reference)
Low	71,645	(85.4)	12,283	(14.6)		1.23	(1.16–1.30)
Moderate	42,567	(84.9)	7565	(15.1)		1.31	(1.24–1.38)
High	88,550	(87.1)	13,152	(12.9)		1.30	(1.23–1.38)
Very high	25,840	(77.3)	7585	(22.7)		1.55	(1.47–1.65)
Occupation					<0.0001		
White collar	73,946	(82.0)	16,188	(18.0)		1.16	(1.12–1.20)
Blue collar	115,906	(86.5)	18,067	(13.5)		1.00	(reference)
Other	52,361	(86.0)	8533	(14.0)		1.06	(1.02–1.11)
Urbanization					<0.0001		
Low	17,323	(90.3)	1858	(9.7)		1.00	(reference)
Moderate	93,336	(87.4)	13,509	(12.6)		1.21	(1.15–1.28)
High	131,554	(82.8)	27,421	(17.3)		1.44	(1.37–1.52)
Density of TCM					<0.0001		
Low	64,074	(88.8)	8117	(11.2)		1.00	(reference)
Moderate	121,661	(84.6)	22,199	(15.4)		1.17	(1.14–1.21)
High	56,478	(81.9)	12,472	(18.1)		1.43	(1.39–1.48)
Mean ± SD	1.6 ± 1.2		1.8 ± 1.3		<0.0001		

*Logistic regression model included sociodemographics and medical conditions; Hosmer-Lemeshow goodness of fit, p-value = 0.0006; c-statistic = 0.71; CI, confidence interval; OR, odds ratio; TCM, traditional Chinese medicine

of acupuncture use in stroke patients increased with the increasing density of TCM physicians. High urbanization was associated with TCM use in a previous survey [17, 24]. Because acupuncture is a subtype of TCM, it is not surprising that we found in the present study that people who lived in an urbanized area were more likely to use acupuncture.

Economic growth is a determinant of physician supply and utilization of medical services [28]. In Taiwan, TCM has become an increasingly popular form of medicine, particularly after the implementation of the National Health Insurance in the medical care system since 1995. In this study, the frequency of acupuncture use and related insurance-paid expenditure were higher in stroke patients with a low income than in those without a low income. Co-payment is considered an important factor in the use of medical services [29]. According to the Ministry of Health and Wealth [17–19], patients with low-income status who do not need to pay a co-payment when receiving medical services may have more medical visits for acupuncture treatment than stroke patients with higher incomes.

Among the stroke patients, diabetes, hypertension, hyperlipidemia, myocardial infarction, and kidney insuffucuency

Table 2 Medical conditions of stroke patients with and without acupuncture treatment in 2000–2008

	Acupuncture				p-value	OR	(95 % CI)*
	No (N = 285329)		Yes (N = 47832)				
Rehabilitation					<0.0001		
No	166,526	(90.7)	17,087	(9.2)		1.00	(reference)
Yes	75,687	(74.7)	25,701	(25.3)		3.20	(3.13–3.27)
Diabetes					<0.0001		
No	172,698	(85.2)	29,983	(14.8)		1.00	(reference)
Yes	69,515	(84.4)	12,805	(15.6)		1.00	(0.98–1.03)
Hypertension					<0.0001		
No	93,695	(86.0)	15,290	(14.0)		1.00	(reference)
Yes	148,518	(84.4)	27,498	(15.6)		1.18	(1.15–1.21)
Hyperlipidemia					<0.0001		
No	219,658	(85.4)	37,503	(14.6)		1.00	(reference)
Yes	22,555	(81.0)	5285	(19.0)		1.30	(1.26–1.35)
MI					<0.0001		
No	236,962	(84.9)	42,037	(15.1)		1.18	(1.09–1.28)
Yes	5251	(87.5)	751	(12.5)		1.00	(reference)
Dialysis					<0.0001		
No	238,140	(84.9)	42,500	(15.1)		2.76	(2.45–3.13)
Yes	4073	(93.4)	288	(6.6)		1.00	(reference)
Type of Stroke					<0.0001		
Hemorrhage	53,950	(83.4)	10,714	(16.6)		1.02	(0.96–1.08)
Ischemia	173,573	(85.2)	30,155	(14.8)		1.21	(1.15–1.28)
Other	14,690	(88.5)	1919	(11.6)		1.00	(reference)
LOS, days					<0.0001		
1–5	84,534	(87.4)	12,172	(12.6)		1.00	(reference)
6–9	63,969	(85.9)	10,499	(14.1)		1.06	(1.03–1.09)
10–14	34,261	(83.8)	6605	(16.2)		1.16	(1.12–1.20)
15–19	16,537	(82.7)	3465	(17.5)		1.22	(1.17–1.28)
≥20	43,092	(81.1)	10,047	(18.9)		1.23	(1.19–1.27)
Mean ± SD	12.8 ± 17.5		14.9 ± 17.0		<0.0001		

*Logistic regression model included sociodemographics and medical conditions; Hosmer-Lemeshow goodness of fit, p-value = 0.001; c-statistic = 0.71;
CI, confidence interval; LOS, length of stay; MI, myocardial infarction; OR, odds ratio

were common coexisting medical conditions that were also considered comorbidities in this study [30]. Acupuncture treatment can lower blood pressure [31, 32]. Moreover, evidence-based studies have shown acupuncture's beneficial effects in addressing physical illness in stroke patients [12–14, 33]. We found that patients with comorbidities of hypertension or hyperlipidemia were more likely to undergo acupuncture treatment. People with more chronic diseases were likely to use TCM, which was confirmed in previous surveys [17, 24].

In this study, we found that stroke patients who used acupuncture were more likely to simultaneously undergo conventional medical rehabilitation. Previous reports showed a high use of CAM in stroke survivors in many

countries [16, 34]. Medical pluralism, such as adopting more than one medical system or the use of both conventional medicine and CAM for health and illness, is also common in Taiwan [35, 36].

Stroke patients with longer hospitalizations were more likely to undergo acupuncture treatment. Stroke patients who had a longer length of hospital stay may have more neurological impairment [37], so they may require more or longer rehabilitation for stroke. Our study showed that the frequency of acupuncture visits and related expenditure were higher in stroke patients after a longer length of hospital stay.

The incidence of ischemia is higher than that of other stroke subtypes [38]; however, subarachnoid hemorrhage

Table 3 Post-stroke visits and expenditure on acupuncture treatment within one year in stroke patients in 2000–2008 by sociodemographics

	n	Medical visits Mean ± SD	p-value	Medical expenditure Mean ± SD	p-value
Sex			0.0155		0.0264
Women	17,225	6.4 ± 7.7		212 ± 258	
Men	25,563	6.5 ± 7.8		219 ± 271	
Age			0.0342		<0.0001
20–29	369	6.4 ± 7.0		219 ± 272	
30–39	1517	6.8 ± 7.8		240 ± 302	
40–49	5298	6.7 ± 8.2		226 ± 279	
50–59	10,054	6.5 ± 7.7		217 ± 267	
60–69	12,374	6.4 ± 7.6		210 ± 254	
70–79	10,424	6.4 ± 7.7		216 ± 263	
≥80	2752	6.2 ± 7.9		208 ± 267	
Income			<0.0001		<0.0001
Very low	12,172	5.0 ± 6.5		168 ± 220	
Low	10,499	5.7 ± 7.1		187 ± 234	
Moderate	6605	6.7 ± 7.9		217 ± 262	
High	3465	7.6 ± 8.4		246 ± 276	
Very high	10,047	8.5 ± 8.9		295 ± 321	
Occupation			<0.0001		<0.0001
White collar	16,188	6.9 ± 8.0		229 ± 276	
Blue collar	18,067	6.1 ± 7.4		203 ± 253	
Other	8533	6.6 ± 7.9		219 ± 269	
Urbanization			<0.0001		<0.0001
Low	1858	5.2 ± 6.8		173 ± 229	
Moderate	13,509	6.0 ± 7.4		202 ± 259	
High	27,421	6.8 ± 8.0		226 ± 270	
Density TCM			<0.0001		<0.0001
Low	8117	5.9 ± 7.2		198 ± 250	
Moderate	22,199	6.5 ± 7.8		215 ± 263	
High	12,472	6.7 ± 7.9		230 ± 279	

TCM, traditional Chinese medicine

Table 4 Post-stroke visits and expenditure on acupuncture treatment within one year in stroke patients in 2000–2008 by medical condition

	n	Medical visits Mean ± SD	p-value	Medical expenditure Mean ± SD	p-value
Rehabilitation			<0.0001		<0.0001
No	17,087	4.8 ± 6.3		157 ± 206	
Yes	25,701	7.6 ± 8.4		256 ± 292	
Diabetes mellitus			0.02		0.01
No	29,983	6.5 ± 7.8		218 ± 268	
Yes	12,805	6.3 ± 7.7		211 ± 259	
Hypertension			0.77		0.93
No	15,290	6.5 ± 7.8		216 ± 269	
Yes	27,498	6.5 ± 7.7		216 ± 263	
Hyperlipidemia			0.35		0.98
No	37,503	6.5 ± 7.8		216 ± 266	
Yes	5285	6.4 ± 7.6		216 ± 259	
MI			0.14		0.15
No	42,037	6.5 ± 7.8		216 ± 266	
Yes	751	6.1 ± 7.0		204 ± 240	
Renal dialysis			0.0002		<0.0001
No	42,500	6.5 ± 7.8		217 ± 266	
Yes	288	5.1 ± 6.1		161 ± 220	
Length of stay, days			<0.0001		<0.0001
1–5	12,172	5.0 ± 6.5		168 ± 220	
6–9	10,499	5.7 ± 7.1		187 ± 234	
10–14	6605	6.7 ± 7.9		217 ± 262	
15–19	3465	7.6 ± 8.4		246 ± 276	
≥20	10,047	8.5 ± 8.9		295 ± 321	
Type of Stroke			<0.0001		<0.0001
Hemorrhage	10,714	7.4 ± 8.5		253 ± 296	
Ischemia	30,155	6.3 ± 7.5		207 ± 256	
Other	1919	4.7 ± 6.3		154 ± 200	

MI, myocardial infarction

resulted in a higher re-admission rate or mortality than ischemic stroke, and patients with a subarachnoid hemorrhage used more medical resources following stroke admission [39]. Conventional therapy with acupuncture treatment for acute ischemic stroke for four weeks has been shown to improve self-care ability and quality of life compared with sham acupuncture [40]. In this study, patients with ischemic stroke were more likely to use acupuncture than those with a subarachnoid hemorrhage. The frequency of acupuncture visits and related expenditures were higher in ischemic stroke patients.

This study had some limitations. First, we used retrospective medical claims data from health insurance claims data that lacked detailed patient information on clinical risk scores (e.g., National Institute of Health Stroke Scale score, Barthel index, and Rivermead index) and lifestyle, physical, psychiatric, and biochemical measures. We were unable to determine whether these factors were causally related to acupuncture use. Second, our study used ICD-9-CM codes claimed by physicians for the diagnosis of stroke without clarifying the severity of disease. Third, information on folk therapy was not available in the National Insurance Research Database. In addition, in-come measurement and out-come measurements of stroke patients are unavailable in this study, which are valuable indicators for efficacy of acupuncture treatment. It is also one of our study limitations. Finally, this study was based on cross-sectional analyses of acupuncture use in stroke patients. Understanding the benefit of acupuncture in stroke patients requires further cohort studies.

Conclusions

In conclusion, the application of acupuncture in stroke patients is well accepted and increasing in Taiwan. The use of acupuncture in stroke patients is associated with sociodemographic factors and clinical characteristics.

Acknowledgments
This study is based in part on data obtained from the National Health Insurance Research Database provided by the Bureau of National Health Insurance, Department of Health and managed by the National Health Research Institutes. The interpretation and conclusions contained herein do not represent those of the Bureau of National Health Insurance, Department of Health, or National Health Research Institutes.

Funding
This study was supported in part by Shuang Ho Hospital, Taipei Medical University (104TMU-SHH-23), Taiwan's Ministry of Science and Technology (MOST105-2629-B-038-001, MOST104-2314-B-038-027-MY2, MOST103-2320-B-214-010-MY2), Taiwan Ministry of Health and Welfare Clinical Trial and Research Center of Excellence (MOHW105-TDU-B-212-133019).

Authors' contributions
All authors contributed substantially toward the design of the study, the analysis and interpretation of the data, drafting and revising the manuscript. All authors approved the final version.

Competing interests
The authors declare that they have no competing interests.

Author details
[1]Graduate Institute of Chinese Medicine, College of Chinese Medicine, China Medical University, Taichung 404, Taiwan. [2]Department of Chinese Medicine, Taichung Hospital, Ministry of Health and Welfare, Taichung 403, Taiwan. [3]Department of Anesthesiology, Taipei Medical University Hospital, Taipei 110, Taiwan. [4]Department of Anesthesiology, School of Medicine, College of Medicine, Taipei Medical University, Taipei 110, Taiwan. [5]Health Policy Research Center, Taipei Medical University Hospital, Taipei 110, Taiwan. [6]Department of Surgery, China Medical University Hospital, Taichung 110, Taiwan. [7]Department of Surgery, University of Illinois, Chicago, Illinois, USA. [8]School of Chinese Medicine for Post-Baccalaureate, College of Medicine, I-Shou University, Kaohsiung City 824, Taiwan. [9]Department of Healthcare Administration, Asia University, Taichung 413, Taiwan. [10]Ph.D. Program for the Clinical Drug Discovery from Botanical Herbs, College of Pharmacy, Taipei Medical University, Taipei 110, Taiwan.

References
1. Harris PE, Cooper KL, Relton C, Thomas KJ. Prevalence of complementary and alternative medicine (CAM) use by the general population: a systematic review and update. Int J Clin Pract. 2012;66:924–39.
2. Barnes PM, Bloom B, Nahin RL. Complementary and alternative medicine use among adults and children: United States, 2007. Natl Health Stat Report. 2008;12:1–23.
3. Hunt KJ, Coelho HF, Wider B, Perry R, Hung SK, Terry R, et al. Complementary and alternative medicine use in England: results from a national survey. Int J Clin Pract. 2010;64:1496–502.
4. Nahin RL, Barnes PM, Stussman BJ, Bloom B. Costs of complementary and alternative medicine (CAM) and frequency of visits to CAM practitioners: United States, 2007. Natl Health Stat Report. 2009;18:1–14.
5. Chon TY, Lee MC. Acupuncture. Mayo Clin Proc. 2013;88:1141–6.
6. Upchurch DM, Rainisch BW. A sociobehavioral wellness model of acupuncture use in the United States, 2007. J Altern Complement Med. 2014;20:32–9.
7. Go AS, Mozaffarian D, Roger VL, Benjamin EJ, Berry JD, Blaha MJ, et al. Heart disease and stroke statistics–2014 update: a report from the American Heart Association. Circulation. 2014;129:e28–292.
8. Luengo-Fernandez R, Gray AM, Rothwell PM. Costs of stroke using patient-level data: a critical review of the literature. Stroke. 2009;40:e18–23.
9. Kumar S, Selim MH, Caplan LR. Medical complications after stroke. Lancet Neurol. 2010;9:105–18.
10. Tong X, Kuklina EV, Gillespie C, George MG. Medical complications among hospitalizations for ischemic stroke in the United States from 1998 to 2007. Stroke. 2010;41:980–6.
11. Ingeman A, Andersen G, Hundborg HH, Svendsen ML, Johnsen SP. In-hospital medical complications, length of stay, and mortality among stroke unit patients. Stroke. 2011;42:3214–8.
12. Sze FK, Wong E, Or KK, Lau J, Woo J. Does acupuncture improve motor recovery after stroke? A meta-analysis of randomized controlled trials. Stroke. 2002;33:2604–19.
13. Wu P, Mills E, Moher D, Seely D. Acupuncture in poststroke rehabilitation: a systematic review and meta-analysis of randomized trials. Stroke. 2010;41:e171–9.
14. Lee JA, Park SW, Hwang PW, Lim SM, Kook S, Choi KI, et al. Acupuncture for shoulder pain after stroke: a systematic review. J Altern Complement Med. 2012;18:818–23.
15. Zhao XF, Du Y, Liu PG, Wang S. Acupuncture for stroke: evidence of effectiveness, safety, and cost from systematic reviews. Top Stroke Rehabil. 2012;19:226–33.
16. Shah SH, Engelhardt R, Ovbiagele B. Patterns of complementary and alternative medicine use among United States stroke survivors. J Neurol Sci. 2008;271:180–5.
17. Liao CC, Lin JG, Tsai CC, Lane HL, Su TC, Wang HH, et al. An investigation of the use of traditional chinese medicine in stroke patients in Taiwan. Evid Based Complement Alternat Med. 2012;2012:387164.
18. Liao CC, Su TC, Sung FC, Chou WH, Chen TL. Does hepatitis C virus infection increase risk for stroke? A population-based cohort study. PLoS One. 2012;7:e31527.
19. Liao CC, Chang PY, Yeh CC, Hu CJ, Wu CH, Chen TL. Outcomes after surgery in patients with previous stroke. Br J Surg. 2014;101:1616–22.
20. Burke A, Upchurch DM, Dye C, Chyu L. Acupuncture use in the United States: findings from the National Health Interview Survey. J Altern Complement Med. 2006;12:639–48.
21. Jong MC, van de Vijver L, Busch M, Fritsma J, Seldenrijk R. Integration of complementary and alternative medicine in primary care: what do patients want? Patient Educ Couns. 2012;89:417–22.
22. Gansler T, Kaw C, Crammer C, Smith T. A population-based study of prevalence of complementary methods use by cancer survivors: a report from the American Cancer Society's studies of cancer survivors. Cancer. 2008;113:1048–57.
23. Zhang Y, Lao L, Chen H, Ceballos R. Acupuncture use among American adults: what acupuncture practitioners can learn from National Health Interview Survey 2007? Evid Based Complement Alternat Med. 2012; 2012:710750.
24. Shih CC, Liao CC, Su YC, Tsai CC, Lin JG. Gender differences in traditional Chinese medicine use among adults in Taiwan. PLoS One. 2012;7:e32540.
25. Knoflach M, Matosevic B, Rücker M, Furtner M, Mair A, Wille G, et al. Functional recovery after ischemic stroke–a matter of age: data from the Austrian Stroke Unit Registry. Neurology. 2012;78:279–85.
26. Chang LC, Huang N, Chou YJ, Lee CH, Kao FY, Huang YT. Utilization patterns of Chinese medicine and Western medicine under the National Health Insurance Program in Taiwan, a population-based study from 1997 to 2003. BMC Health Serv Res. 2008;8:170.
27. Yang CH, Huang YT, Hsueh YS. Redistributive effects of the National Health Insurance on physicians in Taiwan: a natural experiment time series study. Int J Equity Health. 2013;12:13.
28. Cooper RA, Getzen TE, Laud P. Economic expansion is a major determinant of physician supply and utilization. Health Serv Res. 2003;38:675–96.

29. Kiil A, Houlberg K. How does copayment for health care services affect demand, health and redistribution? A systematic review of the empirical evidence from 1990 to 2011. Eur J Health Econ. 2014;15:813–28.

30. Lackland DT, Elkind MS, D'Agostino Sr R, Dhamoon MS, Goff Jr DC, Higashida RT, et al. Inclusion of stroke in cardiovascular risk prediction instruments: a statement for healthcare professionals from the American Heart Association/American Stroke Association. Stroke. 2012;43:1998–2027.

31. Flachskampf FA, Gallasch J, Gefeller O, Gan J, Mao J, Pfahlberg AB, et al. Randomized trial of acupuncture to lower blood pressure. Circulation. 2007; 115:3121–9.

32. Wang J, Xiong X, Liu W. Acupuncture for essential hypertension. Int J Cardiol. 2013;169:317–26.

33. Geeganage C, Beavan J, Ellender S, Bath PM. Interventions for dysphagia and nutritional support in acute and subacute stroke. Cochrane Database Syst Rev. 2012;10:CD000323.

34. Shin YI, Yang CY, Joo MC, Lee SG, Kim JH, Lee MS. Patterns of using complementary and alternative medicine by stroke patients at two university hospitals in Korea. Evid Based Complement Alternat Med. 2008;5:231–5.

35. Shih SF, Lew-Ting CY, Chang HY, Kuo KN. Insurance covered and non-covered complementary and alternative medicine utilisation among adults in Taiwan. Soc Sci Med. 2008;67:1183–9.

36. Shih CC, Su YC, Liao CC, Lin JG. Patterns of medical pluralism among adults: results from the 2001 National Health Interview Survey in Taiwan. BMC Health Serv Res. 2010;10:191.

37. Luengo-Fernandez R, Gray AM, Rothwell PM. Population-based study of determinants of initial secondary care costs of acute stroke in the United Kingdom. Stroke. 2006;37:2579–87.

38. Tsai CF, Thomas B, Sudlow CL. Epidemiology of stroke and its subtypes in Chinese vs white populations: a systematic review. Neurology. 2013;81:264–72.

39. Chang KC, Lee HC, Huang YC, Hung JW, Chiu HE, Chen JJ, et al. Cost-effectiveness analysis of stroke management under a universal health insurance system. J Neurol Sci. 2012;323:205–15.

40. Shen PF, Kong L, Ni LW, Guo HL, Yang S, Zhang LL, et al. Acupuncture intervention in ischemic stroke: a randomized controlled prospective study. Am J Chin Med. 2012;40:685–93.

17

The effectiveness of long-needle acupuncture at acupoints BL30 and BL35 for CP/CPPS

Minjie Zhou[1,5], Mingyue Yang[3], Lei Chen[4], Chao Yu[4], Wei Zhang[1,2], Jun Ji[1,2], Chi Chen[1], Xueyong Shen[2] and Jian Ying[1,4*] (iD)

Abstract

Background: The chronic prostatitis/chronic pelvic pain syndrome (CP/CPPS) is one of the commonest chronic inflammatory diseases in adult men, for which acupuncture has been used to relieve related symptoms. The present study aimed to evaluate the therapeutic effect of the long-needle acupuncture on CP/CPPS.

Methods: A randomized traditional acupuncture-controlled single blind study was conducted on 77 patients who were randomized into long-needle acupuncture (LA) and traditional acupuncture (TA) groups. The patients received six sessions of acupuncture for 2 weeks and a follow-up was scheduled at week 24. The primary outcome was measured by the total National Institutes of Health-Chronic Prostatitis Symptom Index (NIH-CPSI) score at week 2. Four domains of the NIH-CPSI (urination, pain or discomfort, effects of symptoms, and quality of life) and the clinical efficacy score served as the secondary outcome.

Results: The total NIH-CPSI score at week 2 and week 24 was significantly improved in the LA group compared with the TA group. LA significantly improved urination, pain or discomfort, the effects of symptoms, and the quality of life at week 2 and week 24 and patients undergoing LA treatment had a higher clinical efficacy score.

Conclusion: Needling at the BL30 and BL35 using LA benefits patients with CP/CPPS.

Trial registration: The study was registered at the Chinese Clinical Trial Register (ChiCTR-ICR-15006138).

Keywords: BL30, BL35, CP/CPPS, Acupuncture, Long needle

Background

The chronic prostatitis/chronic pelvic pain syndrome (CP/CPPS) is one of the commonest chronic inflammatory diseases in male adults, the prevalence of which is estimated to range from 2% to 10% and the overall lifetime prevalence from 9% to 16% [1]. The symptoms of CP/CPPS manifest as pelvic pain, prostate inflammation, voiding symptoms, and sexual disturbance [1, 2], which differ from the voiding problem in benign prostatic hyperplasia, another common prostatic problem in male

adults [3]. Pain has a significant effect on the quality of life in patients with CP/CPPS. Antibiotics are the most common treatment for patients with CP/CPPS, but the antibiotic regimen remains controversial in clinical practice and the number of prostatic bacteria in patients with CP/CPPS does not differ significantly from that in asymptomatic patients [4]. Fewer than 10% of patients with CP/CPPS are found to have bacteria in their urinary tracts [1], and systematic reviews have shown no sufficient evidence to support the benefits of antibiotics for patients with CP/CPPS [5, 6]. Collective evidence has shown that CP/CPPS is an inflammatory disease [7], for which anti-inflammatory medications are commonly prescribed. However, no large-scale randomized control trials have been conducted to demonstrate the effectiveness of

---
* Correspondence: yingjian03@sina.com
[1]Shanghai Qigong Research Institute, Shanghai, China
[4]The Longhua Hospital Shanghai University of Traditional Chinese Medicine, Shanghai, China
Full list of author information is available at the end of the article

anti-inflammatory medication in these patients [5, 6] and their adverse effects in elderly patients, such as gastro-intestinal disturbance, are a serious concern [4, 7, 8]. Current evidence has not supported the benefits of the commonly used medication, alpha-blockers, in CP/CPPS patients [5, 6] and the unsatisfactory nature of conventional medications leads patients to seek alternative therapies.

Acupuncture has been used to treat CP/CPPS in a few clinical studies [9]. A meta-analysis indicated that acupuncture results in statistical and clinical improvements in the voiding domain of the National Institutes of Health-Chronic Prostatitis Symptom Index (NIH-CPSI) in CP/CPPS patients [10]. The observational studies and randomized controlled trials revealed that acupuncture also reduced pain and improved the immune function in patients with CP/CPPS [11–14]. The efficacy of acupuncture is determined by the various parameters, e.g. the depth of the needles, the number of acupoints, and needle manipulation [15, 16], which need to be optimized to maximize its effectiveness.

In clinical practice, long-needle treatment effectively produces the Deqi sensation in the deep pelvic area and induces the constriction of the deep transverse perineal muscle, which is thought to be effective for CP/CPPS. Previous observational studies revealed that deep needling at BL30 at a depth of 3.5–4.5 cun significantly improved the clinical symptoms of CP [17], as did needling at BL35 at a depth of 2–3 cun [18]. The traditional filiform needle hardly produces the Deqi sensation in the deep pelvic area. The present investigation aimed to evaluate effectiveness of LA at acupoints BL30 and BL35 in CP compared with traditional acupuncture (TA) in a single blind randomized pilot study.

Methods
Setting and study design
A randomized traditional acupuncture-controlled single blind trial was conducted. The study protocol was approved by Long Hua Hospital Medical Ethics Committee, Shanghai University of Traditional Chinese Medicine (2014LCSY31). The random codes were generated by SPSS 16.0., sealed in opaque envelopes in sequence, and kept by the principal investigator (JY). Patients were recruited from the Long Hua Hospital Shanghai University of Traditional Chinese Medicine and the clinics of the Shanghai Qigong Research Institute. Eligible patients received treatment with either long-needle or traditional acupuncture for 2 weeks. The evaluation of efficacy was performed individually by the assessor, who was blind to the type of acupuncture intervention. The acupuncturist was not involved in the evaluation of efficacy, or data processing and analysis.

Subjects
Sample size
The sample size was determined by the significant difference between LA group and TA group with an effect size of 0.7 for a two-sided significance level of 5% (two-tailed) and 0.8 power. Each group required 34 patients. We estimated a 10% drop-out rate and the sample size was set at 76 (38 per group). In the study, the last two patients were recruited from two study sites at the same time, thus a total of 77 patients were recruited.

Inclusion criteria
The patients included (1) were diagnosed with CP/CPPS according to *Urology* (edited by Dr. Jieping Wu) [19];,(2) had the symptoms for more than 3 months, (3) were men aged 20–50 years, and (4) were able to read, understand, and sign the informed consent form.

Exclusion criteria
Patients that were excluded (1) had acute prostatitis, (2) had a prostate tumor, (3) had primary benign prostatic hyperplasia,(4)had urinary tract infections or urethritis, (5) had urinary stones, epididymitis, groin hernia, varicocele, or pelvic pain caused by the colorectal or lumbar diseases, (6) had severe heart, liver, kidney, or hematopoietic problems, psychiatric disorders, or other life-threatening diseases, and (7) were unable to complete all of the treatments.

Intervention
LA treatment
The acupuncture treatment in both groups was performed by licensed acupuncturists with more than 3 years of clinical experience. The patient was placed in the prone position on the acupuncture bed. The bilateral BL30 (Baihuan Shu) and BL35 (Huiyang) acupoints were used for the treatments. BL30 is at 1.5 cun lateral to the midline of the sacral crest and at the level of the fourth posterior sacral foramen. BL35 is at 0.5 cun lateral to the midline and at the level with the tip of the coccyx. The long needle (0.4 × 100 mm) was inserted perpendicularly at BL30 (bilateral) at a depth of 75–90 mm (3 ~ 3.5 cun). The Deqi sensation (the feeling of soreness, numbness, distension, and heaviness) from the local site to the perineum (including the urethra and anus) was achieved by the twirling and lifting-thrusting of the needle. In addition, the long needle (0.4 × 100 mm) was inserted obliquely at BL35 (bilateral) with the pin of the needle pointing to the ischial rectal fossa at a depth of 3 ~ 3.5 cun. The Deqi sensation from the local site to perineum was achieved. Electrical stimulation was applied to the acupoints with the paired ipsilateral BL30 (the anode) and BL35 (the cathode) under a continuous wave of 2.5-Hz frequency current for 30 min

(Yindi KWD-808-I acupuncture device, Jiangsu, China). The intensity of the electrical current was determined by the tolerance of the patients. The treatment was performed three times per week for 2 weeks (six sessions).

TA treatment
Patients received the same procedures for 2 weeks but traditional treatment was applied. Briefly, the traditional filiform needle (0.3 × 40 mm) was inserted perpendicularly into the bilateral BL30 and BL35 at a depth of 25–35 mm. The Deqi sensation was induced at local site only. The intensity of electrical stimulation (2.5-Hz, continuous wave for 30 min) was the same as that received by the treatment group.

Follow-up
A follow-up was scheduled at week 24 after the patients had started the intervention in our study. The assessor evaluated patients over the telephone during both working hours and non-working hours. The patient was defined as lost to follow-up if he could not be contacted by the assessor within 1 week.

Outcome
The NIH-CPSI was used as the primary outcome measurement. Four domains of NIH-CPSI, including pain or discomfort, urination, the effects of symptoms, and quality of life, were evaluated in a secondary analysis.

The clinical efficacy as the secondary outcome was assessed by determining the percentage of the change in the NIH-CPSI score after treatment ((*score after treatment – score before treatment*)/*score before treatment* × 100%).

A 30% of improvement in NIH-CPSI score was considered clinically effective.

The NIH-CPSI assessment was performed at baseline, week 2, and week 24 (follow-up).

Data analysis
SPSS 16.0 was used for data analysis with the intention-to-treat approach. The last observation carried forward approach was used to estimate the missing value. The *t*-test was used for continuous data between two groups or time-points. The Chi-square test was used for evaluating clinical efficacy. All results were reported as the mean ± standard deviation (SD). A *P* value of less than 0.05 was considered to be statistically significant.

Results
Seventy-seven patients were recruited in the study, 39 of whom received the long-needle treatment and 38 traditional acupuncture treatment. The flowchart is shown in Fig. 1.

The baseline characteristics of the two groups with regard to age, disease duration, NIH-CPSI score and its domains (pain or discomfort score, urination, effects of symptoms, and quality of life), and Chinese Medicine symptom score showed no significant difference (shown in Table 1).

Treatment with LA improved the NIH-CPSI scores
After 2 weeks of acupuncture treatment, the total score of the NIH-CPSI and its four domains (pain or discomfort, urination, effects of symptoms, and quality of life) were significantly decreased in patients who received

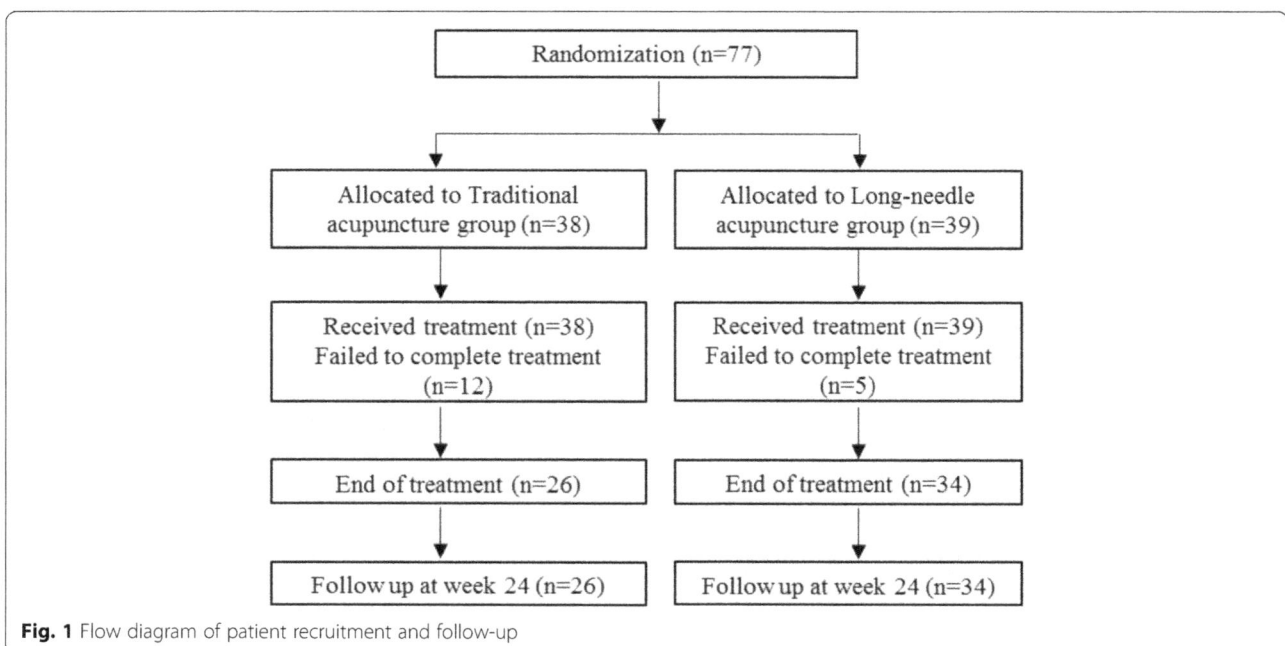

Fig. 1 Flow diagram of patient recruitment and follow-up

Table 1 Baseline characteristics of patients ($\bar{x} \pm S$)

Demographic information	Control group (n = 38)		Treatment group (n = 39)		P value
	Mean ± SD	Range	Mean ± SD	Range	
Age (year)	31.7 ± 6.2	21–44	31.4 ± 7.0	24–50	0.84
Duration (month)	32.4 ± 39.3	3–156	24.3 ± 27.9	3–120	0.31
NIH-CPSI (total)	26.7 ± 4.9	17–37	26.6 ± 5.8	12–37	0.89
Pain or discomfort	11.1 ± 2.8	5–17	11.1 ± 3.1	4–16	1.0
Urination	5.8 ± 2.8	0–10	5.4 ± 3.3	0–11	0.52
Impact of symptoms	5.0 ± 1.0	2–6	5.2 ± 1.1	3–6	0.34
Quality of life	4.9 ± 1.2	2–6	4.9 ± 1.1	3–6	0.84
CM symptom	15.3 ± 7.3	6–34	14.0 ± 5.0	6–24	0.36

either LA or TA ($P < 0.05$) (Table 2). In the LA group, the total score and its four domains were significantly lower than those in the TA group ($P < 0.05$). A 22-week follow-up indicated that the LA treatments reduced the total score and three of its four domains (pain or discomfort, effects of symptoms, and quality of life, but not the urination domain) significantly compared with TA ($P < 0.05$).

LA group had greater improvement in clinical efficacy
After 2 weeks of acupuncture treatment, the Chinese Medicine symptoms in both groups were significantly improved compared with the baselines while the long-needle acupuncture group had a greater reduction from the baseline compared with the TA group (Table 2, CM symptoms). LA had significantly higher clinical effectiveness (30% improvement of NIH-CPSI score) compared to TA ($P = 0.001$) as shown in Table 3.

Discussion
CP/CPPS is the term used in western medicine, but its symptoms were described in ancient books of traditional Chinese medicine as, e.g., the sperm-turbid, white-turbid, and red-turbid. The clinical symptoms of CP are mainly demonstrated in two ways: one is pain in the pelvic cavity and discomfort in other parts and the other is abnormal urination. TA treatment for CP involves

choosing main acupoints in the lower abdomen and lumbosacral region [4], such as RN3 (Zhongji), RN4 (Guanyuan), SP6 (Sanyinjiao), and L23 (Shenshu).

Our previous studies showed that needling at the bilateral BL30 and BL35 significantly improved CP [20, 21]. In Chinese Medicine doctrine, BL30 is an acupoint corresponding to internal essence, where the essence Qi of the human body infuses. This acupoint has the effect of dredging meridians and collaterals, and supplementing the kidney and essence. BL35 was characterized as having the effect of invigorating Qi and removing wet. Acupuncture at the two acupoints could clear dampness-heat, promote blood circulation, and invigorate Qi for the human body. The scientific action mechanism of the electrical deep needling in the study remains largely unexplored. It may be partially associated with the pelvic floor stimulation, which has been used as a physiotherapy to relieve the chronic pelvic pain and incontinence in patients [22–24].

In previous studies, we applied LA with electrical stimulation bilaterally at BL30 and BL35 for CP concurrently with Chinese herbal medicine [20, 21]. We found that needling at BL30 and BL35 could enhance the pudendal nerve stimulation, whereby the concurrent use of acupuncture and Chinese herbal medicine significantly benefited patients with CP/CPPS compared with treatment with Chinese herbal medicine only. In the present

Table 2 NIH-CPSI scores and Chinese Medicine (CM) symptoms after the intervention ($\bar{x} \pm S$)

Scores	TA (n = 38)			LA (n = 39)		
	Pre-treatment	Post-treatment	Follow up	Pre-treatment	Post-treatment	Follow up
NIH-CPSI (total)	26.7 ± 4.9	22.6 ± 5.2*	17.3 ± 9.1*	26.6 ± 5.8	17.0 ± 6.0*△	9.4 ± 8.6*△
Pain or discomfort	11.1 ± 2.8	9.0 ± 2.7*	6.6 ± 4.0*	11.1 ± 3.1	6.5 ± 3.0*△	3.3 ± 3.8*△
Urination	5.8 ± 2.8	5.0 ± 2.0*	3.8 ± 3.1*	5.4 ± 3.3	3.5 ± 2.6*△	2.1 ± 2.6*
Impact of symptoms	5.0 ± 1.0	4.4 ± 1.2*	3.4 ± 1.8*	5.2 ± 1.1	3.5 ± 1.6*△	2.0 ± 1.7*△
Quality of life	4.9 ± 1.2	4.4 ± 1.4*	3.5 ± 1.7*	4.9 ± 1.1	3.5 ± 1.3*△	2.0 ± 1.6*△
CM symptom	15.3 ± 7.3	12.1 ± 5.7*	-	14.0 ± 5.0	8.4 ± 5.3*△	-

*, $P < 0.05$ when comparison the pre-treatment score and post-treatment score in the same group; △, $P < 0.05$ when comparing the long-needle acupuncture group and the conventional acupuncture group. An ITT method was applied for analysis

Table 3 Clinical efficacy in the long-needle acupuncture and traditional acupuncture groups at week 2 (n = 77)

	TA (n = 38)	LA (n = 39)	p-value
Clinical efficacy, No. (%)			
Effective	8 (21.1)	22 (56.4)	0.001
Ineffective	30 (78.9)	17 (43.6)	

LA long-needle acupuncture; TA traditional acupuncture; ITT method and chi-square test was used for the analysis

study, we examined whether needling at BL30 and BL35 had a therapeutic effect compared with the TA treatment. The findings demonstrated that LA had a superior effect than TA, although the change in the absolute value of the NIH-CPSI score was small but significant. For example, the difference in the NIH-CPSI score was 4.7 (4.7/43*100% = 11.9%). Because the control in the study was a positive treatment, the difference between the two treatments is relatively smaller than that which a sham control would provide. However, it pragmatically reflects real clinical practice and evaluates the effectiveness of LA treatment rather than its efficacy. In fact, the change in NIH-CPSI from baseline was 24.1% after long-needle treatment. The clinical efficacy analysis (30% of improvement in NIH-CPSI score) indicated LA is clinically superior to TA.

In the present study, both TA and LA needling at BL30 and BL35 had a therapeutic effect on CP/CPPS. However, when needling at the same acupoints, the deep insertion of the long needle significantly improved CP/CPPS compared with TA. The stimulation of the pudendal nerve by needles may be the key mechanism to the relief of CP/CPPS. The pudendal nerve is the main sensory and motor nerve of the perineum and supplies sensation from the genitalia and control of the urethral sphincter and anal sphincter. Anatomically, the pudendal nerve passes through the tissue under the deep area at BL30 and BL35; therefore, the deep insertion of long needles at these acupoints may enhance the stimulation of the pudendal nerve and thereby promote the inhibition of local sensations passing to the central nervous system [25, 26]. The long-needle manipulation may trigger a stronger contraction of the deep transverse perineal muscle, and consequently improve the local blood circulation of prostate and reduce inflammation in the pelvis [17, 27]. The mechanism needs to be further determined.

In this study, no serious adverse effects were found. Skin bruising and slight bleeding were occasionally observed in both groups and deep needling increases the risk of pelvic injuries. The long-needle treatment should be performed by an experienced acupuncturist. Urinalysis and a fecal occult blood test are recommended to monitor any potential injuries.

The study had limitations. The sample size in the pilot study was small. A large number of patients didn't complete the intervention in the TA and LA groups. One of the reasons for dropping out was that the patients were not tolerant to acupuncture treatment. The majority of reasons for dropping out were not detected as most patients could not be reached by telephone. The study had only one time-point of follow-up while follow-ups need to be made at multiple time-points in the future. Objective parameters, e.g. white blood cells in expressed prostatic secretion, could be used to evaluate chronic prostatitis. As the present study evaluated the effectiveness of acupuncture, the potential placebo effect cannot be excluded. A sham acupuncture can be used to measure the efficacy of acupuncture by excluding the potential placebo effect.

Conclusion

The present study demonstrated that deep needling at BL 30 and BL35 using LA significantly improved CP/CPPS compared with TA. The study supported a large-scale randomized controlled trial to evaluate LA for CP/CPPS.

Acknowledgements
The authors sincerely thank patients for their participation in the study.

Funding
The study was supported by the funds from Shanghai Municipal Health Bureau (No. 20134164) and Shanghai Health and Family Planning Commission Chinese Medicine Research Fund (2014LP061A).

Authors' contributions
JY contributed to the study conception and design, data collection; supervised the study; and drafted and edited the manuscript. MZ, MY, LC, CY, WZ, JJ, CC participated to the study design, study management, and data collection and cleaning. XS contributed to the study conception and design, advised study management, provided logistic support, oversaw data management and analysis, and edited the manuscript. All authors read and approved the final manuscript.

Authors' information
Researchers work at Shanghai Qigong Research Institute, Shanghai, China and the Longhua Hospital Shanghai University of Traditional Chinese Medicine, Shanghai, China.

Competing interests
The authors declare that they have no competing interests.

Author details
[1]Shanghai Qigong Research Institute, Shanghai, China. [2]Graduate School, The Shanghai University of Traditional Chinese Medicine, Shanghai, China. [3]The Department of Pain Management, Luoyang Central Hospital, Luoyang, China. [4]The Longhua Hospital Shanghai University of Traditional Chinese Medicine, Shanghai, China. [5]Shanghai TCM-INTEGRATED Hospital, Shanghai, Shanghai University of Traditional Chinese Medicine, Shanghai, China.

References
1. Strauss AC, Dimitrakov JD. New treatments for chronic prostatitis/chronic pelvic pain syndrome. Nat Rev Urol. 2010;7(3):127–35.
2. Kwon JK, Chang IH. Pain, catastrophizing, and depression in chronic prostatitis/chronic pelvic pain syndrome. Int Neurourol J. 2013;17(2):48–58.

3. Nickel JC. Inflammation and benign prostatic hyperplasia. Urol Clin North Am. 2008;35(1):109–15. vii
4. Pontari MA. Chronic prostatitis/chronic pelvic pain syndrome in elderly men: toward better understanding and treatment. Drugs Aging. 2003;20(15): 1111–25.
5. Le B, Schaeffer AJ. Chronic prostatitis. BMJ Clin Evid. 2011;2011
6. McNaughton C, Mac Donald R, Wilt T. Interventions for chronic abacterial prostatitis. Cochrane Database Syst Rev. 2001;1:CD002080.
7. Duclos AJ, Lee CT, Shoskes DA. Current treatment options in the management of chronic prostatitis. Ther Clin Risk Manag. 2007;3(4):507–12.
8. Udoji MA, Ness TJ. New directions in the treatment of pelvic pain. Pain Manag. 2013;3(5):387–94.
9. Lee SH, Lee BC. Use of acupuncture as a treatment method for chronic prostatitis/chronic pelvic pain syndromes. Current urology reports. 2011; 12(4):288–96.
10. Cohen JM, Fagin AP, Hariton E, Niska JR, Pierce MW, Kuriyama A, Whelan JS, Jackson JL, Dimitrakoff JD. Therapeutic intervention for chronic prostatitis/chronic pelvic pain syndrome (CP/CPPS): a systematic review and meta-analysis. PLoS One. 2012;7(8):e41941.
11. Lee SH, Lee BC. Electroacupuncture relieves pain in men with chronic prostatitis/chronic pelvic pain syndrome: three-arm randomized trial. Urology. 2009;73(5):1036–41.
12. Lee SW, Liong ML, Yuen KH, Krieger JN. Acupuncture and immune function in chronic prostatitis/chronic pelvic pain syndrome: a randomized, controlled study. Complement Ther Med. 2014;22(6):965–9.
13. Lee SW, Liong ML, Yuen KH, Leong WS, Chee C, Cheah PY, Choong WP, Wu Y, Khan N, Choong WL et al: Acupuncture versus sham acupuncture for chronic prostatitis/chronic pelvic pain. Am J Med 2008; 121(1):79 e71–77.
14. Tugcu V, Tas S, Eren G, Bedirhan B, Karadag S, Tasci A. Effectiveness of acupuncture in patients with category IIIB chronic pelvic pain syndrome: a report of 97 patients. Pain Med. 2010;11(4):518–23.
15. Carlsson C. Acupuncture mechanisms for clinically relevant long-term effects–reconsideration and a hypothesis. Acupunct Med. 2002;20(2–3):82–99.
16. MacPherson H, Altman DG, Hammerschlag R, Youping L, Taixiang W, White A, Moher D, Group SR. Revised STandards for reporting interventions in clinical trials of acupuncture (STRICTA): extending the CONSORT statement. PLoS Med. 2010;7(6):e1000261.
17. Ge J, Ge S. Clinical observation on treatment of chronic prostatitis with deeply needling main point Baihuanshu. Chinese Acupuncture & Moxibustion. 2001;21(2):73–4.
18. Zhong W, Yuan Y. Acupunture on Huiyang acupoint (BL35) for chronic prostatitis: a clinical observation of 30 cases. Journal of Clinical Acupuncture and Moxibustion. 2003;19(4):45–6.
19. Wu J. WU Jieping Urology. Jinan: Shandong Science and Technology Press; 2004.
20. Yang MY, Ying J, Li JX, Wang SY, Zhou MJ, Zhang W. Clinical observation of Electroacupuncture at Baihuanshu(BL30) and Huiyang(BL35) for chronic prostatitis. Shanghai Journal of Acupuncture and Moxibustion. 2014;33(10): 913–5.
21. Ying J, Li JX, Wang SY, Yue YM. Zhou Mj, Shang YY: clinical observation of Electroacupuncture at Baihuanshu(BL30) and Huiyang(BL35) for chronic Abacterial prostatitis. Shanghai Journal of Acupuncture and Moxibustion. 2014;33(12):1102–4.
22. Goode PS, Burgio KL, Johnson TM 2nd, Clay OJ, Roth DL, Markland AD, Burkhardt JH, Issa MM, Lloyd LK. Behavioral therapy with or without biofeedback and pelvic floor electrical stimulation for persistent postprostatectomy incontinence: a randomized controlled trial. JAMA. 2011; 305(2):151–9.
23. Doggweiler R, Stewart AF. Pelvic floor therapies in chronic pelvic pain syndrome. Current urology reports. 2011;12(4):304–11.
24. Polackwich AS, Li J, Shoskes DA. Patients with pelvic floor muscle spasm have a superior response to pelvic floor physical therapy at specialized centers. J Urol. 2015;194(4):1002–6.
25. Zheng H. The deep needling at BL29 and BL35 for voiding dysfunctions. Shanghai Journal of Acupuncture and Moxibustion. 1993;12(2):64–5.
26. Chen Y, Shen P, Chen G, Zhang L. Experimental study on the effect of Electroacupuncture of "Huiyang" and "Zhonglushu" on Urodynamics in nonbacterial prostatitis rats. Acupuncture Research. 2001;26(2):127–30.
27. Wang s-y, Chen G-m, Li L-h: "Four sacral needles" therapy for female stress incontinence. Shanghai Journal of Acupuncture and Moxibustion 2006, 25(5):13–15.

18

Optimizing acupuncture treatment for dry eye syndrome

Bong Hyun Kim[1,2], Min Hee Kim[1,3], Se Hyun Kang[1,2] and Hae Jeong Nam[1,2*] (iD)

Abstracts

Background: In a former meta-analysis review, acupuncture was considered a potentially effective treatment for dry eye syndrome (DES), but there were heterogeneities among the outcomes. We updated the meta-analysis and conducted subgroup analysis to reduce the heterogeneity and suggest the most effective acupuncture method based on clinical trials.

Methods: We searched for randomized controlled trials (RCTs) in 10 databases (MEDLINE, EMBASE, CENTAL, AMED, SCOPUS, CNKI, Wangfang database, Oriental Medicine Advanced Searching Integrated System (OASIS), Koreamed, J-stage) and searched by hand to compare the effects of acupuncture and artificial tears (AT). We also conducted subgroup analysis by (1) method of intervention (acupuncture only or acupuncture plus AT), (2) intervention frequency (less than 3 times a week or more than 3 times a week), (3) period of treatment (less than 4 weeks or more than 4 weeks), and (4) acupoints (BL1, BL2, ST1, ST2, TE23, Ex-HN5). The Bucher method was used for subgroup comparisons.

Results: Nineteen studies with 1126 patients were included. Significant improvements on the Schirmer test (weighted mean difference[WMD], 2.14; 95% confidence interval[CI], 0.93 to 3.34; $p = 0.0005$) and break up time (BUT) (WMD, 0.98; 95% CI, 0.79 to 1.18; $p < 0.00001$) were reported. In the subgroup analysis, acupuncture plus AT treatment had a weaker effect in BUT but a stronger effect on the Schirmer test and a better overall effect than acupuncture alone. For treatment duration, treatment longer than 1 month was more effective than shorter treatment. With regard to treatment frequency, treatment less than three times a week was more effective than more frequent treatment. In the acupoint analysis, acupuncture treatment including the BL2 and ST1 acupoints was less effective than treatment that did not include them. None of those factors reduced the heterogeneity.

Conclusions: Acupuncture was more effective than AT in treating DES but showed high heterogeneity. Intervention differences did not influence the heterogeneity.

Keywords: Dry eye syndrome, Acupuncture, Systematic review

Background

Dry eye syndrome (DES) is a multifactorial disease of the tears and ocular surface that can result in ocular discomfort and visual impairment [1]. In recent years, the geriatric proportion of the overall population has increased, and factors causing eye fatigue have diversified (e.g., excessive use of computers or smartphones). In 2011, the prevalence of DES in South Korea was 8.0% [2]. According to statistics from the National Health Insurance Service in South Korea, the prevalence of DES is increasing continuously "(http://opendata.hira.or.kr/home.do)".

Acupuncture can alleviate DES. Some systematic reviews showed that acupuncture is effective for DES [3–5]. However, heterogeneous results from various interventions made it difficult to draw clear conclusions. Each study used different acupoints, durations, and frequencies. An individual treatment strategy according to patient condition is ideal. However, an individual treatment strategy depends on each clinician's subjective experience, which indicates low effectiveness of novice practitioners. An

* Correspondence: ophthrl@khu.ac.kr
[1]Department of Ophthalmology and Otolaryngology of Korean Medicine, College of Korean Medicine, Kyung Hee University, 26, Kyungheedae-ro, Dongdaemun-gu, Seoul 02453, Republic of Korea
[2]Department of Ophthalmology and Otolaryngology of Korean Medicine, Kyung Hee University Korean Medicine Hospital, 23, Kyungheedae-ro, Dongdaemun-gu, Seoul 02447, Republic of Korea
Full list of author information is available at the end of the article

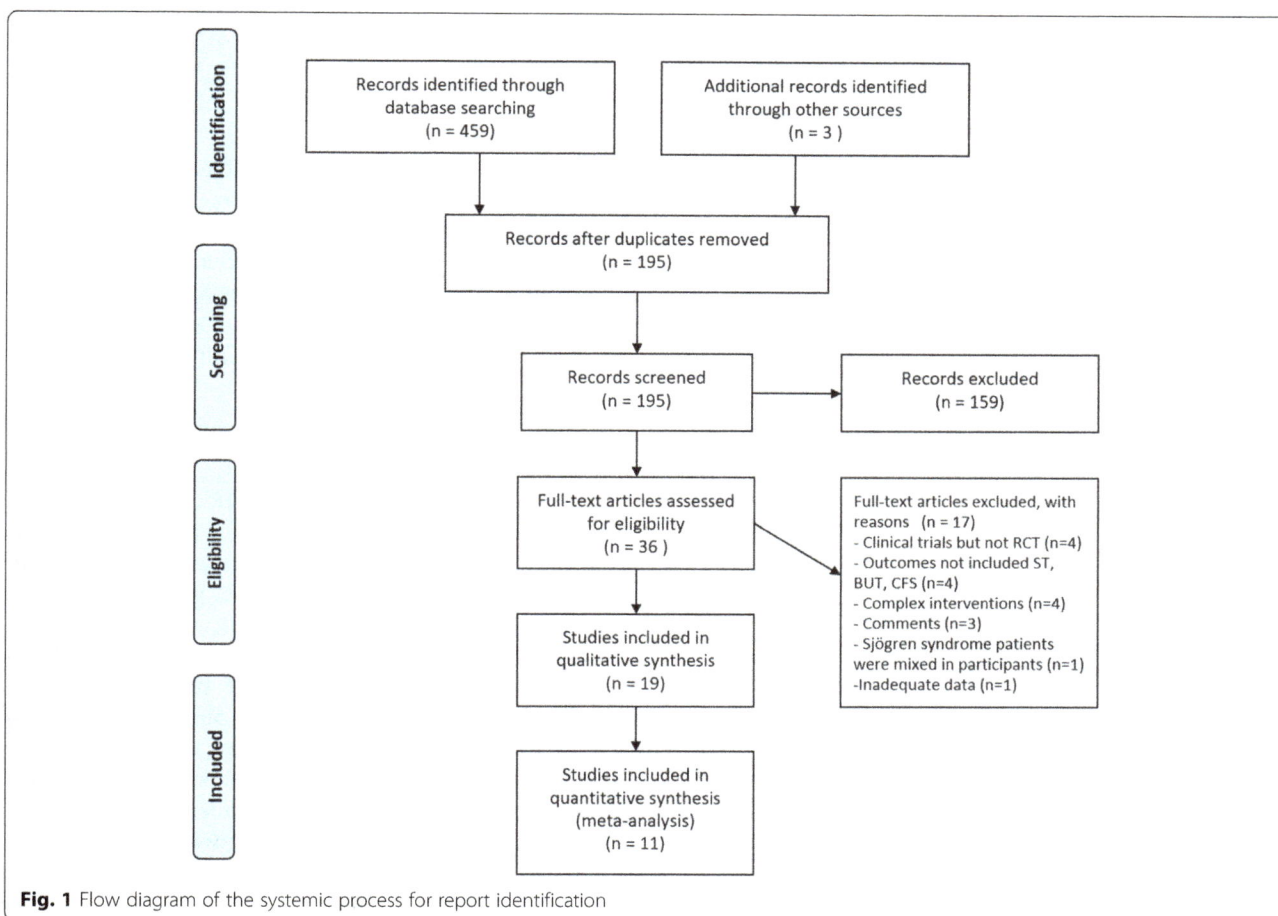

Fig. 1 Flow diagram of the systemic process for report identification

adequate acupuncture dose is needed to standardize and optimize its effects. Also, some standards are required to increase the reproducibility of results. There have been some attempts to define adequate acupuncture treatments for other diseases [6, 7].

Our aim in this study was to evaluate the efficacy of acupuncture using the latest research and to suggest a standard acupuncture treatment for patients with DES, including acupoints, number of sessions, and treatment duration. Therefore, we conducted a systematic review of published acupuncture treatments for DES and analyzed the factors that influence therapeutic effectiveness.

Methods

Search strategy

We searched MEDLINE, EMBASE, CENTAL, AMED, SCOPUS, CNKI, the Wangfang database, the Oriental Medicine Advanced Searching Integrated System (OASIS), Koreamed, and J-stage and conducted manual searches for potentially relevant articles published through July 2017. (CNKI and Wangfang are Chinese databases. OASIS and Koreamed are Korean databases. J-stage is a Japanese database.) The search terms used were 'acupuncture' AND ('dry eye' OR 'xerophthalmia' OR 'keratoconjunctivitis sicca'). In the Chinese databases (CNKI, Wangfang database), we used the Chinese terms ('干眼' AND '针'). There were no limits with regard to publications, other than language limits of English, Chinese, or Korean.

Study selection

The specific inclusion criteria were as follows: (1) clinical trial for DES patients; (2) use of acupuncture or an applied form (e.g., electroacupuncture, pyonex); (3) control group that received appropriate placebo or artificial tears (AT); (4) outcomes included Schirmer's test (ST), break up time test (BUT), or corneal fluorescein staining (CFS); (5) randomized controlled trials (RCT); and (6) full text available. We excluded (1) studies that included Sjögren syndrome patients and (2) interventions combined with other treatments (e.g., herbal medicine, moxibustion). Two researchers (MHK and SHK) carried out the study selection independently and discussed their differences.

Data extraction and assessment of risk of bias

Three independent reviewers (MHK, BHK and SHK) read all selected articles. We extracted publication data, participant information, intervention regime (sites, duration, and frequency), outcome measures, and drop-outs. After extraction, we assessed the risk of bias using the Cochrane Collaboration tool [8].

Data analysis

For our meta-analysis of similar treatment interventions, we used the statistical software provided by the Cochrane Collaboration (RevMan 5.3). The estimated effect of the data was calculated using the weighted mean difference (WMD) and confidence interval (CI). The Q-test or χ^2 was used to evaluate heterogeneity [9]. When the compared populations were homogeneous (Q-test $p > 0.1$), we used the fixed-effect model; when they were heterogeneous ($p < 0.1$), we used the random-effect model. We also performed a sensitivity analysis. Each study was sequentially excluded from the meta-analysis, and the sensitivity was determined from the corresponding heterogeneity results. Funnel plot was conducted for detecting publication bias.

In our subgroup analysis, we used the standard mean difference (SMD) in BUT and ST values to evaluate the overall effects according to the Bucher method. This is one of the most suitable indirect comparisons for RCTs. We applied this method, as there were no direct comparative trials and an indirect method can provide useful information for optimization. This method is supposed that treatments A and C are compared in one RCT and treatments B and C are compared in another RCT, the indirect comparison of A and B is adjusted according to C (common comparator). This method assumes that indirect evidence is consistent with a direct comparison [10].

We analyzed the interventions as follows: (1) method of intervention (acupuncture only or acupuncture plus AT), (2) intervention frequency (less than 3 times a week or more than 3 times a week), (3) treatment duration (less than 4 weeks or more than 4 weeks), and (4) acupoints (BL1, BL2, ST1, ST2, TE23, Ex-HN5). Selection of the acupoints frequently used in clinical trials is explained in a previous study [11].

Results

Literary search

We identified 462 articles of potential relevance. Screening the titles and abstracts yielded 36 studies. After reviewing the full texts, we selected 19 studies. Studies were excluded for the following reasons: (1) not an RCT ($n = 4$); (2) outcomes did not include ST, BUT, or CFS (n = 4); (3) acupuncture was part of a complex intervention (n = 4); (4) comments ($n = 3$); (5) inadequate data ($n = 1$); (6) Sjögren syndrome patients were included as participants (n = 1). The procedure is summarized in Fig. 1.

Study description

We included 19 studies and 1126 subjects in this review. Fourteen studies [12–25] compared manual acupuncture with AT. One study [26] used sham acupuncture as a control group. Four studies [27–30] used an applied form of acupuncture (two studies used electroacupuncture, and two used pyonex). Fifteen of the studies [13, 14, 16–19, 21–25, 27–30] were conducted in China. The study descriptions are given in Tables 1 and 2.

Risk of bias assessment

In 8 studies [14, 16, 19–21, 23, 26, 28], the investigators described a method of random sequence generation (random number table, coin tossing, envelope shuffling, and using a computerized random-number generator). Only 4 studies [16, 20, 26, 28] conducted allocation concealment, and 4 studies [15, 19, 20, 28] used assessor blinding. Drop rates and reasons were reported in 6 studies [19, 20, 23, 26, 28]. Two studies used a study protocol [20, 26]. In 4 studies, we suspected bias: two studies [16, 17] had significant differences between the treatment and control groups at baseline without revision or explanation; in the other two studies, the duration differed between the treatment and control groups [13, 14]. Figure 2 summarizes the risk of bias assessment. Furthermore, there was no evidence of significant publication bias by inspection of the funnel plots.

Meta-analysis between manual acupuncture and artificial tears

In this meta-analysis, we used the results of 11 of 14 studies that recorded both BUT and ST. We excluded Nepp [10] and Gong [15] because the former showed only graph and the later showed change value. We also excluded Zhang [22] through our sensitivity analysis because it presented a heterogeneous result that did not seem to be due to acupuncture. We did not consider CFS results in this meta-analysis because two studies used a dichotomous scale [13, 14], three used a continuous scale [18, 22, 23], and they used different methods of measuring.

In the BUT results, a significant difference was shown between groups (WMD, 0.92; 95% CI, 0.60 to 1.25; $p < 0.00001$), but the heterogeneity was high ($I^2 = 62\%$; $P = 0.003$). The studies that used an acupuncture plus AT intervention did not show a mean difference ($p = 0.21$), but the studies that used only acupuncture did show a significant difference ($p < 0.00001$), including a subgroup difference($p = 0.04$) (Fig. 3).

Table 1 Characteristics of included studies (manual acupuncture vs. artificial tears)

First author	Year	Site	Sample size[a]	Age	Gender (M/F)	Regime (acupoints)	Duration (min)	Frequency (per week)	Total sessions	Outcomes
Nepp [12]	1998	Austria	52 (30/22)	N/A	N/A	GB1, BL2, ST5, EX-HN2, LI4, SI3, LI3, KI6, TE5	30	1	10	ST, BUT, drop frequency
He [13]	2004	China	32 (16/16)	52	12/20	Pattern identification was done by practitioner (ST2, LI20, LI11, LI4, SP6 OR ST2, SP10, SP9, SP6, ST36, KI6)	20–25	3–4 (every other day)	30	ST, BUT, CFS
Wang [14]	2005	China	45(A)15, (B)15/15	51.7	17/28	(A) Pattern identification was done by practitioner (LI11, LI4 SP6, KI3, ST2, LI20 or ST2, SP10, SP9, ST36, SP6, ST40) (B) BL2, TE23, GB14, ST1	20–25	3–4 (every other day)	20	ST, BUT, CFS, RR
Tseng [15]	2006	Taiwan	26 (17/9)	48.9	12/14	Ex-HN5, TE23, GB14, ST2, SP6	20	2	16	ST, BUT, Number of application of artificial tears
Zhang [16]	2009	China	60 (30/30)	44	23/37	ST1, LR3, KI3	20	N/A	N/A	ST, BUT, total symptoms
Gong [17]	2010	China	42 (20/22)	44.8	11/33	BL1, BL2, GB14, SJ23, Ex-HN5, ST2, LI4, LR3, GB37, SP6, GB20	20	3 (every other day)	10	ST, BUT, RBS recording, total score
Gao [18]	2010	China	56 (28/28)	48.9	3/53	BL1, BL2, TE23, GB1,Ex-HN5	30	6	24	ST, BUT, total score
Shi [19]	2012	China	68 (33/35)	49.5	30/38	Ex-HN1, BL1, ST1, Ex-HN5, TE23, LI4, ST36	25	3	9	ST, BUT, tear lactoferrin concentration
Kim [20]	2012	Korea	150 (75/75)	42	41/109	BL2, GB14, TE23, Ex-HN5, ST1, GB20, LI4 LI11, GV23	20	3	12	OSDI, VAS, BUT, ST, MYMOP-2
Nan [21]	2014	China	60 (30/30)	48.1	25/35	Eye acupuncture (liver/gallbladder area, kidney area, spleen stomach area, upper jiao area)	15–20	7	20	ST, BUT, total score
Zhang [22]	2015	China	80 (40/40)	53	28/52	Hair needle therapy (superior and inferior lacrimal puncta)	10	3–4 (every other day)	7	ST, BUT, CFS, total score
Ni [23]	2016	China	93(A)30, (B)32/31	33.3	36/57	(A) BL1, Ex-HN7, SP6, KI3, GV26 (B) BL1, Ex-HN7, SP6, KI3	20	3	9	ST BUT, subjective symptom score
Chao [24]	2016	China	53(A)18, (B)19/16	48.9	15/38	(A), (B) GB20, Ex-HN5, BL2, ST2, LR3, KI3, SP6, SP6, ST36, ST37 (A) applied a qi-absorption needling technique to the GB20	30	7	28	ST, BUT, VAS, CFS total score
Liu [25]	2017	China	28 (14/14)	60.7	0/28	BL2, BL3, TE23, Ex-HN5, ST2, LI4, GB20, GV20, ST1	30	3	24	ST, BUT, OSDI, questionnaire, protein analysis

M/F male/female, ST Schirmer's test, BUT break-up time, CFS corneal fluorescein staining, RBS Rose-Bengal staining, RR response rate, OSDI ocular surface disease index, a questionnaire
[a]Total sample size (number who received manual acupuncture/number who received artificial tears)

Table 2 Characteristics of included studies (other kinds of interventions)

First author	Year	Site	Sample size[a]	Age	Gender (M/F)	Regime (intervention/control group)	Regime (frequency & duration)	Outcomes
Shin [26]	2010	Korea	42 (21/21)	41.6	11/31	Intervention: manual acupuncture GV23, BL2, BL14, TE23, Ex-HN5, ST-1, GB20, SP3, LU9, LU10, HT8 Control: non-acupoints around same site	Needles were retained for 20 min, 3 times a week for a total of 9 times. It takes 3 weeks to complete the treatment.	BUT, SIT, VAS, OSDI
Liu [27]	2012	China	39 (20/19)	32	21/19	Intervention: electro-acupuncture with BL1, Ex-HN5, BL2, TE23, GB1, GB20, KI3, SP6, LR3 Control: Artificial tears	Everyday treatment group undergoes electroacupuncture for 30 min. For a total of 20 sessions.	SIT, BUT
Guo [28]	2013	China	47 (23/24)	52	7/40	Intervention: electro-acupuncture with shang-jingming (Ex), xia-jingming (Ex), GB1, BL2, GB20, LI4, SP6, KI3, LR3 Control: manual acupuncture with the same acupoints	Needles were retained for 20 min, 3 times a week for a total of 12 times. It takes 4 weeks to complete the treatment.	BUT, SIT, VAS
Gao [29]	2016	China	88 (44/44)	41.8	33/55	A: pyonex combined with acupuncture, SP6, ST36, PC6, LR3 are the main points, and pattern identification was done (BL13, LI4 OR BL20, ST40 OR BL18, BL23) B: manual acupuncture with GV20, ST1, BL2, GB20, Ex-HN5, TE23	A: pyonex was embedded for 3 days. The follwing day, it was embedded again. This process was repeated four times and followed by two days free from embedment. After that, another four courses of embedment were conducted. B: needles were retained for 30 min every day for 12 days. Two days rest were followed by another 12 days of treatment.	SIT BUT, total score
Wu [30]	2016	China	40 (20/20)	44.2	10/30	Intervention: BL2, ST2, Ex-HN5 Control: artificial tears	Treatment group undergoes embedding therapy (retained for 24 h) on alternate days for 7 sessions.	BUT, SIT, OSDI

M/F male/female, *ST* Schirmer's test, *BUT* break-up time, *OSDI* ocular surface disease index, a questionnaire
[a]Total sample size (number in intervention group/number in control group)

The ST results also showed a significant difference between manual acupuncture and AT (WMD, 1.98; 95% CI, 0.62 to 3.35; $p = 0.004$), though again, the heterogeneity of the effect was high ($I^2 = 96\%$; $P < 0.00001$). Each of the two subgroups showed significant differences within the groups, but we did not find differences between the subgroups. (WMD, 1.65; 95% CI, 0.37 to 2.92 versus WMD, 2.93; 95% CI, 0.32 to 5.55; $p = 0.39$) (Fig. 4).

Two studies [20, 25] evaluated OSDI scores, and they showed no significant differences between groups (WMD, -5.70; 95% CI, -11.49 to 0.09; $p = 0.05$, Fig. 5).

Subgroup analysis
In treatment duration and frequency, long-term (more than 1 month) and less frequent (less than 3 times a week) treatments were more effective than short-term or

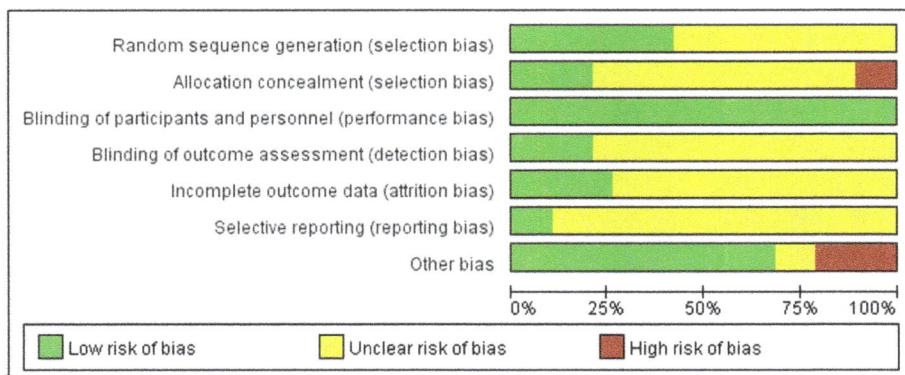

Fig. 2 Risk of bias summary in included studies

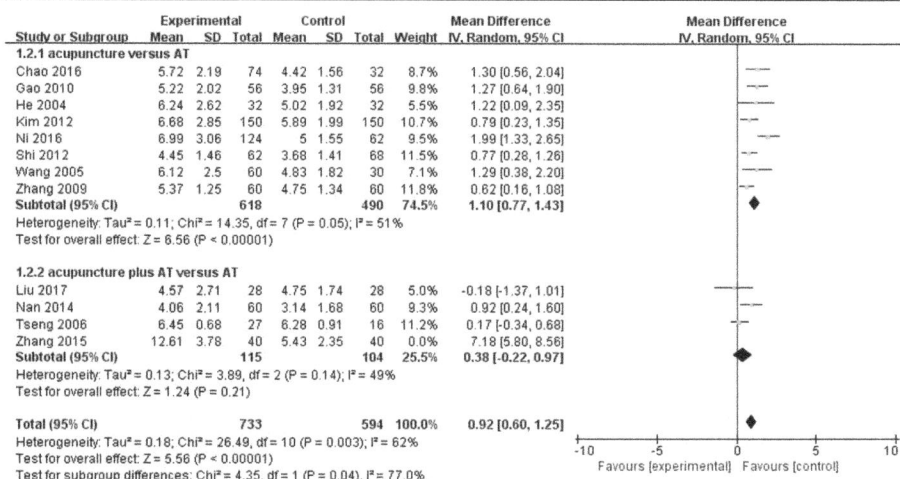

Fig. 3 Break up time (BUT) comparison between acupuncture and artificial tears (AT): Random effect model

intensive treatments, but the difference was not significant. (Table 3).

In acupoint differences, regimes including the BL2 or ST1 acupoints showed significantly weaker effects than regimes that did not include them (BL2; SMD, 0.35 vs 0. 81; $p = 0.03$, ST1, SMD, 0.28 vs 0.91; $p = 0.002$). There were no significantly different values for other acupoints (BL1, TE23, ST2, Ex-HN5, Table 3).

Other interventions

One study compared verum acupuncture with sham acupuncture [26]. In this study, the sham acupuncture was applied to non-acupoints (peri-acupoints). There were no significantly different outcomes between the verum and sham acupuncture groups. Two studies used

electroacupuncture: Liu et al. compared electroacupuncture with AT and found significant ST and BUT effects in the experimental group [27]; Guo et al. compared electroacupuncture at BL1 with manual acupuncture and found minor effects in eye symptoms and ST in the intervention group [28]. Two studies investigated pyonex: one study compared pyonex with manual acupuncture [29], and the other compared it with AT and found limited improvements compared with the control group [30] (Table 2).

Discussion

Some previous systematic reviews have considered the effects of acupuncture in DES [3–5]. In this study, we focused on subgroup analysis to solidify the results and suggest an effective method of acupuncture treatment.

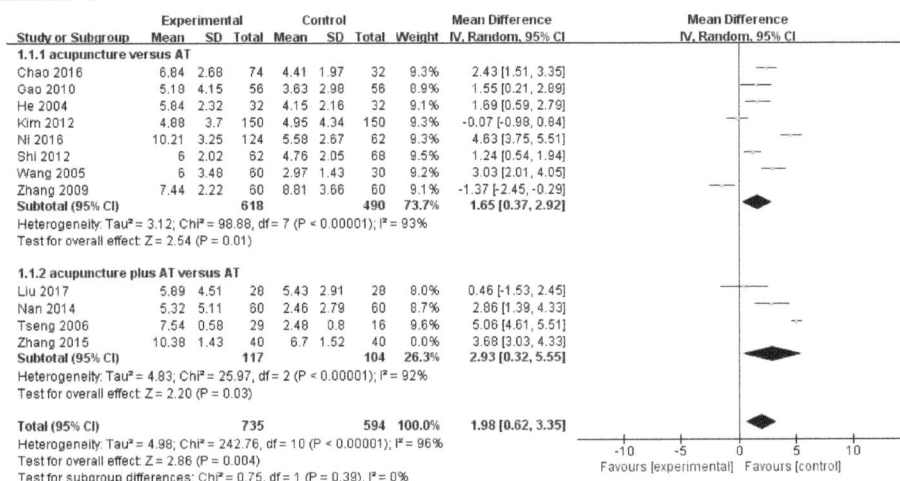

Fig. 4 Schirmer's test (ST) comparison between acupuncture and artificial tears (AT): Random effect model

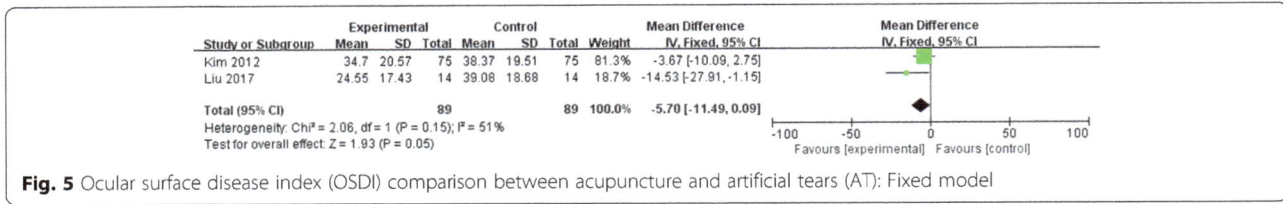

Fig. 5 Ocular surface disease index (OSDI) comparison between acupuncture and artificial tears (AT): Fixed model

We excluded one study [22] for heterogeneity because it showed a unique change and used an unusual intervention: the practitioners treated the superior/inferior lacrimal punctum and proceeded horizontally 5-15 mm through the lacrimal canaliculi, similar to lacrimal probing. This effect focused on penetration, so it was difficult to regard its effects as resulting purely from the acupuncture.

As in former studies, heterogeneity in the effects of manual acupuncture was high; we conducted subgroup analysis for method of intervention, treatment duration, frequency, and acupoints. However, accounting for those factors did not lower the heterogeneity. A high risk of bias can cause heterogeneity. Information about the randomization method, number of and reason for drop outs, statistical analysis methods, and blinding outcome analysis is essential to decrease the risk of bias in a clinical study. However, several studies did not include this data.

Acupuncture combined with AT treatment had a weaker effect on BUT score but a stronger effect on ST score and a better overall effect than acupuncture treatment alone. ST evaluates tear production, and BUT evaluates tear film stabilization. Acupuncture plus AT thus showed a synergetic effect in tear production but not in tear stabilization. Manual acupuncture affected the protein composition in tears [19, 25], but combining with AT, there was no synergetic effect, which clinicians should consider when planning treatments for individual patients.

With regard to duration and frequency, a long period of treatment (more than 1 month) is preferable to a short period (less than 1 month), but frequent treatment does not guarantee better effects. Three times a week showed better effectiveness than 5–6 times a week. Recovery time might be needed to produce optimal effects. Harris et al. said that the effects of acupuncture are dose dependent [31]. Experts recommend at least twice a week to obtain a proper effect [32]. Therefore, 2–3 times a week

Table 3 Results of subgroup analysis by treatment duration, frequency, and specific acupoints

Variables		Number of studies	Number of eyes		SMD	95%CI	Heterogeneity (I^2)	MD (95% CI)
			Acupuncture	AT				
Duration	Short term	7	586	488	0.54	0.30–0.78	86%	−0.41 (−1.10, 0.28)
	Long term	4	148	106	0.95	0.30–1.59	87%	
Frequency	Less frequent	4	250	208	0.49	0.19–0.79	79%	−0.22 (−0.67, 0.22)
	Intensive	7	484	386	0.71	0.37–1.05	90%	
BL1	Included	4	270	214	0.60	0.29–0.91	81%	−0.04 (−0.49, 0.41)
	Not included	7	464	380	0.64	0.32–.96	89%	
BL2[a]	Included	4	264	264	0.35	0.11–0.60	71%	−0.46 (− 0.86, − 0.06)
	Not included	8	470	360	0.81	0.49–1.12	89%	
ST1[a]	Included	5	330	336	0.28	0.01–0.52	77%	−0.63 (−1.02, − 0.24)
	Not included	7	404	288	0.91	0.60–1.22	85%	
ST2	Included	4	148	106	0.95	0.30–1.59	91%	0.41 (−0.28, 1.10)
	Not included	7	586	488	0.54	0.30–0.78	86%	
TE23[a]	Included	6	354	348	0.59	0.25–0.96	88%	−0.10 (− 0.55, 0.35)
	Not included	6	380	276	0.69	0.40–0.99	87%	
Ex-HN5	Included	6	398	350	0.60	0.27–0.93	88%	−0.03 (−0.56, 0.50)
	Not included	5	336	244	0.63	0.30–0.96	86%	

[a]Wang et al. [15] study consists of two different acupuncture group. One group included BL2, ST1, TE23 and the other did not. For the reason, number of studies and number of eyes of AT group was double-counted

could be an optimal frequency to maximize the effects.

Most studies we selected included periorbital acupoints. Thus, the effects of acupuncture in DES are mostly local. According to Shin et al. [26], the effect of acupuncture on DES occurs by dilating blood vessels and increasing the supply of neuropeptides (e.g., Calcitonin gene related peptide). However, our analysis implied positional specificity. The studies that included points BL2 and ST1 were less effective than those that did not include those points. This could be related to the analgesic effect of acupuncture. ST1 is located between the eyeball and the infraorbital ridge, directly below the pupil, and BL2 is located at the medial end of the eyebrow. They are thus near the supraorbital nerve block and infraorbital nerve block sites. Those two nerves innervate the conjunctiva, and decreased conjunctiva sensitivity decreases tear production. Therefore, clinicians should select acupoints according to patient symptoms.

Some of the included studies also considered electroacupuncture and pyonex. Electroacupuncture is commonly considered to be a stronger stimulus than acupuncture. Pyonex is a kind of patch acupuncture known for its long retention. However, only a few studies used those interventions, and they had many limitations in design. Therefore, we did not evaluate the effects of electroacupuncture and pyonex in DES. Well-designed studies are needed to evaluate their effects.

Additionally, Female sex is a risk factor in DES [33]. In our study, there were also female subjects than male subjects. Sex hormone (e.g., androgen) can be a factor in explaining this result. Androgen have a positive effect as anti-inflammatory effect on DES [34, 35]. Acupuncture may modulate sex hormone [36]. However, there was no study focusing on this point. Further study concerning about the hormone is needed to clarify the mechanism of acupuncture.

Our study has several limitations. We conducted indirect comparisons and used the Bucher method to avoid some biases. Indirect comparisons require more caution in interpretation than direct comparisons [37]. Moreover, they require homogeneity for validity. However, the analyzed studies were so heterogeneous in their subgroups that bias was almost inevitable. Nonetheless, even though an indirect analysis is less reliable than a direct comparison, it can allow doctors to make treatment plans for patients and defines a method to improve treatment effects and reproducibility.

Furthermore, some of the reviewed studies have significant weak points. Some studies that we analyzed did not report information necessary to discern the risk of bias. Comparing acupuncture with AT is an open label trial. Therefore, strict randomization, allocation concealment, and blinding of outcome assessments are needed to avoid bias. Furthermore, only two studies conducted [19, 20] follow-up evaluations. Although manual acupuncture was more effective than AT, AT is more convenient to use. Subjects who want to receive acupuncture treatment must go to a clinic and spend time there, which is not necessary for AT treatment. Therefore, acupuncture must have strengths that outweigh the convenience of AT. One study suggested that acupuncture effects last longer than AT [20]. The disadvantage of typical AT is its short persistence. Further studies should include follow-up evaluations to strengthen this conclusion.

Conclusions

Acupuncture is more effective than AT in DES. Treatment duration of more than 1 month and treatment frequency less than 3 times a week could be more effective than shorter or more frequent treatments. Use of the BL2 and ST1 acupoints can reduce the overall effectiveness of acupuncture for DES. Other acupuncture treatments (electroacupuncture, pyonex) could be applicable, but there are not yet enough studies to evaluate their effects.

Authors' contributions
HJN and BHK conceived and designed the protocol. MHK and SHK conducted the article searches, data extraction and assessement of risk of bias with consensus with BHK. BHK performed the statistical analysis and drafted the manuscript. HJN commented on the analytic plan and interpretation. All authors read and approved the final manuscript.

Competing interests
The authors declare that they have no competing interests.

Author details
Department of Ophthalmology and Otolaryngology of Korean Medicine, College of Korean Medicine, Kyung Hee University, 26, Kyungheedae-ro, Dongdaemun-gu, Seoul 02453, Republic of Korea. 2Department of Ophthalmology and Otolaryngology of Korean Medicine, Kyung Hee University Korean Medicine Hospital, 23, Kyungheedae-ro, Dongdaemun-gu, Seoul 02447, Republic of Korea. 3Department of Ophthalmology and Otolaryngology of Korean Medicine, Kyung Hee University Hospital at Gangdong, 892, Dongnam-ro, Gangdong-gu, Seoul, Republic of Korea.

References
1. The definition and classification of dry eye disease: report of the Definition and Classification Subcommittee of the International Dry Eye WorkShop (2007). The ocular surface. 2007;5:75–92.

2.   Ahn JM, Lee SH, Rim THT, Park RJ, Yang HS, Kim TI, et al. Prevalence of and risk factors associated with dry eye: the Korea National Health and nutrition examination survey 2010–2011. Am J Ophthalmol. 2014;158:1205–1214.e7.

3.   Lee MS, Shin B, Choi T, Ernst E. Acupuncture for treating dry eye: a systematic review. Acta Ophthalmol. 2011;89:101–6.

4.   Ba J, Wu Y, Li Y, Xu D, Zhu W, Yu J. Updated meta-analysis of acupuncture for treating dry eye. Med Acupunct. 2013;25:317–27.

5.   Yang L, Yang Z, Yu H, Song H. Acupuncture therapy is more effective than artificial tears for dry eye syndrome: evidence based on a meta-analysis. Evid Based Complement Alternat Med. 2015;2015:143858.

6.   Armour M, Smith CA. Treating primary dysmenorrhoea with acupuncture: a narrative review of the relationship between acupuncture "dose" and menstrual pain outcomes. Acupunct Med: J British Med Acupunct Soc. 2016; 34:416–24.

7.   Vas J, White A. Evidence from RCTs on optimal acupuncture treatment for knee osteoarthritis–an exploratory review. Acupuncture in medicine : journal of the British medical acupuncture society. British Med Acupunct Soc. 2007;25:29–35.

8.   Higgins JP, Green S. Cochrane Handbook for Systematic Reviews of Interventions Version 5.1.0. Collaboration. TC, editor. Wiley; 2011. http://handbook-5-1.cochrane.org/. Accessed Aug 2017.

9.   Higgins JPT, Thompson SG. Quantifying heterogeneity in a meta-analysis. Stat Med. 2002;21:1539–58.

10. Bucher HC, Guyatt GH, Griffith LE, Walter SD. The results of direct and indirect treatment comparisons in meta-analysis of randomized controlled trials. J Clin Epidemiol. 1997;50:683–91.

11. Med S, Jiaojiao W, Weiping G. Literature analysis involving dry eye managed by Chinese medicine. China J Chin Ophthalmol. 2016;26:269–73.

12. Nepp J, Wedrich A, Akramian J, Derbolav A, Mudrich C, Ries E, et al. Dry eye treatment with acupuncture. A prospective, randomized, double-masked study. Advances in experimental medicine and biology. J Nepp, University eye Clinic of Vienna, Austria. 1998;438:1011–6.

13. He H, Wang Z, Hu H, Liu R. Effect of acupuncture on lacrimal film of Xeroma patients. J Nanjing TCM Univ. 2004;20:158–9.

14. Wang Z-L, He H-Q, Huang D, Shi C-G. Effect of integral syndrome differentiation acupuncture on the tear film stability in the patient of xerophthalmia. Chin Acupunct Moxibustion. 2005;25:460–3.

15. Tseng K, Liu H, Tso K, Woung L, Su Y, Lin J. A clinical study of acupuncture and SSP (silver spike point) electro-therapy for dry eye syndrome. Am J Chin Med. 2006;34:197–206.

16. Zhang C, Zhang J, Deng S. Acupuncture treatment for the treatment of 30 cases of dry eye syndrome. Henan Tradit chin Medicine. 2009;29:895–6.

17. Gong L, Sun X, Chapin WJ. Clinical curative effect of acupuncture therapy on Xerophthalmia. Am J Chin Med. 2010;38:651–9.

18. Gao W, Liu M, Zhang Y. Observation on therapeutic effect of dry eye syndrome treated with acupuncture on the acupoints around the eyes. Chinese acupuncture & moxibustion. WP Gao, eye department, first affiliated clinical medical College of Nanjing University of TCM, Nanjing 210029, China. 2010;30:478–80.

19. Shi J, Miao W. Effects of acupuncture on lactoferrin content in tears and tear secretion in patients suffering from dry eyes: a randomized controlled trial. J Chin Integr Med. 2012;10:1003–8.

20. Kim T, Kang J, Kim K, Kang K, Shin M, Jung S, et al. Acupuncture for the treatment of dry eye: a multicenter randomised controlled trial with active comparison intervention (artificial teardrops). Rosenbaum JT, editor. PLoS One 2012;7:e36638.

21. Nan H Ping. Clinical observation of 60 cases of dry eye syndrome by the treatment of eye acupuncture combining the artificial tears. Boading: Hubei university of Chin Med; 2014.

22. Zhang D, Xing Y, Song X, Wang Z. Therapeutic observation of hair needle therapy for dry eye syndrome. Shanghai J Acupunct-moxibustion. 2015;34:1195–7.

23. Ni W, Li J, Ji Q, Song Y, Liu B, Wang G, et al. Clinical efficacy on xerosis conjunctivitis of liver and kidney yin deficiency treated with SHI's acupuncture manipulation. Chin Acupunct Moxibustion. 2016;36:364–8.

24. Chao Y. The clinical observations on efficacy of a qi-absorption needling technique in treating dry eye syndromes. Dalian: Dalian Medical University; 2016.

25. Liu Q, Liu J, Ren C, Cai W, Wei Q, Song Y, et al. Proteomic analysis of tears following acupuncture treatment for menopausal dry eye disease by two-dimensional nano-liquid chromatography coupled with tandem mass

spectrometry. International journal of Nanomedicine. J Yu, Department of Ophthalmology, shanghai tenth People's hospital, shanghai, China. 2017;12: 1663–71.

26. Shin M, Kim J, Lee M, Kim K, Choi J, Kang K, et al. Acupuncture for treating dry eye: a randomized placebo-controlled trial. Acta Ophthalmol. 2010;88:e328–33.

27. Liu Y, Yang L, Yang G. Electro-acupuncture for treatment of dry eyes: clinical observation. Jilin J Tradit Chin Med. 2012;32:1275–6.

28. Guo M, Cui E, Li X, Zong L. Diverse needling methods for dry eye syndrome: a randomized controlled study. J Acupunct Tuina Sci. 2013;11:84–8.

29. Gao H, Zhao X, Ma G, Li H, Liu H. Acupuncture combined with pyonex for xerophthalmia. World J Acupunct Moxibustion. 2016;26:37–42.

30. Jing W, Xiaoyun M, Linping H. Needle embedding therapy on dry eye patients. J Changchun Univ Chin Med. 2016;32:1033–6.

31. Harris RE, Tian X, Williams DA, Tian TX, Cupps TR, Petzke F, et al. Treatment of fibromyalgia with formula acupuncture: investigation of needle placement, needle stimulation, and treatment frequency. J Altern Complement Med (New York, NY). 2005;11:663–71.

32. Smith CA, Zaslawski CJ, Zheng Z, Cobbin D, Cochrane S, Lenon GB, et al. Development of an instrument to assess the quality of acupuncture: results from a Delphi process. J Altern Complement Med (New York, NY). 2011;17: 441–52.

33. Stapleton F, Alves M, Bunya VY, Jalbert I, Lekhanont K, Malet F, et al. TFOS DEWS II epidemiology report. Ocul Surf. 2017;15:334–65.

34. Gibson EJ, Stapleton F, Wolffsohn JS, Golebiowski B. Local synthesis of sex hormones: are there consequences for the ocular surface and dry eye? Br J Ophthalmol. 2017;101:1596–603.

35. Truong S, Cole N, Stapleton F, Golebiowski B. Sex hormones and the dry eye. Clin Exp Optom. 2014;97:324–36.

36. Ren Y, Yang X, Zhang Y, Wang Y, Li X. Effects and Mechanisms of acupuncture and moxibustion on reproductive endocrine function in male rats with partial androgen deficiency. Acupunct Med: J British Med Acupunct Soc. 2016;34:136–43.

37. Glenny AM, Altman DG, Song F, Sakarovitch C, Deeks JJ, D'Amico R, et al. Indirect comparisons of competing interventions. Health Technol Assess (Winch Eng). 2005;9:1–134. iii–iv

19

What intrinsic factors influence responsiveness to acupuncture in pain?: a review of pre-clinical studies that used responder analysis

Yu-Kang Kim[1,4], Ji-Yeun Park[2], Seung-Nam Kim[3], Mijung Yeom[4], Seungmin Lee[5], Ju-Young Oh[1,4], Hyangsook Lee[4], Younbyoung Chae[4], Dae-Hyun Hahm[4] and Hi-Joon Park[4*]

Abstract

Background: Not many studies have investigated individual sensitivity to acupuncture. To explore the intrinsic factors related to individual responses to acupuncture, we reviewed published pre-clinical studies using responder analysis on pain.

Methods: We searched the PubMed and EMBASE databases to June 2015. We included pre-clinical reports describing responders and non-responders to anti-nociceptive and analgesic effects of acupuncture in animal study. We identified the potential intrinsic factors which might be related with the response to acupuncture.

Results: Totally, 216 potentially relevant articles were retrieved and 14 studies met our inclusion criteria. Rat ($n = 1348$) and rabbit ($n = 56$) were used, and only electroacupuncture (EA) was applied as an intervention. Results showed that high levels of cholecystokinin-8 and receptors were associated with poor responsiveness to EA. Endogenous opioids including β-endorphin and met-enkephalin, descending inhibitory norepinephrine and serotonin system, and hypothalamic 5′-AMP-activated protein kinase seemed to be associated with high-level responses. Spinal levels of neurotransmitters and pro-inflammatory cytokines were also differentially expressed depending on the EA sensitiveness. In the central nervous system, hypothalamus, periaqueductal grey, pituitary gland, and spinal cord were suggested to be involved in the EA responsiveness. Identified individual variations did not seem to be accidental, as the responsiveness to EA was replicated over time. However, methodological issues such as reproducibility, cut-off criteria, and clinical relevance need to be further elaborated.

Conclusion: Our study suggests that the identification of the biological factors differentiating responders from non-responders is necessary and it may aid in understanding how acupuncture modulates pain.

Keywords: Acupuncture, Responder, Non-responder, Individual difference, Cholecystokinin

Background

Pain is the most prevalent reason patients seek medical attention in many developed countries [1, 2]. It is a chief complaint in numerous disorders that hinders the individual's daily activities and functions [3, 4]. Analgesics can help alleviate such pain but individual sensitivity to pain and individual responsiveness to pharmaceuticals vary considerably even among patients with the same conditions. In the clinic, for example, although morphine has great analgesic properties, some patients experience inadequate analgesia and demand increased dosage or concurrently suffer from significant side effects [5]. These inter-individual differences in the factors causing pain and in the pain mechanisms per se, are clearly in play and a more individualistic approach, which focuses on the responder and non-responder differences, may be useful in the development of novel analgesic treatment [6–8].

* Correspondence: acufind@khu.ac.kr
[4]Acupuncture & Meridian Science Research Center, Kyung Hee University, 26 Kyungheedae-ro, Dongdaemoon-gu, Seoul 02447, Republic of Korea
Full list of author information is available at the end of the article

Acupuncture, the stimulation of specific acupoints on the body with acupuncture needles, is widely used to relieve persistent pain and to treat many disorders [9–12]. An important feature of acupuncture is that the chosen acupoints and the preferred type of manipulation reflect patients' individual characteristics and/or those of their diseases. Intrinsic patient factors are, therefore, at the forefront when doctors plan overall treatment [13].

For decades, researchers have tried to identify what intrinsic factors may constitute the specific effects of acupuncture. A recent innovative brain imaging study showed that acupuncture-induced analgesia of migraine involves the intrinsic functional connectivity of the right frontoparietal network [14]. However other than this study, most of the previous research has only focused on elucidating acupuncture's therapeutic effects, while individual responsiveness was less considered [15]. Analysis of both responders and non-responders would reap the benefits additional to investigating acupuncture outcomes and developing therapeutic effects.

A few preclinical or human studies have provided significant insight into the differences between responders or non-responders. Electroacupuncture (EA) afforded either excellent or almost no effects in human or animals, i.e., it produced beneficial effects in approximately 70% of subjects and resulted in little changes in the other 30%. [16–18]. Low responsiveness to EA effects was known to be associated with changes in cholecystokinin (CCK) levels [19]. It was also suggested that the degree of responsiveness to acupuncture effects was associated with different neural activation by EA in periaqueductal grey (PAG) or hypothalamus [20, 21]. Thus, further work on the mechanisms involved and specific regulation of intrinsic factors related with high or low responsiveness might allow the therapeutic effects of acupuncture to be better predicted. However, to date, no systematic study has distinguished between responders and non-responders when acupuncture was used to modulate pain.

In this review, we reviewed the relevant published literature of pre-clinical studies to define high and low responsiveness of EA to pain and identify trends in the associated factors, regions, or mechanisms of responders and non-responders.

Methods
Search strategy
We searched the PubMed and EMBASE databases to June 2015. The search term was "acupuncture and (responder* or non-responder*)." Additionally, publications in the reference lists of retrieved papers and relevant reviews were manually retrieved.

Study selection
We first screened the records by title and abstract; we included original English-language reports on animal experiments discriminating responders from non-responders. The exclusion criteria were: 1) use of a language other than English, 2) irrelevance in terms of acupuncture treatment, 3) lack of baseline or outcome data, 4) definition of responders using only a survey or a questionnaire, 5) the absence of any distinction between responders and non-responders to acupuncture, 6) the absence of a focus on differences between responders and non-responders, and 7) not conducted in animal models. We included any form of acupuncture and any animal model. As we sought to define the features of acupuncture associated with a response or a non-response, all included studies had to distinguish between responders and non-responders. Any ambiguities were discussed by three reviewers (Kim YK, Park JY, and Park HJ) until unanimous consensus was attained.

Data extraction
We recorded the first author's name, the year of publication, the country in which the work was performed, the animal used (sex and species), the sample size, whether the animals were healthy or diseased, the type of acupuncture applied, the EA parameters (if relevant), the acupoints used, the cut-offs for identification as responders/non-responders, the numbers of responders and non-responders, the outcomes of any behavioral tests applied, target molecules, regions of interest, the defined functions of target molecules, and the outcomes of EA-sensitivity analysis. Data extraction was performed by one author (Kim YK), but two other authors (Park JY, Park HJ) double-checked this work.

Quality assessment
The included publications were independently assessed by two authors (Kim YK, Park HJ) in terms of the methodological quality using the 9-item checklist modified from the CAMARADES checklist [22, 23]: (1) peer-reviewed publication; (2) detailed statement of acupuncture procedure; (3) objective behavior test applied to classify responder or non-responder; (4) statement of cut-off values for dividing responder or non-responder; (5) notification of the ratio of responder or non-responder to the total; (6) blinded assessment of outcome; (7) reproducibility of EA sensitiveness; (8) compliance with animal welfare regulations; and (9) statement of potential conflict of interests. Each study was recorded a sum quality score out of a possible total of 9 points. Discrepancies were resolved after discussion between the two authors (Kim YK, Park HJ).

Results

An overview of the study

Figure 1 shows how reports were selected. We initially identified 106 and 192 relevant publications in PubMed and EMBASE respectively, and additionally added 14 works via manual searching. Among these 312 records, 96 duplicated articles were removed. We excluded 194 of these 216 papers after screening the abstracts and titles. Ultimately, 22 publications were fully evaluated. We subsequently excluded eight of these because responders were not classified (three studies) or studies did not explore factors associated with individual variations (five studies). Finally, 14 studies met our inclusion criteria.

Characteristics of included studies

Table 1 lists the characteristics of the included studies. A total of 1348 rats and 52 rabbits were used. All studies featured EA of low frequency (1–3 Hz, nine studies), medium frequency (15 Hz, one study), or high frequency (100 Hz, five studies). All studies electrically connected acupoint ST36 with acupoint SP6 (six studies), or the adjacent bilateral or ipsilateral ST36 acupoints (six studies). One study used acupoint TE18 in the rabbit. Only three studies included pain models including neuropathic pain [18], incisional pain [24], and inflammatory pain [25] in their evaluations of pain levels; 13 studies employed normal animals.

Study quality

The quality score of the included studies ranged from 2 to 7 out of a total 9 points. Of the 14 studies, 3 studies got 2 points [19–21], 3 studies got 3 points [17, 26, 27], 3 studies got 4 points [28–30], 1 study got 5 points [31], 2 studies got 6 points [24, 25], one study got 7 points [18], and one study got 8 points [32] (Table 2). All 14 studies were published in peer reviewed journals. Six studies described detailed acupuncture procedure [24–26, 28, 30, 32]. Six studies reported objective behavior test applied to classify responder of non-responder [18, 25, 27, 29, 31, 32]. All 14 studies notified cut-off value for dividing responder or non-responder. None of the studies mentioned blinded assessment of outcome. Two studies confirmed reproducibility of EA sensitiveness [18, 32]. Six studies reported compliance with animal welfare regulations [18, 24, 25, 28, 31, 32]. Four studies contained statement of potential conflict of interests [18, 24, 31, 32].

Cut-off values for EA responses

Thirteen studies used the tail flick latency (TFL) to distinguish between EA responders and non-responders; one employed the paw pressure threshold [25]. However, the criteria used to separate responders and non-responders in terms of EA sensitivity were very different. In 10 studies, percentage changes in pain behavior (from baseline) were calculated: cut-off values in the responder ranged 10–150% increase in TFL or the pressure pain threshold, and those in the non-responders were 0–50%. Three studies defined responders as animals exhibiting statistically significant increases in TFL ($p < 0.05$) compared with baseline [20, 21, 28]. One study defined a non-responder as an animal in which the TFL change was less than the mean value plus three standard deviations [24]. All criteria presented were shown in Table 3, and the proportion of responders according to the

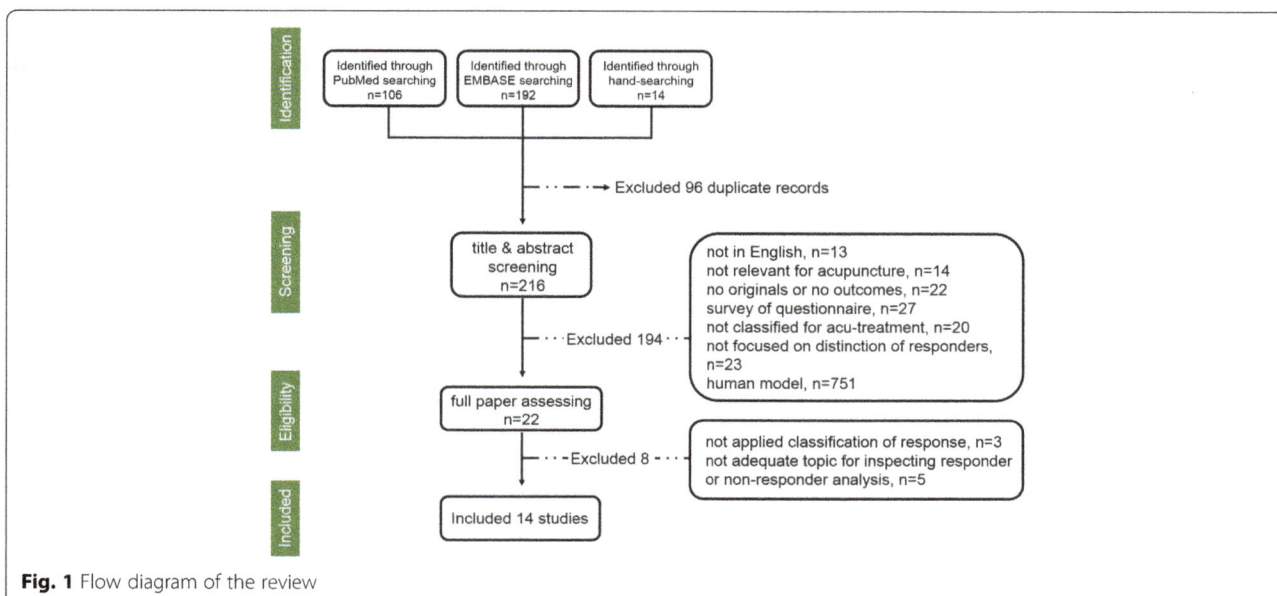

Fig. 1 Flow diagram of the review

Table 1 Experimental index for electroacupuncture

Author (Year, Country)	Animal (sex)	Sample size	Condition	Acupoints (side)	EA Parameters: frequency, amplitude, duration
Kim (2014, Korea)	rats (M)	18	Nor	ST36-subST36 (n.r.)	2 Hz, 0.2–0.3 mA, 20 min
Wang (2012, China)	rats (M)	170	Nor	ST36-SP6 (B)	2 Hz or 100 Hz respectively, 0.5/1.0/1.5 mA, 30 min
Fais (2012, Brazil)	rats (M)	48	Incisional pain	ST36-SP6 (B)	2 Hz, 1.4–1.5 mA, 20 min
Gao (2007, China)	rats (M)	18	Nor	ST36-subST36 (B)	1 Hz, 3.5–5 V, 60 min
Kim (2007, Korea)	rats (M) CCK-AR KO rats (M)	38	Nor / Neur. pain	ST36-subST36 (n.r.)	2 Hz, 0.2–0.3 mA, 20 min
Ko (2006, Korea)	rats (M)	12	Nor	ST36-subST36 (n.r.)	100 Hz, 0.2–0.3 mA, 20 min
Sekido (2003, Japan)	rats (M)	95	Nor / Paw inflam	ST36-subST36 (L)	3 Hz, 1/2/3 mA, 60 min
Lee (2002, Korea)	rats (M)	12	Nor	ST36-subST36 (n.r.)	2 Hz, 0.2–0.3 mA, 15 min
Liu (1999, China)	rats (F)	19	Nor	ST36-SP6 (B)	100 Hz, 1/2/3 mA, 30 min
Tian (1998, China)	rats (F)	193	Nor	ST36-SP6 (n.r.)	100 Hz, 1/2/3 mA, 30 min
Tang (1997, China)	rats (F)	215	Nor	ST36-SP6 (B)	100 Hz, 1/2/3 mA, 30 min
Takeshige (1993, Japan)	rats (M) and rabbits (n.r.)	402 rats and 52 rabbits	Nor	Rats: ST36 (n.r.) Rabbits: TE18 (n.r.)	1 Hz, intensity to cause muscle contraction, 30 min, 45 min or 60 min
Takeshige (1992, Japan)	rats (M)	80	Nor	ST36 (n.r.)	1 Hz, intensity to cause muscle contraction, n.r.
Han (1985, China)	rats (n.r.)	28	Nor	ST36-SP6 (n.r.)	15 Hz, 3 V, 10 min

B bilateral, *CCK-AR KO* cholecystokinin A receptor knockout, *F* female; Incisional pain, mechanical hyperalgesia induced by 1 cm longitudinal incision through skin and fascia and stitches on right hind paw; *M* male, *L* left; *Neur. pain* neuropathic pain; *Nor* normal, *n.r.* not reported; Paw inflam, carrageenan-induced inflammation on the paw; subST36, 5 mm distal from ST36

Table 2 Risk of bias of the included studies

Author (Year)	A	B	C	D	E	F	G	H	I	Total
Kim (2014)	√		√		√			√	√	5
Wang (2012)	√	√	√		√	√	√	√	√	8
Fais (2012)	√	√			√	√		√	√	6
Gao (2007)	√	√			√			√		4
Kim (2007)	√		√		√	√	√	√	√	7
Ko (2006)	√		√		√	√				4
Sekido (2003)	√	√	√		√	√		√		6
Lee (2002)	√				√	√				3
Liu (1999)	√	√			√					3
Tian (1998)	√		√		√					3
Tang (1997)	√	√			√	√				4
Takeshige (1993)	√				√					2
Takeshige (1992)	√				√					2
Han (1985)	√				√					2

Studies fulfilling the criteria of: A: peer reviewed publication; B: detailed statement of acupuncture procedure; C: objective behavior test applied to classify responder or non-responder; D: blinded assessment of outcome E: statement of cut-off value for dividing responder or non-responder; F: notification of the ratio of responder or non-responder to the total; G: reproducibility of EA sensitiveness; H: compliance with animal welfare regulations; I: statement of potential conflict of interests

various criteria are shown in Additional file 1: Fig. S1, in the case of provided information available.

Reproducibility of responsiveness to the anti-nociceptive or analgesic effects of EA

Wang et al. found that EA variance was maintained when TFL was evaluated on two successive days in a physiological state [32]. Kim et al. confirmed that responders exhibiting normal EA-mediated anti-nociception were consistently more sensitive to EA-induced analgesia in a model of neuropathic pain than were non-responders [18]. However, Sekido et al. reported different findings: 50% of normal rats were EA-responders, but all animals (thus both responders and non-responders) were susceptible to EA-induced analgesia after induction of carrageenan-mediated inflammatory pain [25].

Intrinsic factors associated with a poor response to acupuncture

Six studies suggested that the level of CCK or the receptor thereof were related with no or a low response. Han et al. showed that injection of an antibody against the CCK-octapeptide (CCK-8) changed an EA non-response into an apparent response [19], and Tang et al. confirmed that inhibition of brain CCK synthesis rendered non-responders responders [30]. Liu et al. showed that the spinal perfusates of non-responders exhibited a higher level of CCK immunoreactivity than did that of

Table 3 EA response criteria and associated data

Author (Year)	Behavior test for cut off	EA frequency	EA response criteria: Changes from the baseline[a] (n, % = proportion of responder or non-responder)
Kim et al. (2014)	TFL	LF	a) NR (8, n.a.) [discarded] 20% 30% R (10, n.a.)
Wang et al. (2012)	TFL	LF	a) NR (7, 8.8%) 0% R (54, 67.5%) 150% HR (19, 23.8%)
		HF	a) NR (23, 28.8%) 0% R (49, 61.3%) 150% HR (8, 10.0%)
Kim et al. (2007)	TFL	LF	a′) NR (7, 38.9%) 30% R (11, 61.1%)
Ko et al. (2006)	TFL	HF	a′) NR (6, 50.0%) 30% R (6, 50.0%)
Lee et al. (2002)	TFL	LF	a′) NR (5, 41.7%) 30% R (7, 58.3%)
Liu et al. (1999)	TFL	HF	a) LR (10, n.a.) 30% 60% HR (9, n.a.)
Tian et al. (1998)	TFL	HF	a) LR (47, n.a.) 60% HR (43, n.a.)
Tang et al. (1997)	TFL	HF	a) LR 30% (discarded) 60% HR (14, 38.9%)
Han et al. (1985)	TFL	IF	a) NR (28, n.a.) 50%
Sekido et al. (2003)	PPT	LF	a) NR (14, 48.3%) 10% R (15, 51.7%)
Gao et al. (2007)	TFL	LF	a, b) NR (6, n.a.) 25% p=0.05 R (6, n.a.)

Table 3 EA response criteria and associated data *(Continued)*

Takeshige et al. (1993)	TFL	LF	

b) NR (26, n.a.) | R (59, n.a.)
p=0.05

Takeshige et al. (1992)	TFL	LF	

b) NR (15, n.a.) | R (28, n.a.)
p=0.05

Fais et al. (2012)	TFL	LF	

c) NR (48, 32.0%)
+3SD

[a]EA response criteria were differently applied. Researchers assessed with percentage change, *p* values or standard deviation: a) percentage change of during-EA or post-EA from the baseline, a') converted into percentage change after direct contact to the author b) responder = significantly increase ($p < 0.05$ or $p < 0.01$) versus baseline, Non-responder = the others, c) Non-responder = post-EA TFL was less than baseline TFL + 3SD ($p = 0.0014$). *HF*, high frequency; *HR* high-responder, *IF* intermediate frequency, *LF* low frequency, *LR* low-responder, *n.a.* not applicable because of insufficient record, *NR* non-responder, *PPT* paw pressure threshold in normal rats, *R* responder, *SD* standard deviation, *TFL* Tail Flick latency

responders [26]. Lee et al. found that CCK A receptor-encoding mRNA was highly expressed in the hypothalamus of non-responders and suggested that not only the CCK A receptor; CCK B receptor level per se but also that of the CCK receptor played important roles in the insensitivity to pain modulation afforded by EA [17]. Further, Ko et al. showed that the mRNAs encoding both the CCK A and CCK B receptor mRNAs were more highly expressed; these results were in contrast to those reported by Lee et al.. The use of different EA frequencies may explain these discrepancies, as Lee et al. delivered EA at 2 Hz, and the EA of Ko et al. was delivered at 100 Hz. Citing the data of Lee et al., Kim et al. found that CCK A receptor-knockout rats enjoyed significantly higher levels of anti-nociceptive effects after 2 Hz EA. Interestingly, the CCK receptor was more highly expressed in the hypothalamus of the non-responder group [17, 18, 29]. However, Wang et al. found no difference in the level of CCK receptor expression in the spinal dorsal horns of responders and non-responders [32] (Tables 4 and 5).

Intrinsic factors affording a good response to acupuncture

Several intrinsic factors were significant in EA responders. Takeshige et al. showed that the evoked potential in the posterior arcuate nucleus of hypothalamus and the dorsal periaqueductal gray matter of responders differed from that of non-responders [20, 21]. They also reported that administration of morphine (i.p. or microinjection into posterior arcuate nucleus of hypothalamus) increased the anti-nociceptive effects of EA to a level similar to high responders [20], whereas acupuncture-induced anti-nociception in responders remained unchanged. Both

modulation of met-enkephalin [21] and β-endorphin [20, 21] could also convert the response of EA.

Hypophysectomy abolished the EA induced antinociception and evoked potentials of the posterior hypothalamic arcuate nucleus in responders (Tables 4 and 5) [20, 21]. Sekido et al. confirmed that an opioid receptor antagonist, naloxone (i.p.), attenuated EA analgesia in responders (Table 4) [25]. Fais et al. showed that EA combined with inhibition of norepinephrine and serotonin uptake (i.p. and i.t.) converted non-responders into responders (Table 4) [24]. Kim et al. found that hypothalamic 5′-AMP-activated protein kinase (AMPK) gene expression was upregulated after low-frequency EA in responder rats, and hypothalamic microinjection of a dominant-negative AMPK adenovirus, which inhibits AMPK activity, reduced EA analgesia; the wild-type control virus did not do so (Tables 4 and 5) [31].

Additionally, Sekido et al. demonstrated that peripheral inflammation potentiated the EA-induced sensitivity to analgesia; EA responders were about 50% as sensitive to EA analgesia in normal state, but all rats suffering from inflammation were more sensitive to EA. Naloxone, an opioid receptor antagonist, inhibited EA antinociception in normal rats but decreased EA analgesia in rats with inflamed paws in this study (Table 5) [25].

Intrinsic factors influencing both high- and low-level responsiveness to acupuncture

Orphanin FQ (OFQ) influenced the response levels depending on the sites of action; intrathecal injection of anti-OFQ antibody converted responders into non-responders, and intracerebral injection of the antibody converted non-responders into responders (Table 5) [27].

Table 4 Differentially expressed or changed factors between responder and non-responder

Author (Year)	Target regions	Responder > Non-responder	Non-responder > Responder
Low Frequency EA			
Kim (2014)	Hypothalamus	AMPK mRNA expression	
Wang (2012)[a]	Spinal dorsal horn (L5-L6)	- Neurotransmitter receptors-related genes: Aplnr, Gabrg2 (at 24 h) - Regulation of proinflammatory cytokines-related genes: Fcgr2b and Gsk3b	- Neurotransmitter receptors-related genes: Gabrg2 (at 1 h), and Htr1f - Proinflammatory cytokines-related gene expression: C5ar1, IL-6 and TNFα - Neurotransmitter receptors-related genes: Gabra2
Gao (2007)[b]	Hypothalamus	Voltage-gated K+ channels, solute carrier family 8, Synaptic vesicle glycoprotein 2b, glutamatergic A receptor, ghrelin precursor, melanocortin 4 receptor and neuroligin 1	
Lee (2002)	Hypothalamus		CCK-AR mRNA expression, but not CCK-BR
Takeshige (1993)	Dorsal PAG	Neural activity evoked by EA	
Takeshige (1992)	Medial arcuate nucleus of hypothalamus	Neural activity evoked by EA	
High Frequency EA			
Wang (2012)[a]	Spinal dorsal horn (L5-L6)	Aplnr, Gabrg2 (at 24 h)	None
Ko (2006)	Hypothalamus		Both CCK-AR and CCK-BR mRNA expression
Liu (1999)	Spinal perfusate		CCK-8-ir

[a]Through cDNA microarray, Wang (2012) compared the responder group, the non-responder group and the restraint group (not applied EA) at 1 h and 24 h time point after EA stimulation. We selectively reported genes which were significantly different between the responder group and the non-responder group and a more different group from the restraint group was described as the subject. Almost all genes, cited in this table, showed statistical difference at 1 h time point and only Gabrg2 was statistically different between the responder and the non-responder group both at 1 h and at 24 h time point.
[b]We selectively reported statistically different genes through both microarray and RT-PCR. Gao (2007) conducted dissecting hypothalamus immediately after EA stimulation. AMPK, 5'-AMP-activated protein kinase (regulation of energy homeostasis); CCK-8-ir, cholecystokinin octapeptide like immunoreactivity; CCK-AR, cholecystokinin A receptor; CCK-BR, cholecystokinin B receptor; PAG, periaqueductal central gray

Candidate genes affecting EA response from transcriptomic analyses

Transcriptomic analyses revealed that gene expression levels in both the dorsal spinal cord and the hypothalamus varied among animals [28, 32]. Wang et al. profiled gene expression in the spinal dorsal horn after application of 2- and 100-Hz EA and found that the levels of mRNAs encoding neurotransmitter receptors (including the Aplnr, GABAA, glycine, and 5-HT1 receptors) were upregulated in responder (but not non-

Table 5 Biological factors that convert the EA response from responder to non-responder or vice versa

Author (Year)	EA	Factors	
		Responder → Non-responder	Non-responder → Responder
Kim (2014)	LF	Inhibiting AMPK activity in the hypothalamus	
Fais (2012)	LF		Inhibitor of norepinephrine and serotonin uptake at spinal terminals of descending pain inhibitory pathways (amitriptyline, i.p. or i.t)
Kim (2007)	LF		CCK-AR KO
Sekido (2003)	LF	Naloxone (opioid receptor antagonist, i.p.)	
Takeshige (1993)	LF	-Hypophysectomy -Antiserum of β-endorphin (i.c.v.)	Inhibitor of the degrading enzymes of met-enkephalin (DPA, i.p.)
Takeshige (1992)	LF	Hypophysectomy	- Morphine (i.p.) - Morphine (into post. Arcuate nucleus) - β-endorphin (into post. Arcuate nucleus)
Han (1985)	IF		CCK-8 AS (i.c.v. or i.t.)
Tian (1998)	HF	OFQ-Ab (i.t.)	OFQ-Ab (i.c.v.)
Tang (1997)	HF		Antisense CCK (i.c.v.)

AMPK 5'-AMP-activated protein kinase (regulation of energy homeostasis), AS antiserum, CCK cholecystokinin, CCK-8 cholecystokinin octapeptide, CCK-AR cholecystokinin A receptor, DPA D-phenylalanine, i.c.v. intracerebroventricular injection, i.p. intraperitoneal injection, i.t. intrathecal injection, KO knockout, Met-Enk methionine enkephalin, OFQ-Ab orphanin FQ anibody, post. Posterior

responder) rats [32]. They also showed that genes involved in inflammatory modulation were differentially expressed. In non-responder rats, mRNAs encoding proteins associated with the release of proinflammatory cytokines (e.g., IL-6 and TNF-α) were more highly expressed in non-responders than in responders after 2-Hz EA. However, genes inhibiting the release of pro-inflammatory cytokines, including Fcgr2b, GSK3b, and Tsc22d3, were upregulated to a greater extent in responders than in non-responders (Table 4) [32].

Gao et al. observed the changes of hypothalamic gene expressions using microarray analysis. They showed that that several genes including a glutamatergic receptor (Grm6), a precursor of ghrelin (Ghrl), the melanocortin 4 receptor (Mc4r), and neuroligin 1 (Nlgn1) were significantly upregulated in the hypothalamus of responders (Table 4) [28].

Discussion

In this review, we have shown that the levels of signaling molecules associated with acupuncture analgesia (those of the descending inhibitory system, endogenous opioids, and CCK-8 and receptors thereof) may be differentially expressed in responders and non-responders. Also, modulation of such factors may change the response to EA. Responders and non-responders differ in terms of AMPK expression in the hypothalamus and in the levels of neurotransmitter receptors and pro-inflammatory cytokines genes in the spinal cord [31, 32] and such differences may also affect response related to EA (Fig. 2).

Acupuncture analgesia is an integrative process involving both afferent impulses from the acupoints and the painful region [12]. In an early responder study, Takeshige et al. suggested that afferent neural transmission could explain different responses to EA [20, 21]. Upon application of EA, the changes in the neuronal activity in the arcuate nucleus and dorsal PAG differed between responders and non-responders and correlated with the extent of EA-induced analgesia. EA increased neuronal activity in the PAG of responders, irrespective of whether EA was applied ipsilaterally or contralaterally.

As mentioned above, the endogenous descending inhibitory system of the central nervous system (CNS) and various signaling molecules, including opioid peptides, glutamate, and 5-hydroxytryptamine, contribute to acupuncture-induced analgesia [33]. The release of opioid peptides during acupuncture is frequency-dependent. Low- and high-frequency EA release enkephalin/β-endorphin and dynorphin, respectively, in the CNS [34]. Responder analysis has also shown that differences in the expression levels of these factors contribute to individual differences in sensitivity to EA analgesia. Sekido et al. found that intraperitoneal injection of naloxone converted responders to low-frequency EA into non-responders [25]. Injection of anti-β-endorphin antibody into the cerebral ventricles abolished the analgesic effects of low-frequency EA in responders (21). D-phenylalanine, an inhibitor of enzymes degrading met-enkephalin, morphine, and β-endorphin changed the neuronal activity induced by low-frequency EA in non-responders to that characteristic of responders [20,

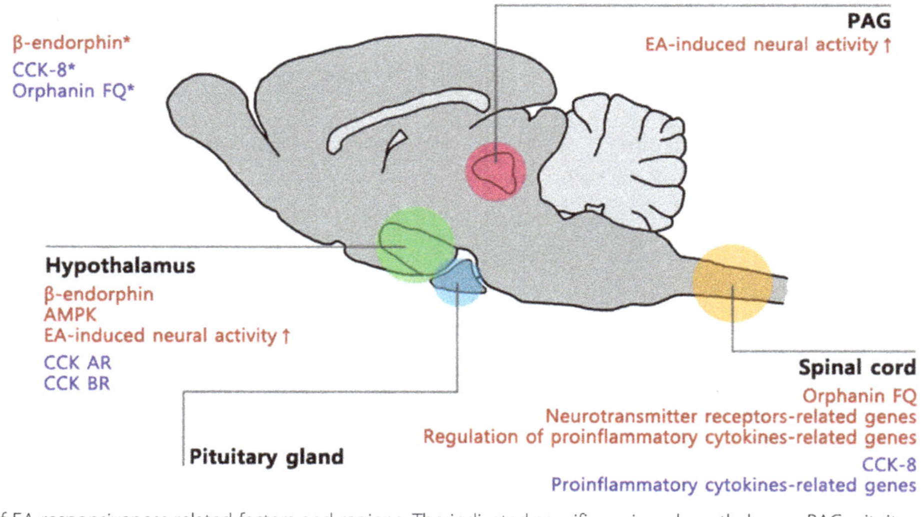

Fig. 2 A scheme of EA responsiveness-related factors and regions. The indicated specific regions, hypothalamus, PAG, pituitary gland and spinal cord, are well-known to be associated with pain regulation, and have been reconfirmed through researches on EA responsiveness. An asterisk implies intracerebroventricular injection. Responder-related factors and non-responder-related factors have been grouped in red and blue letters respectively. CCK AR, cholecystokinin A receptor; CCK BR, cholecystokinin B receptor; CCK-8, cholecystokinin octapeptide; Hypo, hypothalamus; PAG, periaqueductal grey; Pit. g., pituitary gland

21]. The OFQ peptide is involved in many physiological processes, including pain. The effects of the peptide on the nervous system are complex; it is generally accepted that spinal OFQ is anti-nociceptive, while OFQ exerts an anti-opioid action and causes hyperalgesia when injected supraspinally [35]. Tian et al. explored whether OFQ modulated the responses of EA and found that intrathecal injection of an anti-OFQ antibody converted responders to non-responders, whereas intracerebral injection had the reverse effect [27].

Additionally, the norepinephrine and serotonin systems of the descending inhibitory pathway contribute to individual differences in EA analgesia. Fais et al. found that the poor analgesia of non-responders changed to the level of analgesia enjoyed by responders after administration (i.p. and i.t.) of inhibitors of norepinephrine and serotonin uptake at the spinal terminals of the descending inhibitory pathways [24].

Kim et al. suggested that hypothalamic AMPK might be an intrinsic mediator of the EA response [31]. The AMPK enzyme plays roles in cellular energy homeostasis and metabolic stress and was recently shown to modulate both acute and chronic neuropathic pain [36, 37]. Hypothalamic AMPK gene expression was upregulated after low-frequency EA in responder rats, and hypothalamic inhibition of AMPK activity using dominant-negative AMPK adenovirus reduced EA analgesia.

The best-studied intrinsic factors are CCK-8 and receptors thereof. CCK is a CNS neurotransmitter playing roles in pain, satiety, feeding, learning, cognition, and emotion. CCK-8, a major form of CCK, is found predominantly in the CNS [38–40], and has been found to play a role in the development of tolerance to EA; CCK-8 may counter pain alleviation by exerting an anti-opioid action [41]. Liu et al. showed that the extent of CCK-8 immunoreactivity increased in the spinal perfusate of non-responders after high-frequency EA [26]. Intracerebroventricular or intrathecal injection of anti-CCK-8 antibody or antisense CCK-8 converted non-responders into responders [19]. However, the levels of CCK in the spinal dorsal horn were increased in both responders and non-responders after EA [32]. It has been suggested that the CCK receptor isoforms, CCK AR and BR are differentially affected [29]. However, it remains unclear which receptor may be more important in terms of the response to EA analgesia. Upon application of low-frequency EA, the level of CCK AR but not BR mRNA increased [17]. CCK AR-knockout rats exhibited an elevated anti-nociceptive response after low-frequency EA [18]. In contrast, the hypothalamic levels of mRNAs encoding both CCK AR and BR were upregulated after high-frequency EA. A CCK-B antagonist potentiated EA anti-nociception after high-frequency EA [42]. However, no significant changes in the levels of CCK AR or BR

mRNAs were evident in the dorsal horn of the spinal cord [32]. Thus, it seems clear that the CCK system reduces the analgesic effects of EA, regardless of the frequency. However, further research is required to determine whether this is the principal cause of EA non-responsiveness.

Transcriptomic analyses have suggested that the actions of several novel intrinsic factors may explain the different responses to acupuncture. Wang et al. found that the differential regulation of genes encoding neurotransmitters and their receptors indicated that the neurotransmitter system may be more active in responders than in non-responders. Genes involved in the modulation of inflammation were also differentially expressed. In non-responder rats, the levels of mRNAs facilitating the release of proinflammatory cytokines (including IL-6 and TNF- α) were higher in non-responders. In responders, the levels of mRNAs inhibiting the release of proinflammatory cytokines (e.g., Fcgr2b, GSK3b, and Tsc22d3) were higher in responders. It is known that proinflammatory cytokines induce the release of various inflammatory materials and play important roles in the nociceptive and analgesic systems of the CNS. These results suggest that the intrinsic response to spinal cord inflammation may partly explain the different responses to EA [32].

There are several issues to discuss for developing the responder analysis more useful. First, the reproducibility of the EA response is an important consideration. If factors influencing this response are intrinsic, the response must be reproducible. Wang et al. repeated TFL tests on the same rats at 2-day intervals and found that the EA response was maintained [32]. However, most studies have not addressed reproducibility. Additionally, more than 70 % of the included studies measured anti-nociceptive effects in non-diseased normal animals, and it is doubtful that results can be applicable to diseased individuals. Kim et al. explored whether the anti-nociceptive response to EA in non-diseased normal animals was reproduced after induction of neuropathic pain; the responses of both responders and non-responders were in fact maintained [18]. However, Sekido et al. reported a different finding: 50% of non-diseased normal rats were classified as EA responders, but all tested rats, regardless of response status, experienced EA-induced analgesia of carrageenan-induced inflammatory pain [25]. In addition, it should be considered that the ratio of responder and non-responder might be varied across the types of disease. In Li et al.'s study, the number of responder was twice as many as that of non-responder for the modulatory effects of EA (acupoint PC5-PC6) on cardiovascular reflex response [43], while there are not enough data for the responder ratio in other physiological or pathological condition.

Further studies with different pathological models should address this question.

Second, the classification of responders or non-responders needs to set a good validation. The cut-off criteria for responders were extremely variable among the 14 relevant studies, including a 10–150% increase in the TFL or the pressure pain threshold from baseline. The notifying accurate description of classifying responder or non-responder and the use of validated cut-offs is essential in future work. Next, the acupuncture conditions reviewed are very limited; all studies employed very common methods such as EA of acupoint ST36 (100% of studies). There are more than 360 acupoints with various stimulation methods [44]. Thus, caution is required when generalizing the results.

Further, the responder studies in clinical setting are limited. Only a few studies have sought to identify human responders. Chae et al. used a microarray to identify genes differing in expression level between high- and low-responders in 15 healthy volunteers. Genes related with signaling, stress response, transcriptional regulators, and/or regulators of immune function may be relevant, although the "responder" mechanism needs to be clarified further [45]. Genetic factors have been suggested to play roles in individual sensitivity to acupuncture [5, 13, 45]. However, the gap between pre-clinical and clinical researches remains very wide, and further translational clinical studies are essential.

Next, various parameters beyond individual variance can affect the responsiveness of acupuncture. For instance, the selection of acupoints, the number of acupuncture treatments, stimulation modality (manual, EA or others) and intensity, learning from pre-exposed cues, and the condition of the patients can influence the acupuncture effects [34, 46–50]. EA tolerance, which means a gradual decline of EA effects due to the repeated use, is also important to explain the low-responsiveness of EA [51]. It might be interesting how these various factors synergistically contribute to acupuncture effects.

Finally, it is also important to consider how the various intrinsic factors identified can contribute to the elucidating the acupuncture mechanism. Though there are still lots of limitation, the existed evidences suggest this possibility: the factors identified in the low responder (i.e. CCK-8 and spinal OFQ) have shown to be involved in the attenuation of EA analgesia and the induction of EA tolerance [19, 26, 27]; the injection of morphine and β-endorphin could convert non-responder into high-responder, and these results are helpful to understand the involvement of endogenous opioid system in the acupuncture analgesia [20, 21]. Further well designed responder analysis is needed to aid the acupuncture mechanism.

In spite of the several limitations mentioned above, our review of pre-clinical studies is meaningful to show the benefit of responder and non-responder analysis for elucidating the mechanism of acupuncture in pain. Further responder analysis considering the validated cut-off criteria, animal models depicting human disease, and real-world acupuncture methods is recommendable. This kind of approach might help to develop the strategy to enhance the acupuncture effects in pain medicine.

Conclusion

In conclusion, we confirmed that dividing animals into responders and non-responders identified novel candidate mediators of the effects of acupuncture. A number of studies have found that the EA responsiveness could be modifiable by modulating these mediators. Although most included studies regarding EA responsiveness was investigated in the physiological state, and there are several methodological issues to be improved, this study may allow us the development of new strategies potentiating the therapeutic effects of acupuncture.

Additional file

Additional file 1: Fig. S1. Varied ratio of responders according to arbitrary cut-off value. Low frequency EA was arranged on the left and high frequency EA on the right. Since an arbitrary cut-off value can change the allocation of responder rats, we divided absolutely high responsiveness as a genuine responder and relatively high responsiveness as a modifiable responder. This allowed those with relatively high responsiveness not to be misallocated as a responder with a higher cut-off value.

Acknowledgments
The English in this review has been checked by at least two professional editors of Textcheck, both native speakers of English (http://www.textcheck.com/certificate/hsqock). This research was supported by the National Research Foundation of Korea funded by the Korean Ministry of Science (NRF-2015M3A9E052338 and 2017R1A2B4009963).

Funding
This research was supported by the National Research Foundation of Korea funded by the Korean Ministry of Science (NRF-2015M3A9E052338 and 2017R1A2B4009963).

Authors' contributions
Conceived and designed this review: HJP MY DHH YC HL. Extracted the data: YKK JYP SNK. Analyzed the data: YKK JYP SL JYO. Wrote the paper: YKK HJP. All authors read and approved the final manuscript.

Competing interests
The authors declare that they have no competing interests.

Author details
[1]Department of Science in Korean Medicine, Graduate School, Kyung Hee University, 26 Kyungheedae-ro, Dongdaemoon-gu, Seoul 02447, Republic of Korea. [2]College of Korean Medicine, Daejeon University, 62 Daehak-ro, Dong-gu, Daejeon 34520, Republic of Korea. [3]College of Korean Medicine,

Dongguk University. 32, Dongguk-ro, Ilsandong-gu, Goyang-si, Gyeonggi-do 10326, Republic of Korea. [4]Acupuncture & Meridian Science Research Center, Kyung Hee University, 26 Kyungheedae-ro, Dongdaemoon-gu, Seoul 02447, Republic of Korea. [5]Department of Acupuncture and Moxibustion, College of Korean Medicine, Kyung Hee University, Seoul 130-701, Republic of Korea.

References

1. Gereau RW, Sluka KA, Maixner W, Savage SR, Price TJ, Murinson BB, et al. A pain research agenda for the 21st century. J Pain. 2014;15(12):1203–14.
2. Melnikova I. Pain market. Nat Rev Drug Discov. 2010;9(8):589–90.
3. Mills S, Torrance N, Smith BH. Identification and Management of Chronic Pain in primary care: a review. Curr Psychiatry Rep. 2016;18(2):22.
4. Tsang A, Von Korff M, Lee S, Alonso J, Karam E, Angermeyer MC, et al. Common chronic pain conditions in developed and developing countries: gender and age differences and comorbidity with depression-anxiety disorders. J Pain. 2008;9(10):883–91.
5. Ren ZY, Xu XQ, Bao YP, He J, Shi L, Deng JH, et al. The impact of genetic variation on sensitivity to opioid analgesics in patients with postoperative pain: a systematic review and meta-analysis. Pain Physician. 2015;18(2):131–52.
6. Scholz J, Woolf CJ. Can we conquer pain? Nat Neurosci. 2002;5(Suppl):1062–7.
7. Schork NJ. Time for one-person trials. Nature. 2015;520(7549):609–11.
8. Woodcock J, Witter J, Dionne RA. Stimulating the development of mechanism-based, individualized pain therapies. Nat Rev Drug Discov. 2007; 6(9):703–10.
9. Kim TH, Kang JW, Kim KH, Kang KW, Shin MS, Jung SY, et al. Acupuncture for the treatment of dry eye: a multicenter randomised controlled trial with active comparison intervention (artificial teardrops). PLoS One. 2012;7(5): e36638.
10. Lau CH, Wu X, Chung VC, Liu X, Hui EP, Cramer H, et al. Acupuncture and related therapies for symptom Management in Palliative Cancer Care: systematic review and meta-analysis. Medicine (Baltimore). 2016;95(9):e2901.
11. Qin Z, Wu J, Zhou J, Liu Z. Systematic review of acupuncture for chronic prostatitis/chronic pelvic pain syndrome. Medicine (Baltimore). 2016;95(11):e3095.
12. Zhang R, Lao L, Ren K, Berman BM. Mechanisms of acupuncture-electroacupuncture on persistent pain. Anesthesiology. 2014;120(2):482–503.
13. Park HJ, Kim ST, Yoon DH, Jin SH, Lee SJ, Lee HJ, et al. The association between the DRD2 TaqI a polymorphism and smoking cessation in response to acupuncture in Koreans. J Altern Complement Med. 2005;11(3):401–5.
14. Li K, Zhang Y, Ning Y, Zhang H, Liu H, Fu C, et al. The effects of acupuncture treatment on the right frontoparietal network in migraine without aura patients. J Headache Pain. 2015;16:518.
15. Salehi A, Marzban M, Imanieh MH. The evaluation of curative effect of acupuncture: a review of systematic and meta-analysis studies. J Evid Based Complementary Altern Med. 2015;
16. Li P, Ayannusi O, Reid C, Longhurst JC. Inhibitory effect of electroacupuncture (EA) on the pressor response induced by exercise stress. Clin Auton Res. 2004;14(3):182–8.
17. Lee G, Rho S, Shin M, Hong M, Min B, Bae H. The association of cholecystokinin-a receptor expression with the responsiveness of electroacupuncture analgesic effects in rat. Neurosci Lett. 2002;325(1):17–20.
18. Kim SK, Moon HJ, Park JH, Lee G, Shin MK, Hong MC, et al. The maintenance of individual differences in the sensitivity of acute and neuropathic pain behaviors to electroacupuncture in rats. Brain Res Bull. 2007;74(5):357–60.
19. Han JS, Ding XZ, Fan SG. Is cholecystokinin octapeptide (CCK-8) a candidate for endogenous anti-opioid substrates? Neuropeptides. 1985;5(4–6):399–402.
20. Takeshige C, Nakamura A, Asamoto S, Arai T. Positive feedback action of pituitary beta-endorphin on acupuncture analgesia afferent pathway. Brain Res Bull. 1992;29(1):37–44.
21. Takeshige C, Oka K, Mizuno T, Hisamitsu T, Luo CP, Kobori M, et al. The acupuncture point and its connecting central pathway for producing acupuncture analgesia. Brain Res Bull. 1993;30(1–2):53–67.
22. Lu L, Zhang XG, Zhong LL, Chen ZX, Li Y, Zheng GQ, et al. Acupuncture for neurogenesis in experimental ischemic stroke: a systematic review and meta-analysis. Sci Rep. 2016;6:19521.
23. Macleod MR, O'Collins T, Howells DW, Donnan GA. Pooling of animal experimental data reveals influence of study design and publication bias. Stroke. 2004;35(5):1203–8.
24. Fais RS, Reis GM, Rossaneis AC, Silveira JW, Dias QM, Prado WA. Amitriptyline converts non-responders into responders to low-frequency electroacupuncture-induced analgesia in rats. Life Sci. 2012;91(1–2):14–9.
25. Sekido R, Ishimaru K, Sakita M. Differences of electroacupuncture-induced analgesic effect in normal and inflammatory conditions in rats. Am J Chin Med. 2003;31(6):955–65.
26. Liu SX, Luo F, Shen S, Yu YX, Han JS. Relationship between the analgesic effect of electroacupuncture and CCK-8 content in spinal perfusate in rats. Chin Sci Bull. 1999;44(3):240–3.
27. Tian JH, Zhang W, Fang Y, Xu W, Grandy DK, Han JS. Endogenous orphanin FQ: evidence for a role in the modulation of electroacupuncture analgesia and the development of tolerance to analgesia produced by morphine and electroacupuncture. Br J Pharmacol. 1998;124(1):21–6.
28. Gao YZ, Guo SY, Yin QZ, Hisamitsu T, Jiang XH. An individual variation study of electroacupuncture analgesia in rats using microarray. Am J Chin Med. 2007;35(5):767–78.
29. Ko ES, Kim SK, Kim JT, Lee G, Han JB, Rho SW, et al. The difference in mRNA expressions of hypothalamic CCK and CCK-A and -B receptors between responder and non-responder rats to high frequency electroacupuncture analgesia. Peptides. 2006;27(7):1841–5.
30. Tang NM, Dong HW, Wang XM, Tsui ZC, Han JS. Cholecystokinin antisense RNA increases the analgesic effect induced by electroacupuncture or low dose morphine: conversion of low responder rats into high responders. Pain. 1997;71(1):71–80.
31. Kim SK, Sun B, Yoon H, Lee JH, Lee G, Sohn SH, et al. Expression levels of the hypothalamic AMPK gene determines the responsiveness of the rats to electroacupuncture-induced analgesia. BMC Complement Altern Med. 2014;14:211.
32. Wang K, Zhang R, Xiang X, He F, Lin L, Ping X, et al. Differences in neural-immune gene expression response in rat spinal dorsal horn correlates with variations in electroacupuncture analgesia. PLoS One. 2012;7(8):e42331.
33. Zhao ZQ. Neural mechanism underlying acupuncture analgesia. Prog Neurobiol. 2008;85(4):355–75.
34. Han JS. Acupuncture: neuropeptide release produced by electrical stimulation of different frequencies. Trends Neurosci. 2003;26(1):17–22.
35. Di Cesare ML, Micheli L, Ghelardini C. Nociceptin/orphanin FQ receptor and pain: feasibility of the fourth opioid family member. Eur J Pharmacol. 2015; 766:151–4.
36. Melemedjian OK, Asiedu MN, Tillu DV, Sanoja R, Yan J, Lark A, et al. Targeting adenosine monophosphate-activated protein kinase (AMPK) in preclinical models reveals a potential mechanism for the treatment of neuropathic pain. Mol Pain. 2011;7:70.
37. Tillu DV, Melemedjian OK, Asiedu MN, Qu N, De Felice M, Dussor G, et al. Resveratrol engages AMPK to attenuate ERK and mTOR signaling in sensory neurons and inhibits incision-induced acute and chronic pain. Mol Pain. 2012;8:5.
38. Crawley JN, Corwin RL. Biological actions of cholecystokinin. Peptides. 1994; 15(4):731–55.
39. Dockray GJ. Cholecystokinin and gut-brain signalling. Regul Pept. 2009; 155(1–3):6–10.
40. Zhang JG, Liu JX, Jia XX, Geng J, Yu F, Cong B. Cholecystokinin octapeptide regulates the differentiation and effector cytokine production of CD4(+) T cells in vitro. Int Immunopharmacol. 2014;20(2):307–15.
41. Carlino E, Benedetti F. Different contexts, different pains, different experiences. Neuroscience. 2016;
42. Zhou Y, Sun YH, Shen JM, Han JS. Increased release of immunoreactive CCK-8 by electroacupuncture and enhancement of electroacupuncture analgesia by CCK-B antagonist in rat spinal cord. Neuropeptides. 1993; 24(3):139–44.
43. Li M, Tjen ALSC, Guo ZL, Longhurst JC. Electroacupuncture modulation of reflex hypertension in rats: role of cholecystokinin octapeptide. Am J Physiol Regul Integr Comp Physiol. 2013;305(3):R404–13.
44. WHO Western Pacific Region. WHO standard acupuncture point locations in the western Pacific region. In: WHO standard acupuncture point locations in the Western Pacific region; 2008.
45. Chae Y, Park HJ, Hahm DH, Yi SH, Lee H. Individual differences of acupuncture analgesia in humans using cDNA microarray. J Physiol Sci. 2006;56(6):425–31.
46. Lee J, Napadow V, Park K. Pain and sensory detection threshold response to acupuncture is modulated by coping strategy and acupuncture sensation. BMC Complement Altern Med. 2014;14:324.
47. Liu H, Xu JY, Li L, Shan BC, Nie BB, Xue JQ. FMRI evidence of acupoints specificity in two adjacent acupoints. Evid Based Complement Alternat Med. 2013;2013:932581.

48. MacPherson H, Maschino AC, Lewith G, Foster NE, Witt CM, Vickers AJ. Characteristics of acupuncture treatment associated with outcome: an individual patient meta-analysis of 17,922 patients with chronic pain in randomised controlled trials. PLoS One. 2013;8(10):e77438.

49. Prady SL, Burch J, Vanderbloemen L, Crouch S, MacPherson H. Measuring expectations of benefit from treatment in acupuncture trials: a systematic review. Complement Ther Med. 2015;23(2):185–99.

50. Bossut DF, Mayer DJ. Electroacupuncture analgesia in rats: naltrexone antagonism is dependent on previous exposure. Brain Res. 1991;549(1):47–51.

51. Cui L, Ding Y, Feng Y, Chen S, Xu Y, Li M, et al. MiRNAs are involved in chronic electroacupuncture tolerance in the rat hypothalamus. Mol Neurobiol. 2017;54(2):1429–39.

20

Comprehensive evaluation of gene expression signatures in response to electroacupuncture stimulation at Zusanli (ST36) acupoint by transcriptomic analysis

Jing-Shan Wu[1], Hsin-Yi Lo[1], Chia-Cheng Li[1], Feng-Yuan Chen[1], Chien-Yun Hsiang[2]* (iD) and Tin-Yun Ho[1,3]*

Abstract

Background: Electroacupuncture (EA) has been applied to treat and prevent diseases for years. However, molecular events happened in both the acupunctured site and the internal organs after EA stimulation have not been clarified.

Methods: Here we applied transcriptomic analysis to explore the gene expression signatures after EA stimulation. Mice were applied EA stimulation at ST36 for 15 min and nine tissues were collected three hours later for microarray analysis.

Results: We found that EA affected the expression of genes not only in the acupunctured site but also in the internal organs. EA commonly affected biological networks involved in cytoskeleton and cell adhesion, and also regulated unique process networks in specific organs, such as γ-aminobutyric acid-ergic neurotransmission in brain and inflammation process in lung. In addition, EA affected the expression of genes related to various diseases, such as neurodegenerative diseases in brain and obstructive pulmonary diseases in lung.

Conclusions: This report applied, for the first time, a global comprehensive genome-wide approach to analyze the gene expression profiling of acupunctured site and internal organs after EA stimulation. The connection between gene expression signatures, biological processes, and diseases might provide a basis for prediction and explanation on the therapeutic potentials of acupuncture in organs.

Keywords: Electroacupuncture, ST36, Zusanli, Microarray

Background

Acupuncture, a traditional therapy in ancient China over thousands of years, has been widely accepted and used in Western society [1, 2]. Acupuncture is believed to balance Yin-Yang, stimulate the circulation of vital energy (qi) and blood, maintain the body health, and prevent the incidence of illness [3]. Electroacupuncture (EA) is a modification of acupuncture that stimulates acupoints with electrical current and displays reproducible in both research and clinical application. Moreover, EA therapy has been used for postoperative analgesia and

anesthesia, for the treatment of diverse disorders of internal organs, and for the release of pain [4, 5].

In traditional Chinese medicine, ST36 (Zusanli) is a commonly acupoint that modulates the biological activities of gastrointestinal system, immune system, cardiovascular system, and muscular system. Transcutaneous EA at ST36 reduces gastric accommodation and improves impaired gastric motility in patients with functional dyspepsia [6]. Transcutaneous neuromodulation at ST36 also improves the frequency of spontaneous defecation and increases the bowel movements in patients with chronic constipation [7]. Chronic EA at ST36 improves baroreflex function and hemodynamic parameters in rats with heart failure [8]. Long-term EA stimulation at ST36 and DU20 (BaiHui) also relieves the increased mean arterial pressure and cardiovascular abnormality in both structure and function in spontaneously hypertensive rats [9]. ST36 displays the

* Correspondence: cyhsiang@mail.cmu.edu.tw; tyh@mail.cmu.edu.tw
[2]Department of Microbiology, China Medical University, 91 Hsueh-Shih Road, Taichung 40402, Taiwan
[1]Graduate Institute of Chinese Medicine, China Medical University, 91 Hsueh-Shih Road, Taichung 40402, Taiwan
Full list of author information is available at the end of the article

anti-nociceptive and anti-hyperalgesic effect. EA at ST36 reduces postoperative analgesic requirements and associated side effects in patients undergoing lower abdominal surgery [10]. Treatment of EA at ST36 and GN34 also ameliorates L5 spinal nerve ligation-induced neuropathic pain in rats [11]. Moreover, EA at ST36 and CV4 (Guanyuan) improves clinical curative effects in patients with sepsis in a prospective randomized controlled trial via the regulation of immune system [12]. EA at ST36 promotes myofiber regeneration and restoration of neuromuscular junctions in a rabbit gastrocnemius contusion model [13]. Furthermore, EA at ST36 also improves intestinal mucosal immune barrier in sepsis by increasing the concentration of secretory IgA, the percentage of CD3+, γ/δ, and CD4+ T cells, and the ratio of CD4+/CD8+ T cells [14].

ST36 is an acupoint of Foot's Yang Supreme Stomach Meridian that targets at gastrointestinal tract [15]. We wondered whether EA stimulation at ST36 altered molecular events in other organs. The genome-wide analysis of ST36-stimulated region (skin) and distant visceral organs or tissues, including cerebral medulla, cerebral cortex, hippocampus, lung, spleen, kidney, uterus and thigh muscle, was therefore performed. Mice were stimulated by EA at ST36, and gene expression signatures of nine organs or tissues were explored by microarray analysis. The process network and disease connection of gene expression profiles were further analyzed to elucidate the molecular events and effects of organs after ST36 stimulation.

Methods
Animals
Female BALB/c mice (6–8-week-old, 18–22 g) were obtained from National Laboratory Animal Center (Taipei, Taiwan) and maintained in an air-controlled pathogen-free animal facility with a 12-h light/dark cycle at 23 ± 2 °C. Food and water were available ad libitum. Mouse experiments were conducted under ethics approval from China Medical University Animal Care and Use Committee (Permit No. 101–61-N).

EA stimulation
A total of 10 mice was randomly divided into two groups of 5 mice. For control group, mice were anesthetized with isoflurane without ST36 stimulation. For ST36 group, mice were anesthetized with isoflurane, gently immobilized in a plastic restrainer, and applied EA stimulation at ST36 acupoint, which is located at the midpoint of tibialis anterior muscle of hind limbs. Briefly, sterilized acupuncture needle (0.24 × 12 mm, 36 gauge, Yu-Kuang Acupuncture Co., Taipei, Taiwan) was inserted bilaterally into the acupoint, which was 3–4 mm below the knee midline and laterally 1–2 mm at a depth of 2–3 mm. Electrical stimulation pulse with voltage ranging from 3.5 to 5 V, duration

of 0.05 ms, and frequency of 2 Hz was generated from a pulse generator (HANS model, LH202H, Taipei, Taiwan) and applied using two outlets via two needles. The intensity of EA stimulation was determined as the minimum voltage causing moderate muscle contraction for 15 min. Three hours after EA stimulation, mice were sacrificed by carbon dioxide inhalation, and organs were removed for RNA extraction.

Total RNA extraction
Total RNAs from acupunctured site, muscle, cerebral cortex, cerebral medulla, hippocampus, lung, spleen, kidney, and uterus were extracted using RNeasy Mini kit (Qiagen, Valencia, CA, USA). The amount and the integrity of total RNA were quantified and evaluated using a spectrophotometer (Beckman Coulter, Fullerton, CA, USA) and an Agilent 2100 bioanalyzer (Agilent Technologies, Santa Clara, CA, USA), respectively.

Microarray analysis
Microarray analysis was performed as described previously [16, 17]. Briefly, fluorescence-labeled RNA targets were prepared from total RNA using MessageAmp™ aRNA kit (Ambion, Austin, TX, USA) and Cy5 dye (Amersham Pharmacia, Piscataway, NJ, USA). Fluorescent targets were hybridized to the Mouse Whole Genome OneArray (Phalanx Biotech Group, Hsinchu, Taiwan) and scanned by an Axon 4000 scanner (Molecular Devices, Sunnyvale, CA, USA). The Cy5 fluorescent intensity of each spot was analyzed by genepix 4.1 software (Molecular Devices, Sunnyvale, CA, USA). The signal intensity of each spot was normalized by R program in limma package using quantile normalization. Normalized data were analyzed using the "geneSetTest" function implemented in the limma package to detect groups of regulated genes in biological pathways. This function computes a p-value to test the hypothesis that the selected genes tend to be up- or down-regulated. Then, the score of each pathway in EA treatment was defined as score = $-\log(p)$ if p-value ≤0.5 or score = $\log(2(1-p))$ if p-value >0.5. The score more than 0.3, equivalent to p-value less than 0.5, was considered to be statistically significant. A total of 352 pathways was extracted from ArrayTrack (http://www.fda.gov/ScienceResearch/BioinformaticsTools/Arraytrack) and used in this analysis. The scores of pathways were then displayed using TIGR Multiexperiment Viewer (http://mev.tm4.org) [18]. In addition to biological pathways analysis, genes with fold changes ≥1.5 or ≤ −1.5 were selected and used as input genes for the generation of process network and diseases using Enrichment algorithm in MetaCore™ Analytical suit (GeneGo Inc., St. Joseph, MI, USA). All microarray data are MIAMI compliant database (Gene Expression Omnibus accession number GSE73939).

Results

EA affected the expression of genes in distant organs

To explore the molecular events happened in local or distant regions after ST36 stimlation, we applied EA stimulation in BALB/c mice for 15 min and collected ST36-stimulated region (skin) and distant visceral organs or tissues, including cerebral medulla, cerebral cortex, hippocampus, lung, spleen, kidney, uterus and thigh muscle, 3 h later for microarray analysis. BALB/c mice were applied for EA stimulation in this study because BALB/c mice are among the most widely used inbred strains for animal experiments. Moreover, BALB/c mice are useful for researches of immunology and neurobiology, the potent biological activities of ST36 acupoint. As expected, EA affected the expression of genes in the skin at ST36 acupoint (Fig. 1). In a total of 29,922 genes, the transcripts of 169 genes and 231 genes were upregulated and downregulated, respectively, by 1.5 fold in EA-treated skin. In addition to skin, EA affected the expression levels of genes in distant organs. EA regulated the expression of 931 genes in uterus, followed by kidney (743 genes), cerebral medulla (547 genes), muscle (463 genes), spleen (450 genes), lung (303 genes), cerebral cortex (197 genes), and hippocampus (147 genes).

EA affected biological processes in various organs

We further analyzed the canonical pathways affected by EA at ST36 acupoint. "geneSetTest" function was performed to test a set of signaling and metabolic pathways regulated by EA. Scores of pathways were further visualized by TIGR Multiexperiment Viewer. As shown in Fig. 2, a hierarchical clustering of EA-affected canonical pathways displayed varieties among nine organs or tissues, and the number of signaling and metabolic pathways significantly regulated (score ≥ 0.3) by EA in different organs was also

varied. Some pathways, such as oxidative phosphorylation, ribosome, proteasome and serum response factor-mediated pathways, were commonly regulated by EA in organs. However, more pathways were regulated by EA in organs without consistency. About 2/3 pathways in spleen and skin were significantly regulated by EA, while less pathways were regulated by EA in hippocampus.

We further analyzed the process network of protein interactions regulated by EA treatment and classified the process networks into five categories, including cell cycle and apoptosis, inflammation and immune response, signaling transduction, cytoskeleton and cell adhesion, and development. EA treatment affected the process networks in these organs in different ratio (Fig. 3). Cytoskeleton and cell adhesion was the most EA-regulated category in organs, except hippocampus and lung. "Inflammation and immune response" was the most affected category in lung. About 60% of the total number of EA-affected process networks was related to inflammation and immune response. Signaling transduction was the most affected category in hippocampus, and approximately 27% of the total number of affected process networks was involved in signaling transduction. In addition, EA treatment affected some unique process networks in organs (Fig. 4). For example, some neurophysiological processes, such as transmission of nerve impulse and γ-aminobutyric acid-ergic (GABAergic) neurotransmission, were commonly regulated by EA in cerebral cortex, cerebral medulla, and hippocampus, while melatonin signaling, corticoliberin signaling, and long-term potentiation were regulated by EA in cerebral medulla. Moreover, male sex differentiation in kidney, follicle-stimulating hormone-beta signaling pathway in uterus, and blood coagulation in spleens were significantly affected by EA.

Gene expression connection between EA stimulation and diseases in brain and lung

EA stimulation at ST36 regulated the expression of about 300–500 genes in lung and brain. Although the organs with the top two changes in gene expression were uterus and kidney, the ratios of process network categories altered by uterus and kidney were similar to those altered by other organs, except brain and lung. Process network analysis showed that "inflammation and immune response" was the abundant category in lung and neurological processes were unique processes regulated in brain. Therefore, we further analyzed whether genes affected by EA were related to those in diseases. As shown in Table 1, EA stimulation commonly regulated the genes involved in psychiatry and psychology, mental disorders, mood disorders, and heredodegenerative disorders in brain tissues. EA treatment also regulated the expression of genes related to some unique diseases in brain tissues. For

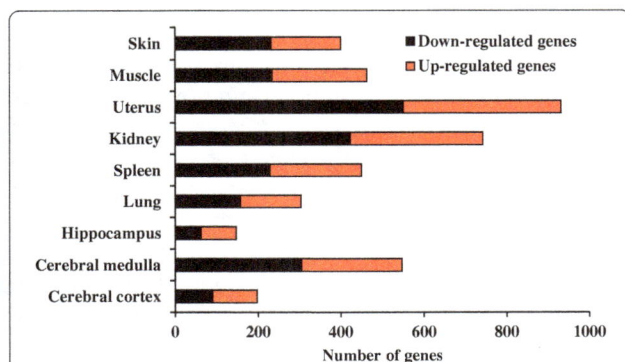

Fig. 1 Number of ST36-regulated genes in various organs. EA stimulation was applied at ST36 acupoint in mice for 15 min. Three hours later, mice were sacrificed and organs were collected for microarray analysis. Data are presented by histograms, and the height of histogram corresponds to the number of upregulated (*red*) and downregulated (*blue*) genes

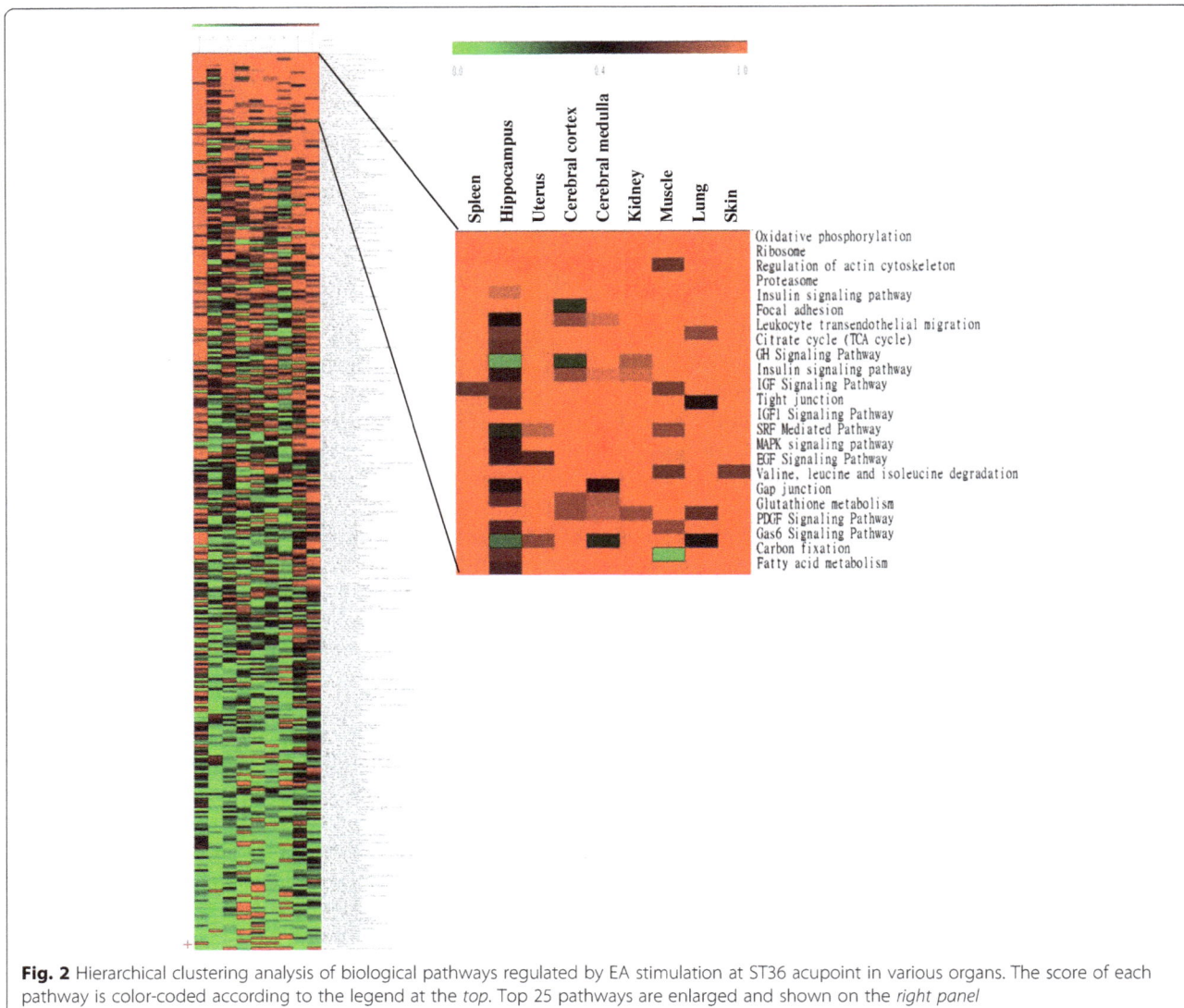

Fig. 2 Hierarchical clustering analysis of biological pathways regulated by EA stimulation at ST36 acupoint in various organs. The score of each pathway is color-coded according to the legend at the *top*. Top 25 pathways are enlarged and shown on the *right panel*

example, genes involved in neurodegenerative diseases, such as Alzheimer's disease, amyloid neuropathies and parkinsonian disorders, were regulated by EA in cerebral medulla. Genes related to endocrine system diseases, such as ovarian diseases, adnexal diseases, ovarian neoplasms, gonadal disorders, and prostatic intraepithelial neoplasia, were regulated by EA in hippocampus. As shown in Table 2, genes involved in obstructive pulmonary diseases, hypersensitivity, such as rheumatic diseases and rheumatoid arthritis, infection, such as bacterial infections and mycoses, and cardiopulmonary diseases, such as cardiovascular diseases, heart diseases and vascular diseases, were affected by EA in lung. These findings suggested that EA stimulation at ST36 acupoint affected the biological process and network in distant organs. Moreover, EA-affected gene expression profiles might be related to diseases states in brain and lung.

Discussion

In this study, we applied transcriptomic analysis to analyze the gene expression signatures in nine organs or tissues responsive to ST36 stimulation. Microarray analysis has been applied to elucidate the effects of various acupoints in specific organs or tissues. For example, acupuncture at GB34 and LR3 acupoints attenuates the decrease of tyrosine hydroxylase and exhibits the protective effects via affecting the expression of degeneration-related genes in the substantia nigra region in Parkinsonism mouse model [19]. Acupuncture at PC6 acupoint up-regulates the expression of Tph1 gene and down-regulates the expression of Olr883 genes in rat brains, suggesting that the therapeutic effect of acupuncture for ischemic stroke may be closely related to the suppression of post-stroke depression and the regulation of olfactory transduction in middle cerebral artery occlusion rat model [20]. Moreover,

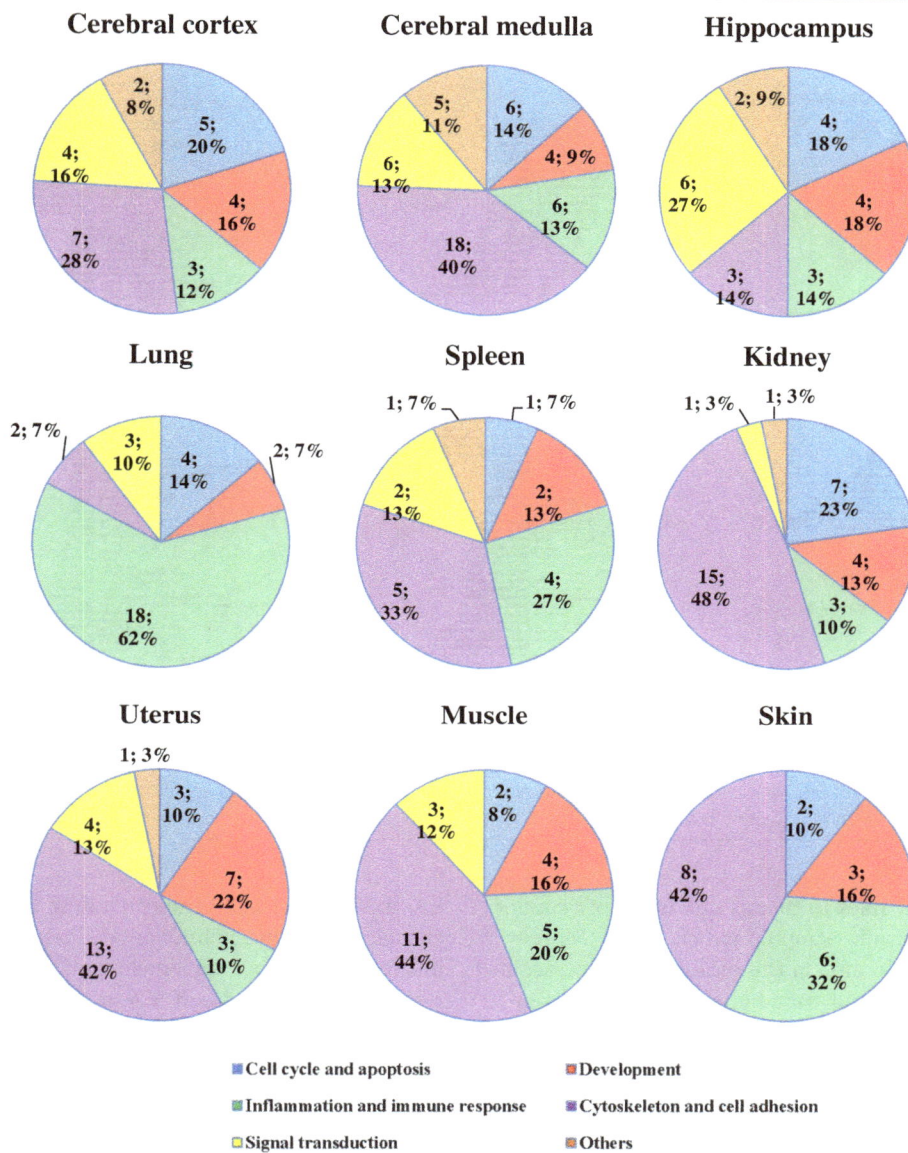

Fig. 3 Process network categories affected by EA stimulation at ST36 acupoint in various organs. Genes with fold changes ≥1.5 or ≤ −1.5 were selected for the generation of process networks using MetaCore Analytical suit. Process networks were sorted into five categories and the categories were illustrated at the *bottom*. The pie chart sectors represent the number and the ratio of process networks in each category

EA at PC3 and PC6 acupoints significantly ameliorates the colonic lesions, and affects both the inflammatory pathways in colons and the immunity-associated pathway in spleens in mice with trinitrobenzene sulfuric acid-induced colitis [21]. Gene expression profiles of specific organs or tissues after EA stimulation at ST36 have also been analyzed. For example, gene expression profiles in periaqueductal gray-spinal dorsal horn region of rats after EA stimulation at ST36 and SP6 show that the modulation of neural-immune interaction in the central nervous system plays an important role during EA analgesia [22]. Gene expression profiling of rat arcuate nucleus region

responsive to EA at ST36 and SP6 shows that the expression levels of genes are effectively regulated by low-frequency EA, compared with high-frequency EA. It might explain the mechanisms of therapeutic effects of the low-frequency EA [23]. In addition to brain tissues, EA at ST36 affects the expression of cell adhesion molecules in muscle, which might be related to the glucose-lowering effect of ST36 in rats with type 1 diabetes [24]. Acupuncture at ST36, CV12 (Zhongwan), and BL20 (Pishu) acupoints down-regulates nuclear factor-κB p65, miRNA-155, and miRNA-21 and up-regulates miRNA-146a expression in chronic atrophic gastritis rats, suggesting that these genes

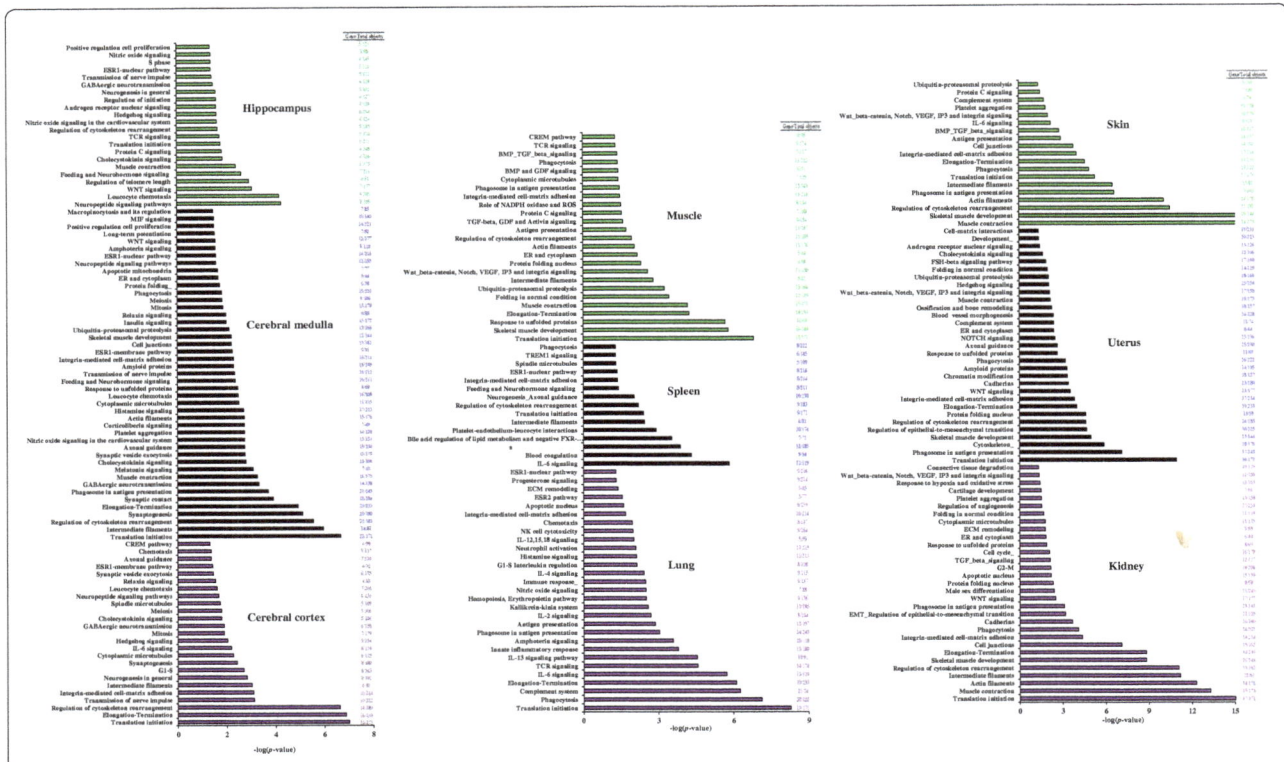

Fig. 4 List of process networks regulated by EA stimulation at ST36 acupoint in various organs. Genes with fold changes ≥1.5 or ≤ −1.5 were selected for the generation of process networks using MetaCore Analytical suit. Data are presented as -log(p-value). The number of affected genes and total objects in each process network is shown on the *right panel*

may play important roles in therapeutic effect of acupuncture in treating chronic atrophic gastritis [25]. Moreover, moxibustion at ST36 affects the biological processes involved in immunity and metabolism in moxibustioned skin under pathological and physiological conditions, respectively [26]. Since ST36 displays various benefit or therapeutic effects in whole bodies, we performed a global and comprehensive study on the gene expression signatures of nine different organs or tissues after ST36 stimulation. Our data showed that EA at ST36 affected the gene expression of different organs or tissues in various degrees. Moreover, EA at ST36 has a more impact on the regulation of gene expression in uterus and has a lesser impact in hippocampus.

By process network and disease connection analysis, we found that EA at ST36 affected the process networks involved in inflammation and immune responses in lung and affected the expression of genes involved in respiratory diseases, such as obstructive pulmonary diseases and microbial infection. Interestingly, a prospective single-blind randomized placebo-controlled study shows that transcutaneous electrical nerve stimulation at ST36, EX-B-1(Dingchuan), BL13 (Feishu), and BL23 (Shenshu) improves lung function on patients with stable chronic obstructive pulmonary disease [27]. Another study shows that

EA at ST36 and BL13 improves lung function of rats with chronic obstructive pulmonary disease and displays an anti-inflammatory effect via downregulation of orexin and its receptor [28]. In addition, EA at ST36 displays a potential protective effect on severe thermal injury-induced remote acute lung injury via the limitation of inflammatory responses in rats [29]. Moreover, EA treatment at ST36 and BL13 attenuates lung injury in rats with endotoxic shock-induced acute lung injury through the activation of NF-E2-related factor pathway and the up-regulation of heme oxygenase-1 expression [30]. Acupuncture at ST36 also regulates the disorders of Fas and Bcl-2 mRNA expression, promotes the apoptosis of eosinophils, and consequently inhibits the development of inflammatory reaction of asthma in rats [31].

Acupuncture has shown some benefit effects on Alzheimer's disease and Parkinson's disease. Lu et al. [32] showed that acupuncture at ST36 increases blood perfusion and glycol metabolism in certain brain areas in Alzheimer's disease rat model by Positron Emission Tomography scanning. ST36 stimulation also induces neurogenesis in adult brains via the up-regulations of brain-derived neurotrophic factor, glial cell line-derived neurotrophic factor, basic fibroblast growth factor and neuropeptide Y, and the activation of the function of

Table 1 Top 20 diseases affected by EA stimulation at ST36 in brain tissues

Diseases	p-value	Gene/Total objects
Cerebral cortex		
Psychiatry and Psychology	4.95E-16	55/1875
Dementia	6.28E-15	47/1480
Central Nervous System Diseases	7.87E-13	65/2983
Mental Disorders	1.65E-12	45/1593
Brain Diseases	1.79E-12	62/2804
Depressive Disorder	3.92E-12	26/557
Neurodegenerative Diseases	1.14E-11	50/2030
Delirium, Dementia, Amnestic, Cognitive Disorders	1.73E-11	15/164
Chorea	2.58E-11	23/467
Dyskinesias	6.16E-11	28/733
Huntington Disease	1.21E-10	22/459
Diabetes Insipidus, Neurogenic	2.95E-10	5/6
Movement Disorders	4.92E-10	29/859
Nervous System Diseases	7.33E-10	86/5368
Mood Disorders	1.55E-09	27/789
Hyponatremia	2.71E-09	42,498
Intellectual Disability	4.60E-09	22/558
Basal Ganglia Diseases	7.57E-09	26/792
Heredodegenerative Disorders, Nervous System	1.03E-08	30/1045
Behavior and Behavior Mechanisms	1.11E-08	20/484
Cerebral medulla		
Mental Disorders	1.15E-32	124/1593
Psychiatry and Psychology	3.08E-32	135/1875
Schizophrenia and Disorders with Psychotic Features	1.99E-29	88/914
Neurodegenerative Diseases	1.50E-19	117/2030
Basal Ganglia Diseases	1.50E-17	64/792
Brain Diseases	3.66E-17	138/2804
Dementia	7.17E-17	91/1480
Movement Disorders	2.13E-16	65/859
Central Nervous System Diseases	1.08E-15	140/2983
Amyloid Neuropathies	3.68E-15	42,655
Tauopathies	1.57E-14	72/1113
Heredodegenerative Disorders, Nervous System	2.17E-13	67/1045
Mood Disorders	1.45E-12	55/789
Neurologic Manifestations	6.85E-12	81/1511
Pathological Conditions, Signs and Symptoms	8.83E-12	169/4334
Alzheimer Disease	1.86E-11	65/110
Parkinsonian Disorders	5.34E-11	35/401

Table 1 Top 20 diseases affected by EA stimulation at ST36 in brain tissues (Continued)

Cerebral Hemorrhage	1.36E-10	15/72
Alzheimer disease, early onset	2.51E-10	12/43
Lewy Body Disease	7.83E-10	12/43
Hippocampus		
Mental Disorders	4.44E-07	27/1593
Psychiatry and Psychology	1.01E-06	29/1875
Schizophrenia and Disorders with Psychotic Features	8.91E-05	16/914
Ovarian Diseases	1.19E-04	34/3046
Adnexal Diseases	1.21E-04	34/3049
Ovarian Neoplasms	1.28E-04	33/2927
Behavioral Symptoms	1.91E-04	6/142
Osteoarthritis, Knee	1.93E-04	4/49
Gonadal Disorders	1.99E-04	34/3128
Behavior	2.76E-04	6/152
Dyskinesias	3.73E-04	13/733
Huntington Disease	3.77E-04	10/459
Prostatic Intraepithelial Neoplasia	3.87E-04	7/227
Heredodegenerative Disorders, Nervous System	4.05E-04	16/104
Chorea	4.31E-04	10/467
Craniofacial Abnormalities	4.64E-04	7/234
Suicide	5.83E-04	5/115
Self-Injurious Behavior	5.83E-04	5/115
Mood Disorders	7.43E-04	13/789
Endocrine System Diseases	9.26E-04	50/5714

primo vascular system [33]. By database searching and screening for articles on clinical trials, Feng et al. [34] found that ST36 combined with GV20 (Baihui) or GV24 (Shenting) is the most frequent and represent potential combination for vascular dementia treatment. In addition, acupuncture at ST36 improves cognitive deficits and increases pyramidal neuron number of hippocampal CA1 area in vascular dementia rats [35]. Moreover, EA at ST36 alleviates dementia via the modulation of interneuron function and the increases of long-term potentiation of hippocampus in rats [36]. By analyzing the gene expression profiling of cerebral cortex, cerebral medulla, and hippocampus after ST36 stimulation, we found that stimulation at ST36 affected the expression of genes involved in neurodegenerative diseases, such as Alzheimer's disease and Parkinsonian disorder, and mental disorders, such as dementia. In addition, neurophysiological processes, such as GABAergic neurotransmission and long-term potentiation, were also regulated by ST36 stimulation in brains. The connection between gene expression signatures in brain and neurological

Table 2 Top 20 diseases affected by EA stimulation at ST36 in lung

Diseases	p-value	Gene/Total objects
Pathologic Processes	7.75E-28	101/2642
Pulmonary Disease, Chronic Obstructive	8.21E-26	57/881
Nutritional and Metabolic Diseases	8.30E-25	105/3099
Metabolic Diseases	4.00E-23	96/2765
Pathological Conditions, Signs and Symptoms	6.83E-23	123/4334
Connective Tissue Diseases	3.75E-21	82/2213
Rheumatic Diseases	2.30E-20	67/1563
Lung Diseases, Obstructive	6.69E-20	68/1640
Bacterial Infections and Mycoses	7.73E-20	60/1293
Arthritis	9.28E-20	68/1650
Arthritis, Rheumatoid	1.83E-19	63/1446
Joint Diseases	2.43E-19	68/1680
Infection	2.11E-18	55/1171
Hypersensitivity	3.60E-18	63/1535
Hypersensitivity, Immediate	4.38E-18	59/1362
Wounds and Injuries	6.15E-18	50/995
Cardiovascular Diseases	8.12E-18	100/3520
Heart Diseases	2.58E-16	56/1351
Vascular Diseases	3.33E-16	91/3179
Fibrosis	5.08E-16	33/475

diseases might provide an explanation on the therapeutic effects of acupuncture for neurological diseases.

In this study, we found that, in addition to brain and lung, EA stimulation at ST36 affected the expression of genes in the local region, such as acupunctured skin, and in the distant regions, like muscle, uterus, kidney, and spleen. How can the stimulation at body surface affect the gene expression in the internal region far from the acupunctured site? Autonomic nervous system is frequently considered to be a mediator of acupuncture. Vagus nerve is a primary target for exploring the possible effect of acupuncture on internal organs because vagus nerve broadly regulates the functions of internal organs. Acupuncture stimulation raises the vagal tone and consequently affects the heart rate and the arterial pressure of cardiovascular system, and the intestinal motility of gastrointestinal system [37]. Acupuncture also exhibits anti-inflammatory effects via vagal modulation of inflammatory responses in internal organs. For example, acupuncture at ST36 activates the splenic nerve via vagus nerve activity to induce anti-inflammatory responses in macrophages of spleens in a lipopolysaccharide-induced inflammation rat model [3]. EA also controls systemic inflammation by inducing vagal activation of aromatic L-amino acid decarboxylase, leading to the production of dopamine in the adrenal medulla and the inhibition of cytokine production

[38]. Some neurotransmitters are involved in the transmission of acupuncture stimulation to nerves. Tjen-A-Looi et al. [39] showed that EA at P5 and P6 acupoints restores the blood pressure in phenylbiguanide-induced hypotension and bradycardia cat models through both opioid and GABAergic processing mechanisms. They also showed that EA at P5 and P6 modulates the cardiovascular depressor responses during gastric distention in rats via GABAergic mechanisms [40]. Our data also showed that gene expression signatures responsive to ST36 stimulation connected to the GABAergic neurotransmission network in brain.

Conclusions

In conclusion, we performed a global comprehensive study on the gene expression signatures of nine different organs or tissues after ST36 stimulation. EA at ST36 affected the expression of genes not only in acupunctured site but also in internal organs. Gene expression signatures showed that stimulation at ST36 acupoint commonly affected process networks involved in cytoskeleton and cell adhesion in these organs. However, EA at ST36 also regulated unique process networks in specific organs or tissues. In addition, ST36 stimulation affected the expression of genes related to various diseases. The connection between gene expression signatures and diseases might provide a basis for the prediction and the explanation on the therapeutic potentials of acupuncture in various organs.

Funding
This work was supported by grants from Ministry of Science and Technology (MOST104–2320-B-039-018-MY3, MOST104–2325-B-039-004, and MOST105–2320-B-039-017-MY3), China Medical University (CMU104-H-01 and CMU104-H-02), and CMU under the Aim for Top University Plan of the Ministry of Education, Taiwan.

Authors' contributions
JSW and HYL carried out animal studies and involved in the interpretation of animal experiment data. CCL and FYC carried out microarray analysis. CYH and TYH involved in conception and design of experiments, obtaining grants and overall coordination of the project, interpretation of data, and preparation of the manuscript. All authors read and approved the final manuscript.

Competing interests
The authors declare that they have no competing interests.

Author details
[1]Graduate Institute of Chinese Medicine, China Medical University, 91 Hsueh-Shih Road, Taichung 40402, Taiwan. [2]Department of Microbiology, China Medical University, 91 Hsueh-Shih Road, Taichung 40402, Taiwan. [3]Department of Health and Nutrition Biotechnology, Asia University, Taichung 41354, Taiwan.

References
1. Ernst E. Acupuncture. Lancet Oncol. 2010;11:20.
2. NIH National Center for Complementary and Integrative Health. Website – introduction. https://nccih.nih.gov/about/plans/2011/introduction.htm. Accessed 1 Mar 2017.

3.   Lim HD, Kim MH, Lee CY, Namgung U. Anti-inflammatory effects of acupuncture stimulation via the vagus nerve. PLoS One. 2016;11:e0151882.

4.   Gao YH, Li CW, Wang JY, Kan Y, Tan LH, Jing XH, Liu JL. Activation of hippocampal MEK1 contributes to the cumulative antinociceptive effect of electroacupuncture in neuropathic pain rats. BMC Complement Altern Med. 2016;16:517.

5.   Cha M, Chae Y, Bai SJ, Lee BH. Spatiotemporal changes of optical signals in the somatosensory cortex of neuropathic rats after electroacupuncture stimulation. BMC Complement Altern Med. 2017;17:33.

6.   Xu F, Tan Y, Huang Z, Zhang N, Xu Y, Yin J. Ameliorating effect of transcutaneous electroacupuncture on impaired gastric accommodation in patients with postprandial distress syndrome-predominant functional dyspepsia: a pilot study. Evid Based Complement Alternat Med. 2015;2015:168252.

7.   Zhang N, Huang Z, Xu F, Xu Y, Chen J, Yin J, Lin L, Chen JD. Transcutaneous neuromodulation at posterior tibial nerve and ST36 for chronic constipation. Evid Based Complement Alternat Med. 2014;2014:560802.

8.   Lima JW, Hentschke VS, Rossato DD, Quagliotto E, Pinheiro L, Almeida E Jr, Dal Lago P, Lukrafka JL. Chronic electroacupuncture of the ST36 point improves baroreflex function and haemodynamic parameters in heart failure rats. Auton Neurosci. 2015;193:31–7.

9.   Huo ZJ, Li Q, Tian GH, Zhou CM, Wei XH, Pan CS, Yang L, Bai Y, Zhang YY, He K, Wang CS, Li ZG, Han JY. The ameliorating effects of long-term electroacupuncture on cardiovascular remodeling in spontaneously hypertensive rats. BMC Complement Altern Med. 2014;14:118.

10. Lin JG, Lo MW, Wen YR, Hsieh CL, Tsai SK, Sun WZ. The effect of high and low frequency electroacupuncture in pain after lower abdominal surgery. Pain. 2002;99:509–14.

11. Li C, Ji BU, Kim Y, Lee JE, Kim NK, Kim ST, Koo S. Electroacupuncture enhances the antiallodynic and antihyperalgesic effects of milnacipran in neuropathic rats. Anesth Analg. 2016;122:1654–62.

12. Yang G, Hu RY, Deng AJ, Huang Y, Li J. Effects of electro-acupuncture at Zusanli, Guanyuan for sepsis patients and its mechanism through immune regulation. Chin J Integr Med. 2016;22:219–24.

13. Yu ZG, Wang RG, Xiao C, Zhao JY, Shen Q, Liu SY, Xu QW, Zhang QX, Wang YT. Effects of Zusanli and Ashi acupoint electroacupuncture on repair of skeletal muscle and neuromuscular junction in a rabbit gastrocnemius contusion model. Evid Based Complement Alternat Med. 2016;2016:7074563.

14. Zhu MF, Xing X, Lei S, Wu JN, Wang LC, Huang LQ, Jiang RL. Electroacupuncture at bilateral Zusanli points (ST36) protects intestinal mucosal immune barrier in sepsis. Evid Based Complement Alternat Med. 2015;2015:639412.

15. Cheng K, Qin Z, Wang J, Zhai L. Lower He-sea sequence and indication specificity analysis regarding Zusanli (ST 36), Shangjuxu (ST 37) and Xiajuxu (ST 39). Zhongguo Zhen Jiu. 2015;35:1167–70.

16. Chou ST, Hsiang CY, Lo HY, Huang HF, Lai MT, Hsieh CL, Chiang SY, Ho TY. Exploration of anti-cancer effects and mechanisms of Zuo-Jin-Wan and its alkaloid components in vitro and in orthotopic HepG2 xenograft immunocompetent mice. BMC Complement Altern Med. 2017;17:121.

17. Chou ST, Lo HY, Li CC, Cheng LC, Chou PC, Lee YC, Ho TY, Hsiang CY. Exploring the effect and mechanism of Hibiscus sabdariffa on urinary tract infection and experimental renal inflammation. J Ethnopharmacol. 2016;194:617–25.

18. Eisen MB, Spellman PT, Brown PO, Botstein D. Cluster analysis and display of genome-wide expression patterns. Proc Natl Acad Sci U S A. 1998;95:14863–8.

19. Yeo S, An KS, Hong YM, Choi YG, Rosen B, Kim SH, Lim S. Neuroprotective changes in degeneration-related gene expression in the substantia nigra following acupuncture in an MPTP mouse model of Parkinsonism: Microarray analysis. Genet Mol Biol. 2015;38:115–27.

20. Zhang C, Wen Y, Fan X, Yang S, Tian G, Zhou X, Chen Y, Meng Z. A microarray study of middle cerebral occlusion rat brain with acupuncture intervention. Evid Based Complement Alternat Med. 2015;2015:496932.

21. Ho TY, Lo JY, Chao DC, Li CC, Liu JJ, Lin C, Hsiang CY. Electroacupuncture improves trinitrobenzene sulfonic acid-induced colitis, evaluated by transcriptomic study. Evid Based Complement Alternat Med. 2014;2014:942196.

22. Wang K, Xiang XH, Qiao N, Qi JY, Lin LB, Zhang R, Shou XJ, Ping XJ, Han JS, Han JD, Zhao GP, Cui CL. Genomewide analysis of rat periaqueductal gray-dorsal horn reveals time-, region-and frequency-specific mRNA expression changes in response to electroacupuncture stimulation. Sci Rep. 2014;4:6713.

23. Wang K, Zhang R, He F, Lin LB, Xiang XH, Ping XJ, Han JS, Zhao GP, Zhang QH, Cui CL. Electroacupuncture frequency-related transcriptional response in rat arcuate nucleus revealed region-distinctive changes in response to low- and high-frequency electroacupuncture. J Neurosci Res. 2012;90:1464–73.

24. Tzeng CY, Lee YC, Chung JJ, Tsai JC, Chen YI, Hsu TH, Lin JG, Lee KR, Chang SL. 15 Hz electroacupuncture at ST36 improves insulin sensitivity and reduces free fatty acid levels in rats with chronic dexamethasone-induced insulin resistance. Acupunct Med. 2016;34:296–301.

25. Zhang J, Huang K, Zhong G, Huang Y, Li S, Qu S, Zhang J. Acupuncture decreases NF-κB p65, miR-155, and miR-21 and increases miR-146a expression in chronic atrophic gastritis rats. Evid Based Complement Alternat Med. 2016;2016:9404629.

26. Yin HY, Tang Y, Lu SF, Luo L, Wang JP, Liu XG, Yu SG. Gene expression profiles at moxibustioned site (ST36): A microarray analysis. Evid Based Complement Alternat Med. 2013;2013:890579.

27. Liu X, Fan T, Lan Y, Dong S, Fu J, Mao B. Effects of transcutaneous electrical acupoint stimulation on patients with stable chronic obstructive pulmonary disease: a prospective, single-blind, randomized, placebo-controlled study. J Altern Complement Med. 2015;21:610–6.

28. Zhang XF, Zhu J, Geng WY, Zhao SJ, Jiang CW, Cai SR, Cheng M, Zhou CY, Liu ZB. Electroacupuncture at Feishu (BL13) and Zusanli (ST36) down-regulates the expression of orexins and their receptors in rats with chronic obstructive pulmonary disease. J Integr Med. 2014;12:417–24.

29. Song XM, Wu XJ, Li JG, Le LL, Liang H, Xu Y, Zhang ZZ, Wang YL. The effect of electroacupuncture at ST36 on severe thermal injury-induced remote acute lung injury in rats. Burns. 2015;41:1449–59.

30. Yu JB, Shi J, Gong LR, Dong SA, Xu Y, Zhang Y, Cao XS, Wu LL. Role of Nrf2/ARE pathway in protective effect of electroacupuncture against endotoxic shock-induced acute lung injury in rabbits. PLoS One. 2014;9:e104924.

31. Wu ZL, Li CR, Liu ZL, Zhang QR. Effects of acupuncture at "Zusanli" (ST 36) on eosinophil apoptosis and related gene expression in rats with asthma. Chin Acupunct Moxibustion. 2012;32:721–5.

32. Lu Y, Huang Y, Tang C, Shan B, Cui S, Yang J, Chen J, Lin R, Xiao H, Qu S, Lai X. Brain areas involved in the acupuncture treatment of AD model rats: a PET study. BMC Complement Altern Med. 2014;14:178.

33. Nam MH, Ahn KS, Choi SH. Acupuncture stimulation induces neurogenesis in adult brain. Int Rev Neurobiol. 2013;111:67–90.

34. Feng S, Ren Y, Fan S, Wang M, Sun T, Zeng F, Li P, Liang F. Discovery of acupoints and combinations with potential to treat vascular dementia: a data mining analysis. Evid Based Complementd Alternat Med. 2015;2015:310591.

35. Li F, Yan CQ, Lin LT, Li H, Zeng XH, Liu Y, Du SQ, Zhu W, Liu CZ. Acupuncture attenuates cognitive deficits and increases pyramidal neuron number in hippocampal CA1 area of vascular dementia rats. BMC Complement Altern Med. 2015;15:133.

36. He X, Yan T, Chen R, Ran D. Acute effects of electro-acupuncture (EA) on hippocampal long term potentiation (LTP) of perforant path-dentate gyrus granule cells synapse related to memory. Acupunct Electrother Res. 2012;37:89–101.

37. He W, Wang X, Shi H, Shang H, Li L, Jing X, Zhu B. Auricular acupuncture and vagal regulation. Evid Based Complement Alternat Med. 2012;2012:786839.

38. Torres-Rosas R, Yehia G, Peña G, Mishra P, del Rocio Thompson-Bonilla M, Moreno-Eutimio MA, Arriaga-Pizano LA, Isibasi A, Ulloa L. Dopamine mediates vagal modulation of the immune system by electroacupuncture. Nat Med. 2014;20:291–5.

39. Tjen-A-Looi SC, Li P, Li M, Longhurst JC. Modulation of cardiopulmonary depressor reflex in nucleus ambiguus by electroacupuncture: roles of opioids and γ-aminobutyric acid. Am J Physiol Regul Integr Comp Physiol. 2012;302:833–44.

40. Tjen-A-Looi SC, Guo ZL, Li M, Longhurst JC. Medullary GABAergic mechanisms contribute to electroacupuncture modulation of cardiovascular depressor responses during gastric distention in rats. Am J Physiol Regul Integr Comp Physiol. 2013;304:321–32.

21

A systematic review of the effects of acupuncture on xerostomia and hyposalivation

Zainab Assy and Henk S. Brand*

Abstract

Background: Saliva is fundamental to our oral health and our well-being. Many factors can impair saliva secretion, such as adverse effects of prescribed medication, auto-immune diseases (for example Sjögren's syndrome) and radiotherapy for head and neck cancers. Several studies have suggested a positive effect of acupuncture on oral dryness.

Methods: Pubmed and Web of Science were electronically searched. Reference lists of the included studies and relevant reviews were manually searched. Studies that met the inclusion criteria were systematically evaluated. Two reviewers assessed each of the included studies to confirm eligibility and assessing the risk of bias.

Results: Ten randomized controlled trials investigating the effect of acupuncture were included. Five trials compared acupuncture to sham/placebo acupuncture. Four trials compared acupuncture to oral hygiene/usual care. Only one clinical trial used oral care sessions as control group. For all the included studies, the quality for all the main outcomes has been assessed as low. Although some publications suggest a positive effect of acupuncture on either salivary flow rate or subjective dry mouth feeling, the studies are inconclusive about the potential effects of acupuncture.

Conclusions: Insufficient evidence is available to conclude whether acupuncture is an evidence-based treatment option for xerostomia/hyposalivation. Further well-designed, larger, double blinded trials are required to determine the potential benefit of acupuncture. Sample size calculations should be performed before before initiating these studies.

Keywords: Acupuncture, Xerostomia, Hyposalivation, Salivary flow rate, Sjögren's syndrome, Radiotherapy, Randomized controlled trials

Background

Saliva is fundamental to our oral health and our well-being [1]. Important functions of saliva are lubrication, digestion, antibacterial/antifungal activity, buffering, remineralization, and production of growth factors and other regulatory peptides [2]. Furthermore, oral functions such as speaking, swallowing and tasting require saliva. When the protective function of saliva becomes insufficient, this has profound negative effects on the oral health. An impaired saliva secretion (hyposalivation) usually results in the feeling of a dry mouth (xerostomia). Other consequences are increased caries formation, increased

rate of acute gingivitis, dysarthria, dysgeusia, increased rate of candidal infection and burning tongue [2]. Other negative effects are taste aberrations, breath malodor and poor denture retention [3, 4]. All these distressing symptoms have a profound negative impact on patients' quality of life [5, 6].

Many factors can impair saliva secretion. The most frequent cause of xerostomia is use of medication. Especially anticholinergic medications (for example tricyclic antidepressants, antipsychotics) are notorious for their xerostomic side effects [7]. The risk of xerostomia increases with the number of medications being taken [8]. Another cause of xerostomia is radiotherapy and chemotherapy. Head and neck malignancies are treated with radiotherapy or chemotherapy or a combination of both. The severity of xerostomia is depending on the total

---
* Correspondence: h.brand@acta.nl
Department of Oral Biochemistry, Academic Centre for Dentistry Amsterdam (ACTA), room 12N-37, Gustav Mahlerlaan 3004, 1081 LA Amsterdam, The Netherlands

exposure of the salivary glands to the radiation or the total number of chemotherapeutic drugs used [7]. Autoimmune disease such as Sjögren's syndrome can also induce xerostomia. Other, less common causes of xerostomia include sarcoidosis, HIV disease and HCV infection.

Various therapeutic strategies are available for xerostomia. To apply the appropriate therapy, the residual secretory capacity of the salivary glands must be assessed. When the salivary glands still can be stimulated, gustatory and/or mechanical stimuli (mint flavoured sucking tablet or sugar free chewing gum) are useful [9]. If these stimuli are not effective, systemic administration of a cholinergic agonist can be considered. A well-known cholinergic agonist is pilocarpine. Pilocarpine can stimulate salivary flow in normal volunteers as well as in patients with xerostomia [2]. However, pilocarpine may have adverse side effects such as nausea, vomiting, increased urinary frequency and headache [10].

When stimulated saliva secretion is much reduced or when stimulation of saliva secretion is impossible, palliative oral care can alleviate xerostomia [9]. Widely used palliative oral care products include mouthwashes, oral gels and saliva substitutes. These products are available over the counter without prescription, and these products can reduce xerostomia symptoms, which in turn may improve the quality of life [1]. However, palliative care products have several limitations. They are removed from the mouth during swallowing, the duration of their effect is short and they also lack the protective effects of saliva [7]. Due to the limitations of the therapies described above, complementary and alternative medicine (CAM) have become more popular among patients suffering from xerostomia [11]. One of the most widely used CAM therapies is acupuncture.

Acupuncture means to 'to puncture with a needle' [12]. Acupuncture treatment involves the insertion of extremely thin solid needles into intradermal or subdermal loci for the therapeutic relief of many symptoms [13]. In 2003, the World Health Organization published a report on the efficacy of acupuncture in the cure or relief of 64 different symptoms [14].

There are several hypotheses how acupuncture can increase the salivary secretion. Acupuncture can stimulate the parasympathetic and sympathetic nervous systems by neuronal activations [12, 15]. Additionally, acupuncture therapy produces the release of neuropeptides such as the vasodilator calcitonin gene-related peptide [12, 15]. These neuropeptides have anti-inflammatory properties and trophic effects on the salivary gland and increase the blood flow in the acini [12]. Another explanation is that acupuncture can directly affect the local blood flow in the proximity of the salivary gland and thereby increase the salivary secretion [16]. Finally, acupuncture therapy may tap into the neuronal circuit, which activates the salivary

nuclei in the pons and subsequently the salivary glands via the cranial nerves [12]. Acupuncture is a low risk therapy [17–20] and significant adverse events of acupuncture are rare (less than 1 per 20,000 individuals) [13].

Several studies have explored the effect of acupuncture on oral dryness [21, 22]. Although some of these studies suggest a positive effect, a systematic review of the effects of acupuncture on salivary secretion or xerostomia symptoms is still lacking. Therefore, the aim of the present is to investigate whether acupuncture is an evidence-based option for the treatment of xerostomia/hyposalivation, and - if this is the case - to ascertain which patients with oral dryness benefit from acupuncture.

Methods

Systematic review of the literature was performed using the databases of Medline/Pubmed and Web of Science till July 2015. The electronic database of Pubmed was searched for articles using keywords related to acupuncture and xerostomia or hyposalivation. An initial search was conducted using the terms (salivary gland diseases) OR (salivary gland disease) OR (salivary glands) OR ("saliva"[MeSH Terms]) OR ("salivation"[MeSH Terms]) OR (saliva secretion) OR (oral dryness) OR (hyposalivation) OR (asialia) OR (dryness of the mouth) OR ("xerostomia"[MeSH Terms]) OR (mouth dryness) OR (dry mouth). For this study MeSH terms were used to increase our search. The initial search was combined with the following terms: AND ("acupuncture"[MeSH Terms]) OR ("acupuncture therapy"[MeSH Terms]) OR (acupuncture) OR ("moxibustion"[MeSH Terms]) OR (moxibustion) OR (electroacupuncture) OR (electro acupuncture) OR ("acupuncture, ear"[MeSH Terms]) OR (ear acupuncture) OR (ear/electro acupuncture). For the search of Web of science exactly the same terms were used, but without MeSH terms. Manual search was carried out to enrol other potentially relevant articles, which could not be found with the electronic search. Therefore, the reference lists of the included articles were checked for further possible trials.

Selection criteria

Two authors (Z.A. and H.B.) independently searched for articles and independently examined the title and abstract of all records identified. The authors assessed each of these articles to determine which met the inclusion criteria for this review. For all articles that seemed to meet the inclusion criteria, a full text version of was retrieved. The inclusion criteria used for the present study were:

- Articles in English or Dutch
- Randomized controlled trials (RCT)
- Patients with dry mouth symptoms (xerostomia) or hyposalivation due to any cause

- Dentate and/or edentulous patients
- Studies using invasive acupuncture
  (acupuncture with needle penetration of the skin)
- Studies using one or more of the following
  parameters for oral dryness were eligible:
  salivary flow rate (unstimulated whole saliva (UWS)
  or stimulated whole saliva (SWS)), salivary gland
  scintigraphy, functional magnetic resonance imaging
  of salivary glands, or subjective parameters (Visual
  Analogue Scale (VAS), Xerostomia Questionaire,
  Quality of life, duration of effectiveness, patient
  satisfaction with treatment) [23, 24].

Excluded were systematic reviews (plus meta-analysis),
cohort studies, case-control studies, in vitro studies, case
reports/series, letters to the editor and studies using
non-invasive acupuncture.

Any disagreement between the two authors was resolved
by discussion.

Quality assessment

The methodological quality of the included randomized
controlled trials (RCT) was assessed using the Cochrane
Collaboration's tool described in Handbook version 5.1.0
[25]. Table 1 shows the potential biases assessed in the
present study. The same authors who conducted the search
for the articles assessed the quality of each RCT. These
authors independently assessed each RCT for the risk of
bias. Differences in rating between authors were resolved
by discussion. Studies with high risk in one or more
domains were rated as high risk of bias (plausible bias that
seriously weakens confidence in the results). Studies were
only rated as low risk of bias (plausible bias unlikely to
seriously alter the results) when the study met the criteria
in all domains. Studies were rated as unclear risk of bias
(plausible bias that raises some doubt about the results) if
there was unclear risk or if there was no clear description
of the implemented method in one or more domains.

Results

The initial search of Pubmed and Web of Science, and
the subsequent manual search resulted in a total of 341

Table 1 Potential risks of bias, assessed in the present study [25]

Random sequence generation	selection bias
Allocation concealment	selection bias
Blinding of participants	performance bias
Blinding of practitioners	performance bias
Blinding of outcome assessment	detection bias
Incomplete outcome data	attrition bias
Selective reporting	reporting bias
Other bias	

possible articles (Fig. 1). After removing duplicates, a
total of 171 articles were initially identified. Based on the
titles and abstracts of these publications, 68 articles were
discarded by the two reviewers as being not related to
this systematic review, because they did not discuss
acupuncture and xerostomia/hyposalivation. One hundred
and three references were retrieved in full text. Of these
references 93 articles were excluded for several different
reasons. The major reason for exclusion was that studies
did not have a RCT design. The language of some articles
(Swedish, Russian, French, Spanish, German, and Czech)
was another reason to exclude these articles. In addition,
several articles describing non-invasive acupuncture
procedures (like acupuncture-like transcutaneous nerve
stimulation, or laser acupuncture) were also excluded. The
use of other outcome measures like blood flux of the skin,
and the salivary concentration of peptides were another
reason to exclude articles. Finally, nine publications were
excluded because of several other reasons: congress
abstracts of included articles ($n = 4$), articles not discussing
a relation between acupuncture and xerostomia/hypo-
salivation ($n = 4$), and a research using healthy volunteers
($n = 1$). After removing all excluded publications, 10 studies
met the inclusion criteria for the systematic review.

Included studies

Characteristic of the trial design and settings

Ten RCTs met the inclusion criteria and were included
in this systematic review. Table 2 summarizes important
characteristics of the included articles. All studies had
a parallel group trial with two arms comparing an
experimental arm (acupuncture) with a control arm.
The experimental groups consisted of the following
acupuncture methods: auriculotherapy [26], acupuncture
according to traditional Chinese medicine [27, 28],
acupuncture according to traditional Chinese and ortho-
dox Western medicine [29], acupoints mainly in the
regions of the parotid, submandibular and labial glands
[30], acupuncture according to traditional Chinese
medicine and biomedicine [31], real acupuncture (using
different body points) [32, 33], acupuncture using standard
and customized anatomic points [34], acupoints in the
bilateral ears, index finger and an additional facial point
[35]. For the control groups, the studies used also different
methods. The following control groups have been used:
placebo auriculotherapy, placebo acupuncture (superficial
needling) [27, 28], no therapeutic modality at all [29, 30],
sham acupuncture (non-acupoints 2 cm away from the
real acupoints) [33], standard care group (oral hygiene)
[31], sham acupuncture (non-penetrating needle device)
[32], usual care (no specific treatment) [34], oral care
sessions (lifestyle and dietary advices) [35]. Only one study
used a cross-over design [35], with crossover 4 weeks after
the end of the first intervention (acupuncture or oral care

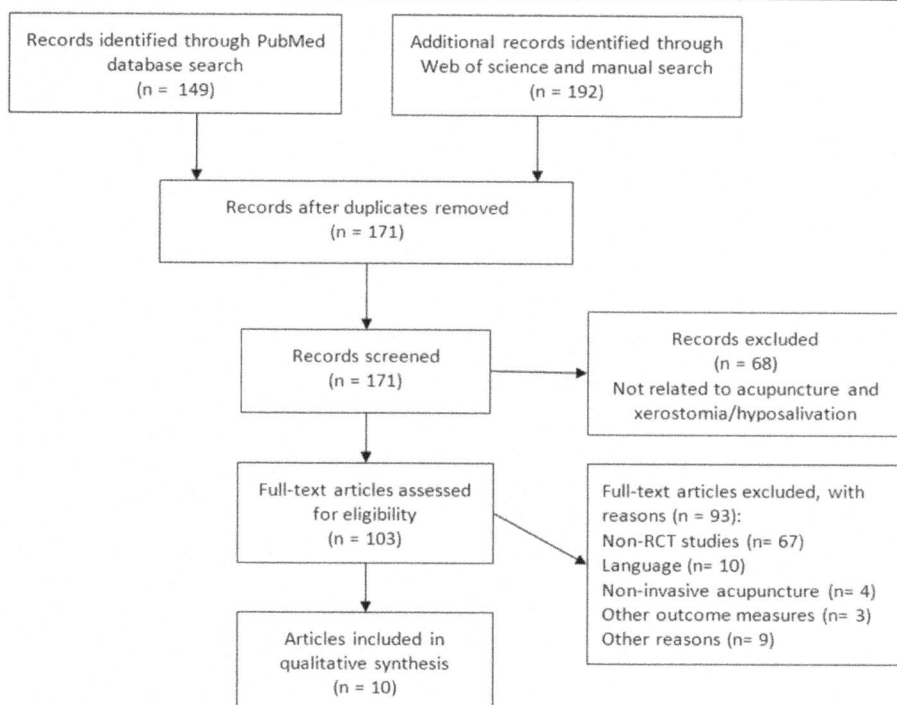

Fig. 1 Prisma flow diagram of the systematic review process

sessions). One study had a mixed design of a RCT and a cohort study [30]. Patients were first randomized between acupuncture and the control group. After finishing a 10 weeks' period the control group were treated with acupuncture as well. Three trials studied the preventive effect of acupuncture in minimizing/preventing xerostomia among cancer patients before and during radiation therapy [29, 31, 32]. Three trials were conducted in Sweden [27, 28, 30], two in China [31, 32], one in France [26], one in Brazil [29], one in South Korea [33], one in the USA [34], and one in the UK [35]. All studies were single centre studies, except the study in the UK, in which seven oncology centres participated [35].

Six studies were funded solely by research grants from publicly funded bodies [28, 30–33, 35]. The remaining four trials did not state the sources of funding for the studies [26, 27, 29, 34].

Characteristics of the participants
A total of 503 participants took part in the ten trials with a mean of 62 participants per trial and a range of 12 to 175. All participants were adults with different causes of xerostomia. One study included only patients with primary Sjögren's syndrome [30]. In seven trials the cause of xerostomia was radiotherapy for head and neck cancer [26, 28, 29, 31–33, 35], sometimes in combination with chemotherapy. Furthermore, one study included patients who had undergone neck dissection and

radiotherapy for cancer [34]. In the remaining study participants suffered from a variety of causes of xerostomia, including primary and secondary Sjögren's syndrome, radiotherapy and hypothyroidism [27].

Characteristics of the intervention
All the trials evaluated acupuncture. Only one study used both manual stimulation and electrical stimulation of two acupuncture points [30]. Five trials compared acupuncture to sham/placebo acupuncture [26–28, 32, 33]. Four trials compared acupuncture to oral hygiene/usual care [29–31, 34]. The patients in the control group of oral hygiene/usual care did not receive any therapeutic modality. Only one clinical trial used oral care sessions as control group [35]. During these sessions dietary and lifestyle advices to improve xerostomia where given to patients. The duration of acupuncture treatment varied between the clinical trials. The acupuncture treatment lasted for 6 weeks in most of the included studies [27, 28, 32, 33], separated in one study [28] by a 2 weeks resting period. Other studies used 4, 7, 8 (two studies) or 10 weeks of acupuncture treatment [26, 30, 31, 34, 35]. In one study the experimental period varied between 8 and 10 weeks [29].

Characteristics of the outcomes
Six studies used a combination of objective and subjective outcome measures. Two studies used the salivary flow rate

Table 2 This table shows the characteristics of the included randomised controled trials

Articles	Year	Country	Type of patients	Total of patients	Type of acupuncture	Type of control group	Studying preventive acupuncture effect	Outcome measures
Alimi [26]	2012	France	Receiving radiotherapy for head and neck cancer	60	Auriculotherapy acupuncture	Sham/placebo acupuncture	No	VAS scores
Blom [27]	1992	Sweden	Variety of patients	21	Traditional Chinese medicine acupuncture	Sham/placebo acupuncture	No	SFR and changes in subjective symptoms
Blom [28]	1996	Sweden	Receiving radiotherapy for head and neck cancer	41	Traditional Chinese medicine acupuncture	Sham/placebo acupuncture	No	SFR and changes in subjective symptoms
Braga [29]	2011	Brazil	Receiving radiotherapy for head and neck cancer	24	Traditional Chinese and orthodox Western medicine acupuncture	Oral hygiene/usual care	Yes	SFR and VAS scores
Cho [33]	2008	South Korea	Receiving radiotherapy for head and neck cancer	12	real acupuncture	Sham/placebo acupuncture	No	SFR and XQ scores
List [30]	1998	Sweden	Sjögren's syndrome patients	21	Parotid, submandibular and labial glands acupuncture	Oral hygiene/usual care	No	SFR and VAS scores
Meng [31]	2012	China	Receiving radiotherapy for head and neck cancer	86	Traditional Chinese medicine and biomedicine acupuncture	Oral hygiene/usual care	Yes	SFR and XQ scores
Meng [32]	2012	China	Receiving radiotherapy for head and neck cancer	23	Real acupuncture	Sham/placebo acupuncture	Yes	SFR and XQ scores
Pfister [34]	2010	USA	Receiving neck dissection and radiotherapy for cancer	70	Standard and customized anatomic points acupuncture	Oral hygiene/usual care	No	Xerostomia Inventory
Simcock [35]	2012	UK	Receiving radiotherapy for head and neck cancer	145	Bilateral ears, index finger and an additional facial point acupuncture	Oral care sessions	No	SFR. Quality of Life Questionnaire and the Head and Neck subscale

SFR salivary flow rate, *UK* United Kingdom, *USA* United States of America, *VAS* visual analogue scale, *XQ* xerostomia questionnaire

(unstimulated as well as stimulated) in combination with a VAS xerostomia questionnaire to measure the effect of acupuncture [29, 30]. Three studies [31–33] used a combination of salivary flow rates and Xerostomia Questionnaire (XQ) to assess dry mouth. Finally, one study measured the unstimulated and stimulated flow rates in combination with the European Organisation for Research and Treatment of Cancer Quality of Life Questionnaire and the Head and Neck subscale as subjective outcome measures [35].

Four studies used either objective or subjective outcome measures [26–28, 34]. Alimi et al. [26] used a VAS for dry mouth, while Pfister et al. [34] used the Xerostomia Inventory, a validated questionnaire. In the two studies by Blom and co-workers [27, 28], the unstimulated and stimulated salivary flow rates were reported, as well as changes in subjective symptoms and changes in the medication during or after the acupuncture procedure. *Risk of bias in included studies* (Table 3).

Allocation

With the exception of one study [29] all studies have adequate sequence generation (Table 3). Four did not describe an adequate allocation of concealment [27–30] and therefore these trials were assessed as high risk of selection bias.

Table 3 The risk of bias in all the included studies (top-down) according to Cochrane Collaboration's biases tool (from left to right). The plus sign indicating low risk of bias whereas the minus sign indicates high risk of bias. The question mark indicates an unknown risk of bias

	Random sequence generation (selection bias)	Allocation concealment (selection bias)	Blinding of participants (performance bias)	Blinding of practitioners (performance bias)	Blinding of outcome assessment (detection bias)	Incomplete outcome data (attrition bias)	Selective reporting (reporting bias)	Other bias
Alimi 2012 [26]	+	+	+	–	+	+	–	+
Blom 1992 [27]	+	–	+	–	+	–	+	–
Blom 1996 [28]	+	–	+	–	+	–	+	–
Braga 2011 [29]	–	–	–	–	–	+	+	–
Cho 2008 [33]	+	+	+	–	+/?	+	+	–
List 1998 [30]	+	–	–	–	–/+	–	–	–
Meng 2012 [31]	+	+	–	–	–/?	–	+	+
Meng 2012 [32]	+	+	+	–	+/?	–	+	+
Pfister 2010 [34]	+	+	–	–	–	+	+	–
Simcock 2013 [35]	+	+	–	–	–	–	+	+

+ = low risk of bias
- = high risk of bias
? = unknown risk of bias

Blinding

Blinding of participants to the allocated treatment by the use of placebo acupuncture (sham acupuncture) was done in five of the included studies [26–28, 32, 33]. These trials were assessed as low risk of performance bias. The other five studies were assessed as high risk of performance bias, because the participants were not blinded to the allocated treatment.

Blinding of the practitioner was not observed in any study. For this reason, all the included studies had high risk for this part of performance bias.

The outcome assessors (the patient or the examiner) were blinded with regard to the treatment in three trials [26–28] and these trials were assessed as low risk of detection bias. Three other studies did not blind the outcome assessors and were judged as high risk of detection bias [29, 34, 35]. The remaining studies did not report clear information concerning the blinding of the outcome assessors.

The study of Cho et al. [33] had a low risk and an unknown risk of detection bias. In this study, the patients were blinded to the allocated treatment, so when they administer the self-reported XQ-questionnaire, no risk of bias would be expected, as the patients did not know which treatment they received. However, the publication did not mention whether the outcome assessor was also blinded to the allocated treatment. Therefore, the risk of detection bias for this part of the study is unclear. The study of List et al. [30] had a high and a low risk of detection bias. The participants were not blinded with regard to their treatment. Because the participants were aware of their treatment this results in a potential detection bias for the VAS questionnaire. The

salivary secretion rate was measured by one person while the acupuncture treatment was performed by another person. Therefore, this part of the study was assessed as low risk of detection bias. Meng et al. [31] had a high risk and an unknown risk of detection bias. In this study the patients were not blinded to the allocated treatment, resulting in a potential detection bias for the Xerostomia Questionnaire, because the participants were aware of their treatment. It was unclear from the publication who measured the salivary secretion rate and subsequently the risk of detection bias for that part of the study was assessed as unknown. Meng et al. [32] had a low and unknown risk of detection bias. In this study, the participants were blinded to the allocated treatments resulting in a low risk of detection bias for the Xerostomia Questionnaire. However, in this study it was unclear who measured the salivary secretion rate, the reason why for that part of the study the risk of detection bias was assessed as unknown.

Incomplete outcome data

Four trials [26, 29, 33, 34] were assessed as low risk of attrition bias, because no drop out was reported or the intention to treat principle had not been used to evaluate the outcome data. The other six trials were assessed as high risk of attrition bias: Blom et al. [27] did not mention why some patients did not complete the treatment and some data with regard to the salivary flow rate are missing without any explanation. Four studies [28, 30, 31, 35] had a high risk of attrition bias because there was selective drop out in either the experimental group or the control group. Although Meng et al. [32] had similar numbers of dropouts in both arms of the trial, the initial dropout rate was high for the participants in both groups. Hence this article was assessed as high risk of attrition bias.

Selective reporting
Eight publications articles were assessed as low risk of reporting bias. Alimi et al. [26] reported that they used VAS to measure dry mouth and pain. However, no data were reported about pain. On the other hand, they reported results of mouth moistening (in liters!) and effectiveness of the acupuncture needles over time. For these reasons this publication was assessed as high risk of reporting bias. List et al. [30] reported in their methods that labial salivary gland biopsy data would be collected. As these data were not reported, this article is also assessed as high risk of reporting bias.

Other sources of bias
Four of the included trials [26, 31, 32, 35] were assessed as low risk of other bias. The remaining six trials were assessed as high risk of other bias. The most common source for bias was inconsistent acupuncture protocol. Blom et al., Pfister et al. [27, 28, 34] did not use the same number of acupuncture points in all patients. The number of acupuncture points used depended on the patients' particular complaints and their general health. On the other hand, Braga et al. [29] gave the patients different numbers of acupuncture sessions (16–20 sessions). Another point for high risk was inconsistent penetration depth of the acupuncture needles. Blom et al., Braga et al., Pfister et al. [27–29, 34] did not use a similar depth for the acupuncture needles. Cho et al. [33] did not have a standardized depth (less than 0,5 cm) of the acupuncture needles for the control group (sham acupuncture). In Blom et al. [27, 28] the distance between the classical acupuncture point and the placebo acupuncture point was not standardized but varied between 1 and 2 cm. Another problem in some acupuncture protocols was electric stimulation of some acupuncture points. In the publication by List and co-workers [30] one group got electrical stimulation of 2 acupuncture points while another group only received manual stimulation of all the acupuncture points.

A concerning point about the trial of Pfister and co-workers [34] is the study participants would not return to complete the final assessments, a fifth acupuncture treatment was added to enhance compliance.

The use of block randomization was another point of bias. In the study of Cho et al. [33] this resulted in an uneven distribution of subjects with regard to disease characteristics. This unbalanced grouping was the result of the use of block randomization.

Overall risk of bias
All of the included trials in this review had at least one domain where risk of bias was high (see Table 3). Consequently, all the trials were assessed as high risk of bias. The lowest risk of bias was observed for the study by Alimi et al. [26], the highest for the study by List and co-workers [30].

Effects of the intervention
In this section, acupuncture compared to other interventions will be discussed. These interventions include sham/placebo acupuncture, regular (oral) care and other treatments. The outcomes measures are unstimulated saliva secretion rate, stimulated saliva secretion rate and subjective outcome measures.

Acupuncture versus sham/placebo acupuncture
Unstimulated saliva Four trials with high risk of bias reported data for the unstimulated secretion rate. Meng et al. [32] investigated the effect of acupuncture before and during treatment with radiotherapy. During a period of 11 weeks the unstimulated salivary flow rate decreased significantly over time. After 3 weeks there was no difference between acupuncture and sham procedure. After 6 weeks real acupuncture-treated patients had an approximately 50% higher salivary flow rate compared to sham acupuncture patients, but this difference was not statistically significant.

The three other studies [27, 28, 33] investigated the effect of acupuncture in patients that had been treated with radiotherapy in the past or in patients suffering from severe xerostomia associated with a systemic disease. Cho et al. [33] measured the salivary flow rate for a period of 6 weeks. Blom et al. [27, 28] measured the flow rates for a longer period (12 months).

Using acupuncture, Cho et al. [33] noticed that after 3 weeks the unstimulated flow rate had increased by 55% compared to baseline and after 6 weeks with 75%. However, acupuncture only significantly improved saliva secretion at 6 weeks. In the sham treated population, after 3 and 6 weeks the unstimulated salivary flow rate was 2 and 15% higher, respectively, than the base line. Although these values suggest that patients benefit more from acupuncture, the differences between the two experimental groups were not significant at any time point.

Blom et al. [27] reported a significant increase of the unstimulated flow rate versus baseline in the acupuncture group at all time points from 7 to 64 weeks. In the placebo group a significant increase versus baseline was observed only at 16 weeks. After 28 weeks and 40 weeks the difference in salivary flow rate was significant in favour of acupuncture.

In the trial of Blom et al. [28], both acupuncture and placebo showed a significant effect on the unstimulated salivary flow rate at all the time points compared to baseline, except for 6 months in the placebo group, which did not reach any statistical significance. When comparing acupuncture and placebo, the differences were not statistically significant.

Stimulated saliva In the study of Meng et al. [32] on the effect of acupuncture before and during radiotherapy, a significant decrease of the stimulated flow rate over time was observed in both the treatment and control group. At baseline, week 3 and week 6, the average flow rate of the acupuncture group was 24, 0 and 36%, respectively, higher than that of the sham-treated group. There was no statistical significant difference, however, at any time point. At the end (week 11) there was only 8% difference between acupuncture and sham procedure.

Cho et al. [33] noticed that after 3 weeks the stimulated flow rate of patients with radiation-induced xerostomia increased by 3% compared to baseline using acupuncture and after 6 weeks the flow rate had increased with 20% compared to baseline. The sham procedure induced a decrease in salivary flow rate: at week 3 and 6 the flow rate had decreased respectively 9 and 5% compared to baseline. However, the difference between the two treatments was not significant.

Blom et al. [27] reported an increase of the stimulated flow rate both in the acupuncture and in the placebo group. When comparing acupuncture and placebo, significant differences in favour of acupuncture were seen at all time points, except 16 weeks. The acupuncture group showed significant differences at all time points versus baseline. In contrast, in the placebo group no significant differences were found.

The other study of Blom et al. [28] included only patients who had all or some of their salivary glands irradiated. In this study a significant increase was observed for the stimulated flow rate for most of the time points versus the baseline flow rates in both the acupuncture and the placebo group. Only at week 8 and 12 the flow rate of the placebo group did not differ significantly from the baseline value. Although acupuncture seemed to be better compared to placebo, no significant effect was seen between the two groups at any time point.

Perceived dry mouth Alimi et al. [26] measured variations in the intensity of dry mouth using a VAS. Acupuncture induced a significant 66% improvement of the VAS score compared to 4% for the sham procedure.

Meng et al. [32] quantified the dry mouth feeling using the Xerostomia Questionnaire (XQ). The sham group had after 3 and 6 weeks significantly higher XQ scores

than the acupuncture group, respectively 37 and 43% in favour of acupuncture. The greatest difference was seen at week 11: 56%.

Cho et al. [33] also used the Xerostomia Questionnaire. In both the treatment and the placebo group the subjective dry-mouth complaints improved compared to the baseline. However, no statistical difference in XQ score between the two groups was found at any time point.

Blom et al. [27, 28] did not use a questionnaire to quantify the dry mouth feeling but reported any changes of subjective symptoms during or after the treatment. Blom et al. [27] noted that in the experimental group two patients reported that they had less viscous saliva while in the control group none of the patients reported such change. Blom et al. [28] reported that many patients (number not reported) experienced a decrease of mucus secretion and a more fluid saliva. Some patients also reported improved taste, diminished pain of the tongue and less hoarseness. Those changes were somewhat slower and weaker in the control group, but these changes were not quantified.

Acupuncture versus regular (oral) care

Unstimulated saliva Three trials with high risk of bias reported data on the effect of acupuncture on unstimulated saliva secretion. Braga et al. [31] and Meng et al. [29] investigated the effect of acupuncture before and during radiotherapy for a period of 8 to 10 weeks, and for a period of 6 month, respectively. In the study of Meng et al. [31] the unstimulated salivary flow rate decreased over time during radiotherapy. The acupuncture group had significantly higher flow rates from week 3 up to week 11 when compared to standard oral hygiene, with the greatest group difference at week 7 (group difference of 0.06 g/min). However, after 6 months, the difference between the two groups was no longer statistically significant.

Braga et al. [29], who did not monitor the salivary flow rate over time reported a significant difference between the acupuncture group and the control group of 425% in favour of acupuncture.

The follow up period in the trial of List et al. [30] in patients with Sjögren's syndrome was 10–20 weeks. No significant effects versus baseline were found for both the acupuncture and the control group, and no significant differences between the two groups were observed.

Stimulated saliva The trial of Meng et al. [31] showed that patients receiving radiotherapy treated with acupuncture had significantly higher flow rates compared to standard oral hygiene from week 4 that remained through till 6 months. The greatest group differences were observed at week 7 (group difference of 0.112 mL/min).

Also Braga et al. [29] found significant changes between the acupuncture–treated and the control group. After radiotherapy the differences in stimulated flow rate between these groups were 308% in favour of acupuncture.

In the trial of List et al. [30] the median of the salivary flow rate increased with 100% in patients with Sjögren's syndrome after acupuncture treatment compared with baseline. However, no statistical significant differences between the acupuncture group and the control group were observed.

Preceived dry mouth Pfister et al. [34] measured the dry mouth symptoms using the Xerostomia Inventory (lower scores indicate a better outcome). The follow up period lasted for 4 weeks. After 4 weeks, there was a decrease of 12% for the XI scores in the acupuncture group versus baseline. For the control group (usual care) a decrease of 2% was seen after 4 weeks. The differences between these two groups were statistically significant.

Meng et al. [31] measured the dry mouth feeling using the Xerostomia Questionnaire. Starting in week 3, the control group had significantly higher XQ scores than the acupuncture group. This difference lasted for 6 months. The absolute differences between the groups increased over time with the greatest difference observed at week 7 (group difference of 10.3). After 7 weeks the difference between the two groups was still significant and the group difference was comparable with week 7.

Braga et al. [29] used a VAS to score the following dry mouth symptoms: 'difficulty in speaking', 'difficulty of swallowing', 'quantity of saliva in the mouth' and 'dryness of the mouth'. The VAS scores of these items revealed statistically significant differences between the acupuncture group and the control group. The score for the item 'difficulty in speaking' was in the control group 57% higher than in the treated group. The scores for 'difficulty swallowing' and 'the dryness of the mouth' were 57 and 47%, higher in the treatment group compared to the acupuncture group. The largest difference between the two groups was found for the item 'quantity of saliva in the mouth', which scored in the acupuncture group 239% higher than in the control group. This indicates that acupuncture treatment had a positive effect on the perceived quantity of saliva in the mouth. List et al. [30] evaluated dry mouth symptoms in the experimental and control groups with VAS items exploring discomfort caused by dryness of the mouth and the eye, and by a burning sensation of the mouth. The scores of eye dryness will not be included in this review. In the test group the perceived mouth dryness decreased significantly versus baseline (the median decreased with 24%), whereas in the control group no significant differences were found (the median increased with 8%). When comparing the acupuncture group with the control group, no significant differences were found after acupuncture treatment (a difference of 19% of the median between the two groups). No effect of acupuncture treatment on the sensation of burning mouth was found. After 10 weeks the control group also received acupuncture. Subjective evaluation of discomfort caused by mouth dryness, eye dryness and burning sensation in the mouth was performed. In addition, reduction in speech, chewing ability and the effect of dry mouth on daily activities were evaluated. Acupuncture treatment had no effect on any of these subjective outcomes.

Acupuncture versus other treatments
Unstimulated and stimulated saliva The trial of Simcock et al. [35] was the only trial (with high risk of bias), which compared acupuncture with another treatment. In this study acupuncture was compared with oral care sessions. During oral care sessions lifestyle and dietary advice were given to patients. Additionally, this was the only study which had a cross-over design. Group one started with oral care sessions first and after a wash out period of 4 weeks they got the acupuncture treatment. Group two started with the reverse order of interventions.

There were no significant changes in either unstimulated saliva or stimulated saliva over time or by intervention.

Preceived dry mouth In the same study [35] subjective dry mouth symptoms were evaluated using the Quality of Life Questionnaire and the Head and Neck subscale. Dry mouth symptoms were explored with questions about, "dry mouth", "sticky saliva", "need to sip liquids to relieve a dry mouth", "need to sip to swallow food", "dry lips" and "waking up at night because of need to drink". For every item, the odds ratio of reduced symptoms following acupuncture versus oral care were given. Significant odds ratios were found for dry mouth symptoms (2.01), sticky saliva (1.67) the need to sip to swallow food (2.08) and waking up at night to drink (1.71). No significant effect of acupuncture was seen on the odds ratio for dry lips (1.65) and sipping of liquids to relieve a dry mouth (1.59).

Discussion
Summary of main results
The ten studies included in this review were classified into three categories based on the comparison groups: sham acupuncture, regular oral care or other treatment. The quality for all the main outcomes has been assessed as low. Although some publications suggest a positive effect of acupuncture on either salivary flow rate or subjective dry mouth feeling, the studies are inconclusive about the potential effects of acupuncture.

Quality of evidence

None of the trials included in this review are at low risk of bias. There was a huge difference in number of participants per trial (varying from 12 to 145 participants). Only one study [34] reported a power analysis. As most other studies did not report sample size calculations these studies are likely to lack statistical power to detect differences between both arms of the trial. This can result in a type II error, the erroneous conclusion of no effect between treatments arms [36, 37]. In trials where several primary outcome measures are studied, such as salivary flow rate as well as xerostomia symptoms, the power needs to be set at a higher level (> 90%) for each endpoint [38].

In one study [29] randomization and concealment of allocation was not performed. This can introduce selection bias with significant effects on the results of a study. It has been reported that lack of random allocation with adequate concealment can have effects as large or larger than the expected effects of the intervention [39].

Blinding of the participants, practitioners and/or outcome assessor was not done in most of the studies. If bias is introduced during a trial because of differential treatment of groups or biased assessment of outcomes, no analytical techniques can correct for this limitation. Subsequently the results from unblinded trials should be interpreted with caution [40]. In a systematic review of 250 RCTs identified from 33 meta-analyses, researchers observed a significant difference in the size of the estimated treatment effect between trials that reported "double-blinding" compared with those that did not (p = 0.01) [41]. Another study of Jüni et al. showed that the results for double blinded studies were more heterogeneous [42]. A meta-analysis of four empirical studies relating key aspects of methodological quality to the effect estimates of controlled trials, revealed that that estimates were on average moderately biased in open trials (odds ratio of 0.83 and 0.88). In contrast, of the two smaller studies, one did not report an effect (odds ratio 1.11), whereas the other concluded that lack of double blinding introduced substantial bias (odds radio 0.56) The combined odds ratio for bias associated with the lack of double blinding is 0.86, further supporting the importance of blinding in a RCT [42]. On the other hand, Balk and co-workers in their meta-analyses of RCTs did not find any consistent associations between double blinding and the magnitude of the treatment effect [43].

Although sham acupuncture seems to be a good placebo procedure to blind the participants, several authors of included studies suggests that the sham procedure itself can have a beneficial effect on dry mouth. According to the philosophy of traditional Chinese medicine, there could be some positive effect of an acupuncture needle even when the needle is not placed accurately [27]. Blom and co-workers expressed that sham acupuncture with superficial needling could not be considered a placebo procedure and should be considered a different type of acupuncture treatment with less sensoric stimulation [28]. Another study of Vincent et al. shows that undifferentiated peripheral stimulation (needling) may have certain therapeutic effects, for example in pain reduction [44]. If sham acupuncture also has effects, its use as a comparison condition with true (point-specific) acupuncture may impose an unrealistic burden of proof upon the latter. This has important implications for the setup of such studies since very high subject numbers are required in order to be able to reveal a small additional effect of true acupuncture over sham treatment [44]. Thomas et al. conducted a controlled study investigating the effect of acupuncture on chronic nociceptive low back pain. They also conclude that 'placebo' acupuncture is a contradiction, since any sensory stimulus provokes a physiological response and thus cannot be inert [45]. This means that consideration should be given to designing a different control intervention.

Blinding of the practitioners was not done in any of the included studies, so performance bias can have influenced the effects in all included studies. Some of the studies [29–31, 34, 35] also did not blind the outcome assessors. Blinding of outcome assessors can be especially important for assessment of subjective outcomes, such as dry mouth symptoms. When no blinding of outcome assessor is done, detection bias may affect the results. Hróbjartsson conducted a systematic review of randomized clinical trials with both blinded and non-blinded assessment of the same measurement scale outcome. They included 16 trials with subjective outcomes. Their study provides empirical evidence for observer bias in randomized clinical trials with subjective measurement scale outcomes. Non-blinded assessors exaggerated the pooled effect size by 68% (95% CI 14% to 230%) [46]. Another study reached a similar conclusion for binary subjective outcomes. Non-blinded assessors of subjective outcomes generated substantially biased effect estimates in randomised clinical trials, exaggerating odds ratios by 36% [47]. The exaggerating of odds ratios in studies with patients being outcome assessors, as in the studies of our review, is unknown, but might be comparable to that of physicians.

Withdrawals from the study lead to incomplete outcome data, which can cause attrition bias. Attrition bias can affect the strength of a trial's findings [48]. Of the studies in this review, Meng et al. [31] showed the highest dropout rate (22%), without disclosing how these were distributed over the two groups. Uneven distribution of dropouts over the different arms of a study population, potentially invalidates the conclusions of a study. Another factor which may negatively impact the reliability of an RCT is the lack of a standard acupuncture protocol. This is a problem potentially affecting the quality of the majority of the included studies. Only four studies [26, 31, 32, 35] used a standard acupuncture protocol for treatment of the participants. Of these four studies only one [31] showed a significant effect of acupuncture on the salivary flow rate. When looking to the other six studies using a non-standardized protocol, two studies [27, 29] show a significant effect on salivary flow rate.

Overall completeness and applicability of evidence

An important consideration is the variation between the participants in these trials. The nature and extent of the salivary gland disease is likely to vary between participants with resultant variations in residual gland function, disease history and prognosis among the participants. Only trials that included patients treated with radiotherapy and trials with a heterogeneous group of patients show a significant effect of acupuncture. A trial that included a heterogeneous group of participants [27] did report a significant effect on the salivary flow rate, but it is unclear whether subgroups of patients in this study - which included radiotherapy patients, Sjögren patients and patients suffering from hypothyroidism - are responsible for this effect. The trial that included patient with Sjögren's disease only, did not report a significant effect of acupuncture. Notably, studies using other forms of acupuncture did report effects in Sjögren's patients. For instance, in a randomized placebo controlled study a positive effect of laser acupuncture was reported on the salivary flow rate in patients with Sjögren's syndrome compared to that in the control group (sham treated laser acupuncture) [49].

Blom et al. measured the effect of acupuncture on local blood flux in patients suffering from Sjögren's syndrome [16]. Patients with Sjögren's syndrome showed an increase in the peripheral vascular flux, which may be an important factor in relief of xerostomia [16].

A factor which complicates the comparison of the outcomes of different studies in cancer patients are differences in treatment modality, e.g. type of radiotherapy, radiation dose, or the type of chemotherapy. A source of variation is the type of radiotherapy that patients received who participated in these studies. In all but three studies [32, 34, 35] the radiotherapy technique used was not specified precisely. Knowledge of the type of radiotherapy patients underwent is important, because late toxicities, including xerostomia and Quality of Life are dependent on the treatment modality [50]. Meng et al. [32] only included patients treated with Intensity-Modulated Radiation Therapy (IMRT). This radiation technique minimizes the dose to surrounding normal tissue [51]. Duarte et al. showed that IMRT patients

exhibited significantly less xerostomia compared with those treated with conventional radiation therapy [52]. This may explain why this study did not find any effect of acupuncture on the salivary flow rate.

Another potential source of variation between studies is the impact of treatment modality. Only four studies [29, 32, 33, 35] clearly mentioned which treatment modality (chemoradiation or only radiation) the patients received. Treatment modality is important because it effects the acute (as example mucositis and dermatitis) and late toxicity (as example dysphagia and xerostomia). The incidences of late toxicity side effects were significantly increased in patients treated by chemoradiation, compared to radiation alone [53]. On multivariate analysis, chemotherapy and radiation technique showed a significant correlation with the incidence of late toxicity [53].

Potential biases in the review process

We conducted a broad search of two different databases and placed restrictions on the language of publication when searching the electronic databases or reviewing reference lists of the included studies. Subsequently it is likely that other studies, published in Chinese journals, may not have been identified for this review. Morrison et al. found no evidence of a systematic bias in conventional medicine studies from the use of language restrictions in systematic review-based meta-analyses [54]. Pham et al. also found the same for conventional medicine. However, the results of systematic reviews of complementary and alternative medicine do substantially alter when language restrictions are used [55, 56]. However, a team of authors based in China identified the same four RCTs that we included in this review, although they searched both English and Chinese databases [23]. This makes it unlikely that Chinese publications on acupuncture would have altered the conclusions of the present systematic review.

We decided to include cross-over studies in this review. A systematic review about non-pharmacological interventions for the management of dry mouth excluded cross-over studies [24], because the beneficial effects of acupuncture might last for weeks or months after the end of the treatment. A non-RCT retrospective study of Blom et al. confirms these results [4]. This non-RCT study shows that acupuncture treatment results in statistically significant improvements in salivary flow rate in patients with xerostomia up to 6 months. It even suggests that additional acupuncture therapy can maintain this improvement in salivary flow rate for up to 3 years. This means that inclusion of cross-over is an important potential limitation of the present review, as the washout period (4 weeks) in the included cross-over study of Simcock et al. [35] was relatively short.

Agreement and disagreement with other studies reviews

Several other studies have investigated the effect of acupuncture on healthy subjects. Dawidson et al. investigated the influence of acupuncture on the salivary flow rates of healthy students or dentists [57]. Unstimulated salivary flow rate showed a significant increase both during and after acupuncture stimulation compared to baseline levels, while stimulated salivary flow rates did not show any significant changes [57]. Deng et al. conducted a randomized, sham acupuncture controlled, subject blinded trial [58]. They included 20 healthy volunteers who received true and sham acupuncture in random order. True acupuncture led to a significantly higher saliva production compared to sham acupuncture [58]. These studies suggest that acupuncture also can have an effect on the saliva secretion of healthy subjects.

Some patients with dry mouth symptoms might benefit from acupuncture, but in absence of good evidence of their effectiveness their clinical relevance is questionable. Especially the costs of acupuncture make wide use less favourable. Based on current practice rates in the US, the cost of acupuncture are estimated at $400–$600 per treatment course [59]. Taken together, this does not seem to justify the use of acupuncture outside clinical trial setting at this moment.

Conclusions

All the included studies had a high risk of bias affecting the evidence of the studies. There is some evidence that acupuncture can increase salivary flow rate and/or alleviate dry mouth symptoms in patients following radiotherapy or in a heterogeneous group of patients. These results need to be interpreted with caution because of the high risk of bias in the included studies (low quality evidence). Overall there is insufficient evidence to determine the effect of acupuncture on dry mouth or hyposalivation symptoms. Acupuncture did not show any significant effect on the saliva production or dry mouth symptoms in patients with Sjögren's syndrome.

Further well-designed, double blinded trials with sufficient number of participants are required to determine the potential benefit of acupuncture. Sample size calculations should be done before before initiating the study. Trials should be designed and conducted according to SPIRIT 2013 statement guidelines and reported according to the CONSORT 2010 statement guidelines. These trials should not only include salivary secretion rates and validated xerostomia questionnaires,

but also other important outcomes like dry mouth symptoms, quality of life, duration of effectiveness and patient's satisfaction with the intervention. During these clinical studies, acupuncture could be compared with other promising potential treatments for hyposalivation e.g. low-laser therapy [60].

Abbreviations
ACTA: Academic Centre for Dentistry Amsterdam; CAM: Complementary and Alternative Medicine; CI: Confidence interval; CONSORT: Consolidated Standards of Reporting Trials; HCV: Hepatitis C Virus; HIV: Human Immunodeficiency Virus; IMRT: Intensity-Modulated Radiation Therapy; MeSH: Medical Subject Headings; RCT: Randomized controlled trials; SPIRIT: Standard Protocol Items: Recommendations for Interventional Trials; SWS: Stimulated Whole Saliva; UK: United Kingdom; US: United States; USA: United States of America; UWS: Unstimulated whole saliva; VAS: Visual Analogue Scale; XI: Xerostomia Inventory; XQ: Xerostomia Questionnaire

Acknowledgements
Not applicable.

Funding
University funding (ACTA). Both authors are staff members of the Academic Centre for Dentistry Amsterdam, and this study was performed as part of their regular research activities.

Authors' contributions
ZA searched for articles, assessed the quality of the included randomised controlled trials and wrote the draft version of the manuscript. HB searched for articles and assessed the quality of the included randomised controlled trials. Both authors read and approved the final manuscript.

Competing interests
The authors declare that they have no competing interests.

References
1. Wolff A, Fox PC, Porter S, Konttinen YT. Established and novel approaches for the Management of Hyposalivation and Xerostomia. Curr Pharm Des. 2012;18:5515–21.
2. Berk LB, Shivnani AT, Small W. Pathophysiology and management of radiation-induced xerostomia. J Support Oncol. 2005;3:191–200.
3. Rydholm M, Strang P. Acupuncture for patients in hospital-based home care suffering from xerostomia. J Palliat Care. 1999;15(4):20–3.
4. Blom M, Lundeberg T. Long-term follow-up of patients treated with acupuncture for xerostomia and the influence of additional treatment. Oral Dis. 2000;6(1):15–24.
5. Bruce SD. Radiation-induced xerostomia: how dry is your patient? Clin J Oncol Nurs. 2004;8:61–7.
6. Hanchanale S, Adkinson L, Daniel S, Fleming M, Oxberry SG. Systematic literature review: xerostomia in advanced cancer patients. Support Care Cancer. 2015;23(3):881–8.
7. Porter SR, Scully C, Hegarty AM. An update of the etiology and management of xerostomia. Oral Surg Oral Med Oral Pathol Oral. 2004;97:28–46.
8. Guggenheimer J, Moore PA. Xerostomia: etiology, recognition and treatment. J Am Dent Assoc. 2003;134(1):61–9.

9. Nieuw Amerongen AV, ECI V. Current therapies for xerostomia and salivary gland hypofunction associated with cancer therapies. Support Care Cancer. 2003;11:226–31.

10. Kahn ST, Johnstone PA. Management of xerostomia related to radiotherapy for head and neck cancer. Oncology (Williston Park). 2005;19(14):1827–32. discussion 1832–4, 1837–9

11. Cohen AJ, Menter A, Hale L. Acupuncture: role in comprehensive cancer care–a primer for the oncologist and review of the literature. Integr Cancer Ther. 2005;4(2):131–43.

12. Naik PN, Kiran RA, Yalamanchal S, Kumar VA, Goli S, Vashist N. Acupuncture: an alternative therapy in dentistry and its possible applications. Med Acupunct. 2014;26(6):308–14.

13. Sagar SM. Acupuncture as an evidence-based option for symptom control in cancer patients. Curr Treat Options in Oncol. 2008;9(2–3):117–26.

14. Lin J-G, Chen Y-H. The role of acupuncture in cancer supportive care. Am J Chin Med. 2012;40(02):219–29.

15. O'Regan D, Filshie J. Acupuncture and cancer. Auton Neurosci Basic Clin. 2010;157(1–2):96–100.

16. Blom M, Lundeberg T, Dawidson I, Angmar-Månsson B. Effects on local blood flux of acupuncture stimulation used to treat xerostomia in patients suffering from Sjögren's syndrome. J Oral Rehabil. 1993;20(5):541–8.

17. Deng G, Cassileth B. Acupuncture in cancer care. Integr Oncol. 2011;173(10):744.

18. Standish LJ, Kozak L, Congdon S, Kramer S. Acupuncture is underutilized in hospice and palliative medicine. Dtsch Zeitschrift fur Akupunkt. 2009;52(1):54–5.

19. Lu W. Acupuncture for side effects of chemoradiation therapy in cancer patients. Semin Oncol Nurs. 2005;21:190–5.

20. Deng G, Vickers A, Yeung KS, Cassileth BR. Acupuncture: Integration into cancer care. J Soc Integr Oncol. 2006;4(2):86–92.

21. Braga FP, Sugaya NN, Hirota SK, Weinfeld I, Magalhaes MH, Migliari DA. The effect of acupuncture on salivary flow rates in patients with radiation-induced xerostomia. Minerva Stomatol. 2008;57(0026–4970): 343–8.

22. Simcock R, Fallowfield L, Jenkins V. Group acupuncture to relieve radiation induced xerostomia: a feasibility study. Acupunct Med. 2009;27(3):109–13.

23. Zhuang L, Yang Z, Zeng X, Zhua X, Chen Z, Liu L, et al. The preventive and therapeutic effect of acupuncture for radiation-induced xerostomia in patients with head and neck cancer: a systematic review. Integr Cancer Ther. 2012;12(3):197–205. https://doi.org/10.1177/1534735412451321.

24. Furness S, Bryan G, McMillan R, Worthington HV. Interventions for the management of dry mouth: non-pharmacological interventions. Cochrane Database Syst Rev. 2013;8(9):CD009603.

25. Higgins JPT, Green S (editors). Cochrane Handbook for Systematic Reviews of Interventions Version 5.1.0 [updated March 2011]. The Cochrane Collaboration. 2011. Available from www.handbook.cochrane.org.

26. Alimi D, Poulain P, Cornillot P. Étude contrôlée randomisée évaluant l'action de l'auriculothérapie dans la xérostomie induite par la radiothérapie des tumeurs de la tête et du cou. Randomized controlled study assessing the action of auricular acupuncture in xerostomia induced by ra. Rev Odontostomatol. 2012;41:245–59.

27. Blom M, Dawidson I, Angmar-Månsson B. The effect of acupuncture on salivary flow rates in patients with xerostomia. Oral Surg Oral Med Oral Pathol. 1992;73(3):293–8.

28. Blom M, Dawidson I, Fernberg JO, Johnson G, Angmar-Månsson B. Acupuncture treatment of patients with radiation-induced xerostomia. Eur J Cancer Part B Oral Oncol. 1996;32(3):182–90.

29. do Braga FP, Lemos Junior CA, Alves FA, Migliari DA. Acupuncture for the prevention of radiation-induced xerostomia in patients with head and neck cancer. Braz Oral Res. 2011;25(2):180–5.

30. List T, Lundeberg T, Lundström I, Lindström F, Ravald N. The effect of acupuncture in the treatment of patients with primary Sjögren's syndrome. A controlled study. Acta Odontol Scand. 1998;56(2):95–9.

31. Meng Z, Kay Garcia M, Hu C, Chiang J, Chambers M, Rosenthal DI, et al. Randomized controlled trial of acupuncture for prevention of radiation-induced xerostomia among patients with nasopharyngeal carcinoma Zhiqiang. Cancer. 2012;118(13):3337–44.

32. Meng Z, Kay Garcia M, Hu C, Chiang J, Chambers M, Rosenthal DI, et al. Sham-controlled, randomised, feasibility trial of acupuncture for prevention of radiation-induced xerostomia among patients with nasopharyngeal carcinoma. Eur J Cancer. 2012;48(11):1692–9.

33. Cho JH, Chung WK, Kang W, Choi SM, Cho CK, Son CG. Manual acupuncture improved quality of life in cancer patients with radiation-induced xerostomia. J Altern Complement Med. 2008;14(5):523–6.

34. Pfister DG, Cassileth BR, Deng GE, Yeung KS, Lee JS, Garrity D, et al. Acupuncture for pain and dysfunction after neck dissection: results of a randomized controlled trial. J Clin Oncol. 2010;28(15):2565–70.

35. Simcock R, Fallowfield L, Monson K, Solis-Trapala I, Parlour L, Langridge C, et al. Arix: a randomised trial of acupuncture V oral care sessions in patients with chronic xerostomia following treatment of head and neck cancer. Ann Oncol. 2013;24(3):776–83.

36. Heidel RE. Causality in statistical Power : isomorphic properties of measurement, research design, effect size, and sample size. Scientifica (Cairo). Hindawi Publishing Corporation. 2016;2016(1):5.

37. Tsang R, Colley L, Lynd LD. Inadequate statistical power to detect clinically significant differences in adverse event rates in randomized controlled trials. J Clin Epidemiol. 2009;62:609–16.

38. Sjögren P, Hedström L. Sample size determination and statistical power in randomized controlled trials. Oral Surg Oral Med Oral Pathol Oral Radiol Endod. 2010;109(5):652–3.

39. Odgaard-Jensen J, Vist G, Timmer A, Kunz R, Akl EA, Schünemann H, Briel M, Nordmann AJ, Pregno S, Oxman AD. Randomisation to protect against selection bias in healthcare trials (review). Cochrane Database Syst Rev. 2011;13(4):MR000012.

40. Karanicolas PJ, Farrokhyar F, Bhandari M. Blinding: who, what, when, why, how? Can J Surg. 2010;53(5):345–8.

41. Schulz KF, Chalmers I, Hayes RJ, Altman DG. Empirical evidence of bias. Dimensions of methodological quality associated with estimates of treatment effects in controlled trials. JAMA. 1995;273(5):408–12.

42. Jüni P, Altman DG, Egger M. Assessing the quality of controlled clinical trials. Br Med J. 2001;323(July):42–6.

43. Balk EM, Bonis PAL, Moskowitz H, Schmid CH, Ioannidis JPA, Wang C, et al. Correlation of quality measures with estimates of treatment effect in meta-analyses of randomized controlled trials. JAMA. 2002;287(22):2973–82.

44. Vincent C, Richardson P. The evaluation of therapeutic acupuncture: concepts and methods. Pain. 1986;24(1):1–13.

45. Thomas M, Lundberg T. Importance of modes of acupuncture in the treatment of chronic nociceptive low back pain. Acta Anaesthesiol Scand. 1994;38(1):63–9.

46. Hróbjartsson A, Thomsen ASS, Emanuelsson F, Tendal B, Hilden J, Boutron I, et al. Observer bias in randomized clinical trials with measurement scale outcomes: a systematic review of trials with both blinded and nonblinded assessors. CMAJ. 2013; https://doi.org/10.1503/cmaj.120744.

47. Hróbjartsson A, Thomsen ASS, Emanuelsson F, Tendal B, Rasmussen JV, Hilden J, et al. Observer bias in randomized clinical trials with binary outcomes: systematic review of trials with both blinded and non-blinded outcome assessors. BMJ. 2012;344:e1119. https://doi.org/10.1136/bmj.e1119.

48. Dumville JC, Torgerson DJ, Hewitt CE. Reporting attrition in randomised controlled trials. BMJ Br Med J. 2006;332(7547):969–71.

49. Cafaro A, Arduino PG, Gambino A, Romagnoli E, Broccoletti R. Effect of laser acupuncture on salivary flow rate in patients with Sjögren's syndrome. Lasers Med Sci. 2014;30(6):1805–9. https://doi.org/10.1007/s10103-014-1590-8.

50. Huang TL, Chien CY, Tsai WL, Liao KC, Chou SY, Lin HC, et al. Long-term late toxicities and quality of life for survivors of nasopharyngeal carcinoma treated with intensity-modulated radiotherapy versus non-intensity-modulated radiotherapy. Head Neck. 2015;38(Suppl 1):E1026–32. https://doi.org/10.1002/hed.24150.

51. Vissink A, van Luijk P, Langendijk JA, Coppes RP. Current ideas to reduce or salvage radiation damage to salivary glands. Oral Dis. 2015;21(1):e1–10.

52. Duarte VM, Liu YF, Rafizadeh S, Tajima T, Nabili V, Wang MB. Comparison of dental health of patients with head and neck cancer receiving IMRT vs conventional radiation. Otolaryngol Head Neck Surg. 2014;150(1):81–6.

53. Al-Mamgani A, van Rooij P, Verduijn GM, Mehilal R, Kerrebijn JD, Levendag PC. The impact of treatment modality and radiation technique on outcomes and toxicity of patients with locally advanced oropharyngeal cancer. Laryngoscope. 2013;123(2):386–93.

54. Morrison A, Polisena J, Husereau D, Moulton K, Clark M, Fiander M, et al. The effect of English-language restriction on systematic review-based meta-analyses: a systematic review of empirical studies. Int J Technol Assess Health Care. 2012;28(2):138–44.

55. Pham B, Klassen TP, Lawson ML, Moher D. Language of publication restrictions in systematic reviews gave different results depending on

whether the intervention was conventional or complementary.
J Clin Epidemiol. 2005;58:769–76.

56. Moher D, Pham B, Lawson ML, Klassen TP. The inclusion of reports of randomised trials published in languages other than English in systematic reviews. Health Technol Assess. 2003;7:1–90.

57. Dawidson I, Blom M, Lundeberg T, Angmar-Månsson B. The influence of acupuncture on salivary flow rates in healthy subjects. J Oral Rehabil. 1997;24(3):204–8.

58. Deng G, Hou BL, Holodny AI, Cassileth BR. Functional magnetic resonance imaging (fMRI) changes and saliva production associated with acupuncture at LI-2 acupuncture point: a randomized controlled study. BMC Complement Altern Med. 2008;8(37):1–7.

59. Sasportas LS, Hosford DN, Sodini MA, Waters DJ, Zambricki EA, Barral JK, et al. Cost-effectiveness landscape analysis of treatments addressing xerostomia in patients receiving head and neck radiation therapy. Oral Surg Oral Med Oral Pathol Oral Radiol. 2013;116(1):e37–51.

60. Dabic DT, Jurisic S, Boras VV, et al. The effectiveness of low-level laser therapy in patients with drug-induced Hyposalivation: a pilot study. Photomed Laser Surg. 2016;34(9):389–93.

22

Hemodynamic changes caused by acupuncture in healthy volunteers: a prospective, single-arm exploratory clinical study

Tae-Hun Kim[1†], Boncho Ku[2†], Jang-Han Bae[2], Jae-Young Shin[3], Min-Ho Jun[2], Jung Won Kang[4], Junghwan Kim[4], Jun-Hwan Lee[3] and Jaeuk U. Kim[2*] ⓘ

Abstract

Background: Radial pressure pulse wave (RPPW) examination has been a key diagnostic component of traditional Chinese medicine. The objective of this study was to investigate the changes in RPPW along with various hemodynamic variables after acupuncture stimulation and to examine the validity of pulse diagnosis as a modern diagnostic tool.

Methods: We conducted acupuncture stimulation at both ST36 acupuncture points in 25 healthy volunteers. We simultaneously assessed the RPPW by pulse tonometry; heart rate variability (HRV) by electrocardiogram; photoplethysmogram (PPG) signals, respiration rate, peripheral blood flow velocity and arterial depth by ultrasonography; and cardiac output by impedance cardiography, before, during and after a session of acupuncture stimulation.

Results: We observed consistent patterns of increased spectral energy at low frequency (<10 Hz) and pulse power using RPPW examination and in the amplitude and systolic area of the PPG signal during the entire acupuncture session. The low- and high-frequency domains of HRV increased and decreased, respectively, during the acupuncture session. The peripheral blood velocity rose shortly after needle insertion, reached a maximum in the middle of the session and decreased afterwards. The augmentation index (AIX) and pulse transit time (PTT) obtained from RPPW did not change significantly.

Conclusion: Acupuncture stimulation at ST36 in healthy subjects increased the peripheral pulse amplitudes (pressure pulse wave (PPW) and PPG), blood flow velocity (ultrasonography) and sympathetic nerve activity (HRV). The lack of changes in the AIX and PTT suggests that the increased pulse amplitudes and blood flow velocity may result from increased cardiac output.

Trial registration: Clinical Research Information Service (KCT0001663).

Keywords: Acupuncture, Radial artery pressure pulse wave, Radial artery ultrasonography, KIOM-PAS, Hemodynamic variables

Background

Pulse diagnosis is a specific diagnostic and prognostic method used in traditional East Asian medicine (TEAM), including traditional Chinese medicine, traditional Korean medicine, and traditional Kampo medicine. Examining the pressure pulse wave (PPW) along arteries, especially along the radial artery, using the index, middle and ring fingers is a common practice in TEAM clinics [1]. Pulse diagnosis is a key to understanding TEAM medical theory and practice. Although there have been marked quantitative and qualitative improvements in the development of scientific imaging devices and laboratory tests, pulse diagnosis has occupied an important position in TEAM diagnosis. However, despite its clinical importance, very little is known about the physiological and pathological mechanisms underlying pulse diagnosis.

* Correspondence: jaeukkim@kiom.re.kr
†Equal contributors
2KM Fundamental Research Division, Korea Institute of Oriental Medicine, Daejeon 34054, South Korea
Full list of author information is available at the end of the article

From the viewpoint of modern medicine and biological science, the pulse is understood as a quantity that primarily reflects cardiac and hemodynamic activities [2]. The PPW is a wave that propagates along arteries and originates from the periodic blood pumping of the heart and vasodilation: the PPW travels approximately 15 times faster than the flow of the blood in the aorta. The PPW travels from the aortic arch to the peripheral arteries and carries vital information, such as heartbeat, blood pressure, arterial stiffness and aging [2]. These vital signs are affected by various body conditions. For instance, arterial endothelial function [3], the severity of arteriosclerosis [4], obesity [5] and sympathetic tone [6] have been identified as significant factors affecting PPW changes. Nevertheless, many research groups have attempted to reveal more complex factors related to PPW that can reflect health status either directly or indirectly.

Revealing the connection between the behavior of the PPW and various body conditions is a way to modernize and revitalize the pulse diagnosis of TEAM. Investigating the relationship between PPW and other cardiac and hemodynamic bio-signals may elucidate the underlying mechanism of pulse diagnosis and will help promote it as a modern scientific diagnostic method. In this sense, studying the continuous and simultaneous assessments of various hemodynamic factors associated with PPW changes is an important research agenda for understanding and modernizing the pulse diagnosis of TEAM.

A popular treatment modality that affects the characteristics of the PPW is acupuncture. According to the emperor's inner canon (Huangdi Neijing), "The key to acupuncture treatment is Qizhi, which brings about the therapeutic effect of acupuncture," where Qizhi may refer to the changes in the pulse wave [7]. Therefore, the effectiveness of acupuncture in a patient's treatment should be observable by pulse diagnosis and should modify the characteristics of the pulse wave. Indeed, several studies have reported that acupuncture can affect various bio-signals, such as heart rate variability (HRV) [8] and arterial blood flow [9], as well as the PPW [10]. These studies discussed changes in only one or two hemodynamic variables in relation to the acupuncture treatment, and so far no study analyzed various bio-signals simultaneously to investigate integrative hemodynamic phenomena occurred by acupuncture treatment. The objective of this study was to assess the radial PPW (RPPW) and several other bio-signals to obtain an overall picture of the hemodynamic changes in the human body caused by acupuncture stimulation and to help provide a comprehensive understanding of the mechanism underlying the pulse diagnosis of TEAM. The present study experimentally assessed changes in various bio-signals before, during and after ST36 acupuncture stimulation. Healthy young participants attended a single acupuncture session, and bio-signals including radial artery pulse pressure, blood flow and cardiac output were assessed approximately 7 times during the acupuncture session.

Methods

This study was a prospective, single-arm, exploratory clinical study to observe the effect of acupuncture stimulation on various hemodynamic variables, such as RPPW, in healthy young participants. This study was conducted at the Korean Medicine Clinical Trial Center, Kyung Hee University Korean Medicine Hospital, Seoul, South Korea, from October 2015 to December 2015. The study protocol was approved by the Institutional Review Board of Kyung Hee University Korean Medicine Hospital, Seoul, Korea (KOMCIRB-150818-HR-030) and was registered with the Clinical Research Information Service (registration number: KCT0001663) before the first participant was included. Written informed consent was obtained from each participant prior to study participation. Twenty-five healthy adults were recruited through advertisements on bulletin boards at the local hospital and university. Through history taking and assessment of vital signs including blood pressure, respiratory rate, pulse rate and body temperature, we evaluated general health status of the potential participants. The detailed protocol for the study is described in Shin et al. [11].

Inclusion criteria

The following inclusion criteria were applied as follows: healthy participants aged between 20 and 30 years old who had provided signed written informed consent.

Exclusion criteria

Participants who met the following criteria were excluded from this study:

(1) Use of medications within 1 month before participation, including antihypertensives, hypoglycemic agents, narcotics, tranquilizers, antithrombotic or antiplatelet agents, anticoagulants, or hormone drugs
(2) Pregnancy or lactation
(3) Korean Medicine College students or Korean medical doctors
(4) Acupuncture treatment within the last 4 months
(5) Inability to undergo evaluation with the pulse tonometric device or ultrasonography
(6) A history of heart disease or transplanted devices such as pacemakers
(7) Participation in other clinical trials within the last 3 months
(8) Communication disorder
(9) Drug addiction or alcohol abuse
(10) Conditions where acupuncture might not be safe, such as metal allergy

(11) Refusal to participate in the trial or provide informed consent

(12) Exclusion at the investigator's discretion

Study procedures

For preparation, the participants were not allowed to overeat, perform physical exercise or undergo emotional excitement for 1 week before the assessment, and smoking, and any caffeinated drinks such as coffee or Coke were prohibited on the assessment day. The participants who were included in this study after the screening test underwent several sessions of assessments of various bio-signals before, during and after a one-time acupuncture needling at ST36 on both legs during the procedure (Fig. 1). First, the Global Physical Activity Questionnaire (GPAQ) and the Credibility/Expectancy Questionnaire (CEQ) were completed before the assessment. After a 20-min bed rest, the spectral energy from 10 to 30 Hz ($SE_{10-30Hz}$), spectral energy from 0 to 10 Hz (SE_{0-10Hz}), pulse power index (PPI), pulse depth index (PDI), and pulse volume index (PVI) were measured on the left wrist of each subject with an appropriate pulse tonometric device (KIOM-PAS, Korea Institute of Oriental Medicine, Daejeon, Korea; Fig. 2). HRV, photoplethysmogram (PPG) signals, cardiac output (CO), and respiration (RSP) were measured using a physiological data acquisition system on the chest and nasal openings (Biopac module, Biopac MP150, Biopac Systems Inc., USA). The velocity of the blood flow and the diameter and depth of the blood vessel were measured using ultrasonography (Voluson 730 Pro, GE Healthcare Austria GmbH & Co OG, Austria) on the right wrist.

After assessing these bio-signals, the physician conducted the acupuncture procedure at both ST36 points, which were located according to the 'WHO Standard Acupuncture Point Location in the Western Pacific Region' [12]. A 0.16 mm × 40.0 mm disposable stainless steel acupuncture needle (Seirin Co. Ltd., Shizuoka, Japan) was used for needling. The Deqi sensation was induced through bidirectional rotation at a right angle (90°) for 18 s, and the needles were retained for 20 min before removal. Certified Korean Medicine Doctors (KMDs) with more than 10 years of clinical experience and 6 years of education performed the acupuncture treatments. All measurements were performed six times in total. After the measurements were complete, the subjects were given the Acupuncture Sensation Questionnaire (ASQ) [13], and adverse events related to the acupuncture and the measurement of each outcome were assessed.

Outcomes

The medical history of the participants, including their current medication status, surgical history, presence of other diseases, and the results of electrocardiography and pregnancy tests were recorded at baseline. Data regarding lifestyle factors, including exercise, smoking, caffeine intake, and alcohol consumption, were documented. Hypertension, height, weight, and other demographic data were also obtained.

GPAQ is an instrument for assessing physical activity. This questionnaire collects information on physical activity participation in three settings (or domains) and on sedentary behavior using 16 questions (P1-P16). The domains are "activity at work," "travel to and from places," and "recreational activities" [14]. CEQ was recently developed as a measure of treatment credibility and expectancy. This questionnaire consists of 1 question that reflects the expectations for acupuncture and rates on a scale of 1–9 [15]. ASQ was developed by the Department of Applied Korean Medicine, Kyung Hee University, Seoul, Korea, for the measurement of acupuncture sensation. This questionnaire consists of 3 parts: the sensations during the insertion (SIA), manipulation (SMA), and maintenance of the acupuncture needle (SM). The questionnaire consists of 33 items for SIA, 59 for SMA, and 29 for SM, and each

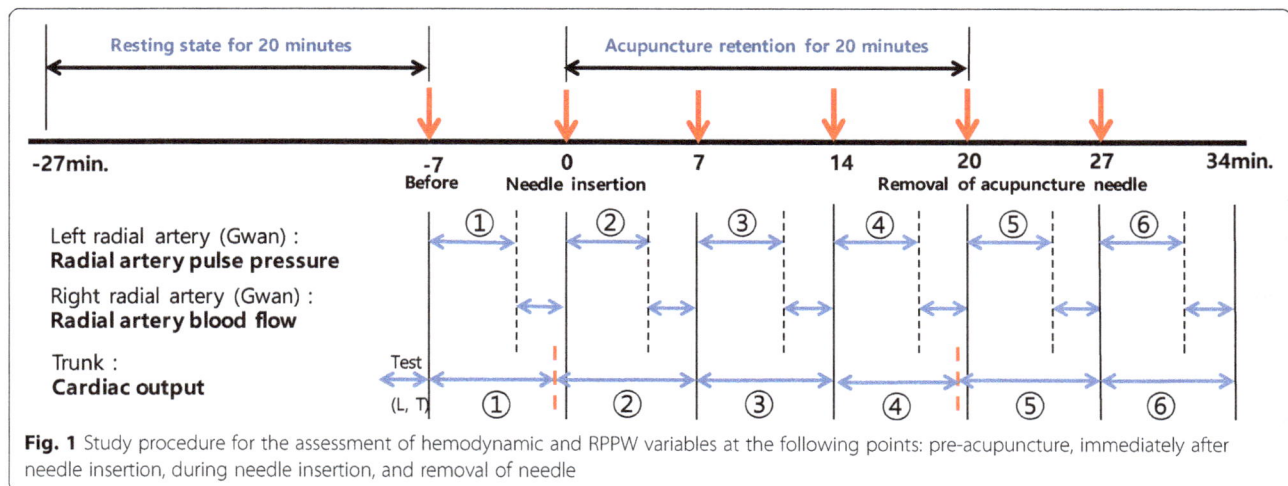

Fig. 1 Study procedure for the assessment of hemodynamic and RPPW variables at the following points: pre-acupuncture, immediately after needle insertion, during needle insertion, and removal of needle

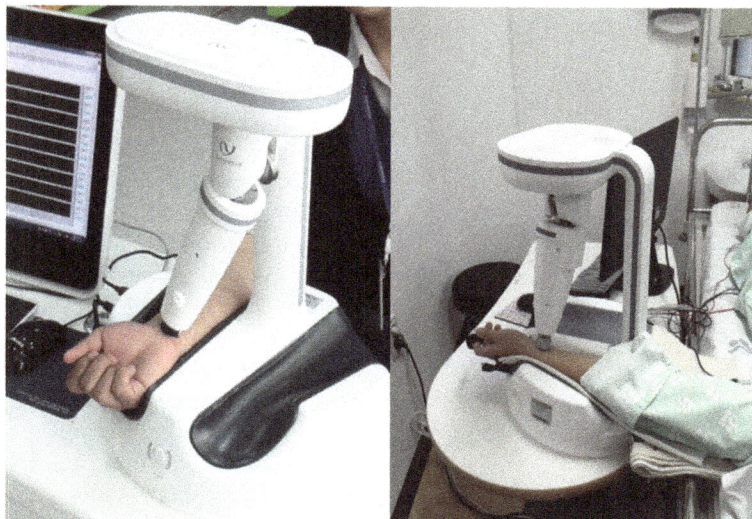

Fig. 2 The overall features of KIOM-PAS for the assessment of radial artery pulse pressure in different positions (*left*: sitting position, *right*: lying position). The figure was epitomized from the previous article that described the study protocol of this study [11]

sensation of acupuncture is evaluated with a 10-cm visual analog scale (VAS) for every item [13]. GPAQ, CEQ and ASQ were all used after acupuncture needling.

Details of RPPW and other bio-signal parameters are presented in Table 1. To assess the RPPW, we used KIOM-PAS, a pulse tonometric device developed at the Korea Institute of Oriental Medicine; this device is used for the assessment of radial artery pulse pressure [16]. KIOM-PAS consists of a main body and a sensing body composed of a piezoresistive 7-channel sensor with the sensors arranged in a row. In this study, the operator measured the pulse signals at Guan during the procedure. $SE_{10-30Hz}$ (the primary outcome of this study), SE_{0-10Hz}, PPI, PDI, PVI, systolic area, diastolic area, subendocardial viability ratio (SEVR) and radial augmentation index (AIX) were extracted from the KIOM-PAS for every measurement.

Bio-signal variables, including HRV, CO, PPG and respiration rate, were assessed using a Biopac MP150 (Biopac module, Biopac Systems Inc., USA). Specifically, the electrocardiogram (ECG) signal was recorded using an ECG100C module with lead II to analyze HRV, and the impedance cardiography signal was recorded using a NICO100C module to calculate the stroke volume (SV) and CO. The PPG signal was acquired using a PPG100C module to determine the average amplitude and average systolic area, and the RSP signal was acquired using an SKT100C module to calculate the respiration rate. Finally, the pulse transit time (PTT) was calculated by analyzing the time delay between the ECG and the RPPW.

For ultrasonography, a medical ultrasound scanner (Voluson 730 Pro, GE Medical, USA) was used with a 12 L

probe. The diameter of the artery was measured in the B mode, and the maximum and average of the blood flow velocity were measured in color Doppler mode. The angle of incidence for the ultrasound was maintained at 60° in the color Doppler mode and 20° in the B mode.

All unexpected responses related to the acupuncture treatment and measurements (adverse events) were reported to the investigators by the participants or were examined by an investigator. Adverse events were evaluated by investigators as mild, moderate, or severe according to the World Health Organization Draft Guidelines for Adverse Event Reporting [17] and Spilker's criteria [18].

Statistical analysis

All statistical analyses were performed using the current version of R statistical software [19]. The sample size was determined based on the results of a previous study performed by Huang et al. [20]. In this study, the spectral energy of 13 to 50 Hz ($SE_{13-50Hz}$) showed a significant mean change between pre- and post-acupuncture stimulation. Based on this result, we derived a mean change of 3.38 and a common standard deviation of 5.23 using the sample size and p-value presented in this paper. We planned to recruit 25 participants to detect differences with a 5% type I error, 80% power and 5% dropout rate. The significance level for all tests was set to 0.05 (two-sided). The baseline characteristics of the participants were described with the available data. Categorical outcomes were represented as the numbers of participants and percentages, and continuous variables were summarized as the means and standard deviation for normal data and the medians and interquartile

Table 1 Description of parameters related with the radial artery pulse-pressure wave and other bio-signal characteristics

Variable (units)	Description
Radial pressure pulse wave	
$SE_{0\text{-}10Hz}$ (V_{rms}^2, 10^{-1})	Sum of the spectral energy within 0–10 Hz
$SE_{10\text{-}30Hz}$ (V_{rms}^2, 10^{-3})	Sum of the spectral energy within 10–30 Hz
PPI (V)	Pulse power index; Maximum amplitude of the voltage response in radial artery pulse
PDI (mm)	Pulse depth index; measure of the pulse depth based on the sensor displacement in the direction normal to the skin surface
Systolic area (Vs)	Area of systolic phase in average pulse
Diastolic area (Vs)	Area of diastolic phase in average pulse
SEVR (%, 10^{-2})	Subendocardial viability ratio; ratio between the diastolic and systolic area
AIX (%)	Radial augmentation index normalized to a heart rate of 75 bpm; (late systolic pressure/systolic pressure) × 100
Heart rate variability	
NN (s)	Normal to normal interval
SDNN (ms)	Standard deviation of the NN interval
RMSSD (ms)	Square root of the mean squared differences of NN intervals
TF (ms^2)	Total frequency power within 0–0.4 Hz
LF (ms^2)	Low frequency power within 0.04–0.15 Hz
HF (ms^2)	High frequency power within 0.15–0.4 Hz
nLF (%)	LF power in normalized units; LF/(LF + HF)
nHF (%)	HF power in normalized units; HF/(LF + HF)
LF/HF	Ratio of low to high frequency components; LF/HF
Photoplethysmogram signals	
PPG amplitude (V)	Maximum amplitude in average PPG
PPG systolic area (Vs)	Area of systolic phase in average PPG
Respiration signals	
Respiration rate (bpm)	Number of respirations per minute.
Impedance cardiography	
SV (ml)	Stroke volume: volume of blood pumped from the left ventricle per beat
CO (ml/min)	Cardiac output: volume of blood being pumped from the heart per minute; stroke volume × heart rate
Combined variable from radial pressure pulse wave and electrocardiography	
PTT (ms)	Time delay between the R-peak of the ECG and the peak of the RPPW

range (25th and 75th quartiles) for skewed data. The Shapiro-Wilk test was used to verify the normality of the quantitative measures. Analyses of the primary and secondary outcomes were conducted on a full analysis set on the basis of the intention-to-treat principle and on per-protocol subsamples for the purpose of sensitivity analyses. The last

observation carried forward (LOCF) method was used to impute missing data.

Although the sample size in this study was obtained from $SE_{13\text{-}50Hz}$, it had almost the same properties as those obtained from $SE_{10\text{-}30Hz}$ [21]. Thus, the primary outcome was chosen as the change in $SE_{10\text{-}30Hz}$ between pre- and post-acupuncture stimulation measured at the baseline and at the end, respectively.

A paired two-sample t-test was used to determine the significance of the change induced by the acupuncture stimulation. The results of the analysis were presented as the means, standard deviation, 95% confidence intervals (CI), t-values and p-values. The changes in $SE_{10\text{-}30Hz}$ at six time points (before acupuncture stimulation, immediately during needle insertion, during the stimulation at 7 and 14 min after needle insertion, and immediately and 7 min after removing acupuncture stimulation) were investigated using a linear mixed-effect model (LMM) as a secondary analysis. The LMM included covariates (sex, age, BMI, pulse rate, GPAQ, CEQ and ASQ scale effects) and interaction terms between sex and time effects. The model was modified by excluding the interaction term if it was not significant. The ANOVA table for the model was provided, and the least square mean, standard error, and 95% CI were provided for each time point. Differences in a value between a given time point and baseline (before acupuncture) were examined using Dunnett's test.

Results
From October to December 2015, 25 healthy volunteers participated in this study, including 13 female and 12 male young adults (average age 23.3 years, standard deviation (SD) 2.4 years). No participants dropped out due to compliance problems related to acupuncture stimulation or repeated assessments (Fig. 3). Most participants had low to moderate levels of physical activity (64%). The participants were of average fitness or were slightly underweight (average body mass index (BMI) of 21.7 (2.5)). Nineteen participants had a previous acupuncture experience (76%). The expectation of the effect of acupuncture was considerably high (mean 6.5, SD 5.6, Table 2).

Effect on the radial artery pressure pulse wave
Significant increases in $SE_{0\text{-}10Hz}$ were observed as the acupuncture session progressed. There was no difference between baseline and immediately after needle insertion (MD 0.49, 95% CI [−0.33, 1.31]), but the differences increased continuously after 7 min (MD 0.95, 95% CI [0.13, 1.76]) and 14 min (MD 1.20, 95% CI [0.38, 2.02]), immediately after needle removal (MD 0.139, 95% CI [0.58, 2.23]) and 7 min after needle removal (MD 1.79, 95% CI [0.98, 2.61]). $SE_{10\text{-}30Hz}$, however, did not show any differences between before and after acupuncture needling, except at the final assessment (MD −0.77, 95% CI [−1.44, −0.11]).

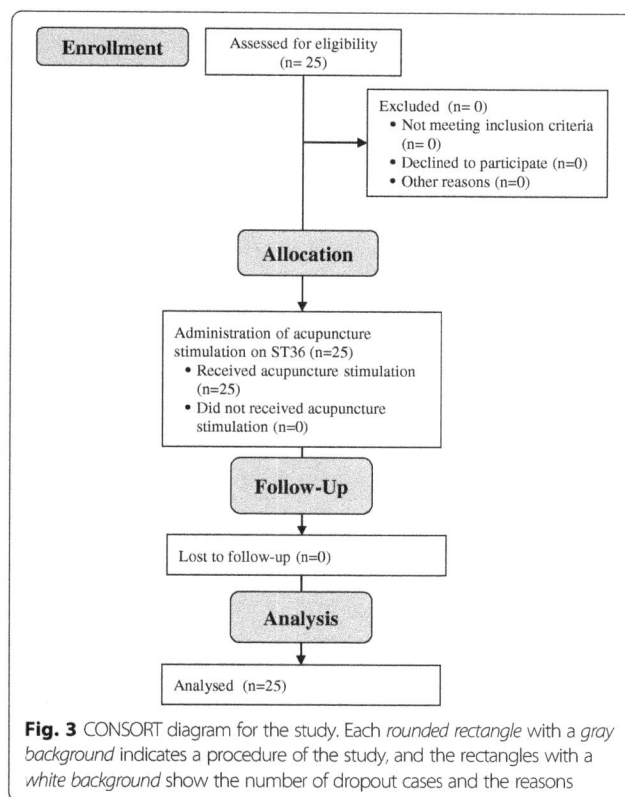

Fig. 3 CONSORT diagram for the study. Each *rounded rectangle* with a *gray background* indicates a procedure of the study, and the rectangles with a *white background* show the number of dropout cases and the reasons

PPI also showed an increasing pattern in the difference between the baseline and after needling values. No significant differences were observed immediately after needling (MD 0.12, 95% CI [−0.05, 0.28]) or 7 min after needling (MD 0.12, 95% CI [−0.05, 0.28]), but the differences increased gradually after 14 min (MD 0.24, 95% CI [0.08, 0.41]), at needle removal (MD 0.27, 95% CI [0.11, 0.44]) and 7 min after needle removal (MD 0.31, 95% CI [0.15, 0.48]). The PDI values did not show significant differences for any measurement. The PVI values showed significant increases in the measurements 7 min after (MD 0.46, 95% CI [0.16, 0.71]) and 14 min after needle insertion (MD 0.32, 95% CI [0.03, 0.61]).

The systolic area and diastolic area also showed an increasing pattern during the procedure. Significant differences were observed 14 min after needle insertion (MD 54.50, 95% CI [15.50, 93.51]), at needle removal (MD 61.68, 95% CI [22.68, 100.68]), and at the final assessment (MD 92.49, 95% CI [53.48, 131.49]) for the systolic area and at needle removal (MD 12.19, 95% CI [0.03, 24.35]) and at the final assessment (MD 18.09, 95% CI [5.93, 30.25]) for the diastolic area. SEVR showed an opposite decreasing tendency after needle insertion, and significant differences were observed 14 min after needle insertion (MD −2.58, 95% CI [−5.04, −0.12]) and immediately after (MD −2.48, 95% CI [−4.94, −0.02]) and 7 min after needle removal (MD −3.35, 95% CI [−5.81, −0.89]). AIX and PTT

Table 2 Demographic characteristics of the participants

Characteristics	Value (Total number = 25)
Sex (n, %)	
Female	13 (52.0)
Male	12 (48.0)
Smoking (n, %)	
None	2 (8.0)
Former smoker	23 (92.0)
Caffeine (n, %)	
None	12 (48.0)
Former user	1 (4.0)
Current user	12 (48.0)
Alcohol (n, %)	
None	15 (60.0)
Former consumer	1 (4.0)
Current consumer	9 (36.0)
Level of physical activity (n, %)[a]	
Low	15 (60.0)
Moderate	1 (4.0)
High	9 (36.0)
Experience of Acupuncture (n, %)	
No	6 (24.0)
Yes	19 (76.0)
Age (mean, SD)	23.3 (2.4)
Height (mean, SD)	168.0 (8.9)
Weight (mean, SD)	61.7 (11.3)
BMI (mean, SD)	21.7 (2.5)
Systolic BP (mean, SD)	111.6 (10.3)
Diastolic BP (mean, SD)	73.6 (5.6)
Pulse (mean, SD)	74.8 (5.6)
Body temperature (mean, SD)	36.3 (0.2)
Expectation for acupuncture (mean, SD)[b]	6.5 (0.8)
Acupuncture-sensational score (mean, SD)[c]	1.5 (1.6)

[a]Physical activity level was assessed through the global physical activity questionnaire
[b]Expectation for acupuncture was assessed through the credibility/expectancy questionnaire
[c]Acupuncture sensation was assessed through the acupuncture sensation questionnaire

did not show significant differences between baseline and any assessment (Table 3).

Effects on bio-signal variables
For HRV, the variables showed significant differences from the baseline value only at the last measurement session. The variables were NN (MD −0.02, 95% CI [−0.05, −0.00]), HF (MD −97.81, 95% CI [−190.71, −4.90]), nLF (MD 9.50, 95% CI [1.26, 17.74]), nHF (MD −9.40, 95% CI [−17.22, −1.58]) and LF/HF (MD 0.98, 95% CI [0.02, 1.95]). Similarly,

Table 3 Results of assessments on the variables related to the radial artery pressure-pulse wave

Variables	Assessment schedule					
	−5 min	0	+7 min	+14 min	+20 min	+27 min
	Baseline (Reference)[a]	Needle insertion[a]	During needle retention[a]		Needle removal[a]	Final[a]
$SE_{10-30Hz}$ (10^{-3}·Vrms^2)	1.76 (−0.39, 3.92)	−0.05 (−0.71, 0.61)	−0.45 (−1.11, 0.21)	−0.26 (−0.92, 0.40)	−0.34 (−1.00, 0.32)	−0.77* (−1.44, −0.11)
SE_{0-10Hz} (10^{-1}·Vrms^2)	7.78 (5.37, 10.19)	0.49 (−0.33, 1.31)	0.95* (0.13, 1.76)	1.20** (0.38, 2.02)	1.39*** (0.58, 2.21)	1.79*** (0.98, 2.61)
PPI (V)	3.20 (2.68, 3.71)	0.12 (−0.05, 0.28)	0.12 (−0.05, 0.28)	0.24** (0.08, 0.41)	0.27*** (0.11, 0.44)	0.31*** (0.15, 0.48)
PDI (mm)	6.96 (4.98, 8.94)	0.08 (−0.44, 0.59)	−0.22 (−0.73, 0.29)	−0.22 (−0.73, 0.30)	−0.45 (−0.96, 0.06)	−0.34 (−0.85, 0.17)
PVI (mm)	2.51 (1.99, 3.03)	0.21 (−0.08, 0.51)	0.46*** (0.16, 0.71)	0.32* (0.03, 0.61)	0.13 (−0.16, 0.42)	0.27 (−0.03, 0.56)
Systolic area (Vs)	575.61 (490.04, 661.18)	32.09 (−6.91, 71.10)	23.72 (−15.29, 62.72)	54.50** (15.50, 93.51)	61.68*** (22.68, 100.68)	92.49*** (53.48, 131.49)
Diastolic area (Vs)	220.79 (196.43, 245.15)	3.76 (−8.40, 15.92)	2.39 (−9.77, 14.55)	10.25 (−1.91, 22.41)	12.19* (0.03, 24.35)	18.09** (5.93, 30.25)
SEVR (%)	39.33 (33.43, 45.23)	−1.58 (−4.04, 0.88)	−1.60 (−4.06, 0.86)	−2.58* (−5.04, −0.12)	−2.48* (−4.94, −0.02)	−3.35** (−5.81, −0.89)
AIX (%)	39.28 (28.40, 50.17)	1.81 (−5.98, 9.60)	0.49 (−7.30, 8.28)	−2.93 (−10.72, 4.86)	1.12 (−6.66, 8.91)	1.70 (−6.09, 9.49)
PTT (ms)	284.97 (267.79, 302.15)	0.67 (−5.18, 6.52)	3.17 (−2.69, 9.02)	1.80 (−4.05, 7.65)	4.87 (−0.99, 10.72)	4.22 (−1.64, 10.07)

$SE_{10-30Hz}$ spectral energy of 10 to 30 Hz, SE_{0-10Hz} spectral energy of 0 to 10 Hz, *PPI* pulse power index, *PDI* pulse depth index, *PVI* pulse volume index, *SEVR* subendocardial viability ratio, *AIX* radial augmentation index, *PTT* pulse transit time
[a]Values represent adjusted mean differences between the baseline and each assessment during the needling procedure as well as their 95% CI based on the result of LMM for each parameter. Mean differences were adjusted for age, sex, height, pulse rate, BMI, GPAQ, CEQ and experience of acupuncture. Dunnett's test was applied to control the family-wise error rate due to the multiple comparisons of the mean difference between baseline and each assessment stage for each variable. The statistical significance was indicated with asterisks: ***,$p < 0.001$; **,$p < 0.01$; *,$p < 0.05$

PPG systolic area showed a significant increase from the baseline only at the last measurement session (average systolic area, MD 12.00, 95% CI [2.57, 21.43]).

CO and SV, which were estimated with the impedance cardiography device, did not present any significant change between baseline and any measurement throughout the entire procedure. Lastly, respiratory rate also did not show any significant changes during the study (Table 4).

Effects on the variables of radial artery ultrasonography

The diameter of the radial artery did not show significant changes throughout the entire procedure. However, the maximum blood velocity increased immediately after needle insertion (MD 2.30, 95% CI [1.46, 3.15]), reached the maximum value 7 min after needling (MD 2.46, 95% CI [1.62, 3.31]), and subsequently decreased significantly until 14 min after needling (1.35, 95% CI [0.50, 2.19]); subsequently, no differences were observed immediately after needle removal or 7 min after needle removal (0.54, 95% CI [−0.30, 1.39] and 0.19, 95% CI [−0.66, 1.03], respectively). The average blood flow velocity showed a similar pattern as the maximum velocity. Significant increases were observed immediately after needling (MD 4.09, 95% CI [2.60, 5.59]) and during needle retention (MD 4.52, 95% CI [3.02, 6.01] after 7 min and MD 2.45, 95% CI [0.96, 3.95]

after 14 min), but there were no differences immediately after needle removal (1.10, 95% CI [−0.40, 2.59]) or 7 min after needle removal (0.30, 95% CI [−1.19, 1.80], Table 5).

Discussion

We found that RPPW and various hemodynamic variables, including peripheral blood velocity, HRV and PPG, followed consistent patterns during the acupuncture session at ST36 (Fig. 4). In the RPPW analysis, significant increases were observed in the low-frequency domain of the power spectral density (SE0-10 Hz), pulse power index (PPI), and systolic and diastolic area, while a decreasing pattern was observed for SEVR (Additional file 1: Figure S1). Likewise, the amplitude and systolic area of the PPG signal showed a continuously increasing pattern during the entire session. Peripheral blood velocity, which was assessed by ultrasonography, began to rise shortly after needle insertion, reached its maximum in the middle of the session and decreased during the rest of the retention period and after needle removal. Together, these changes indicate that the acupuncture stimulation at ST36 induced an increase in blood flow velocity (Additional file 1: Figure S3) and, consequently, pulse pressure (PPI and SE0-10 Hz). This increase was mostly driven by the enhanced systolic blood pressure (SEVR and PPG).

Table 4 Results for the bio-signal variables

Variables	Assessment schedule					
	−5 min	0	+7 min	+14 min	+20 min	+27 min
	Baseline (Reference)[a]	Needle insertion[a]	During needle retention[a]		Needle removal[a]	Final[a]
Heart rate variability (HRV)						
NN (s)	0.89 (0.81, 0.96)	0.01 (−0.02, 0.03)	−0.01 (−0.03, 0.01)	−0.01 (−0.04, 0.01)	−0.02 (−0.04, 0.01)	−0.02* (−0.05, −0.00)
SDNN (ms)	60.89 (49.54, 72.24)	2.97 (−5.84, 11.78)	0.82 (−7.98, 9.63)	3.22 (−5.59, 12.02)	1.41 (−7.40, 10.22)	4.26 (−4.54, 13.07)
RMSSD (ms)	41.51 (28.39, 54.63)	0.76 (−4.56, 6.09)	−2.21 (−7.53, 3.12)	−1.44 (−6.76, 3.88)	−3.15 (−8.47, 2.17)	−3.19 (−8.51, 2.13)
TF (ms^2)	1407.53 (816.28, 1998.78)	−190.15 (−617.85, 237.55)	−91.18 (−518.88, 336.52)	−69.81 (−497.51, 357.89)	−13.75 (−441.45, 413.96)	26.67 (−401.03, 454.37)
LF (ms^2)	432.39 (246.02, 618.75)	−54.68 (−203.00, 93.64)	−45.23 (−193.55, 103.09)	−45.86 (−194.18, 102.45)	−12.04 (−160.36, 136.27)	77.89 (−70.42, 226.21)
HF (ms^2)	256.67 (25.13, 488.20)	−17.95 (−110.86, 74.96)	−42.69 (−135.60, 50.22)	−62.72 (−155.63, 30.18)	−68.12 (−161.03, 24.79)	−97.81* (−190.71, −4.90)
nLF (%)	53.03 (43.27, 62.79)	−2.90 (−11.14, 5.34)	5.01 (−3.23, 13.25)	4.26 (−3.97, 12.50)	7.10 (−1.13, 15.34)	9.50* (1.26, 17.74)
nHF (%)	43.72 (34.52, 52.93)	2.39 (−5.43, 10.21)	−5.11 (−12.92, 2.71)	−4.31 (−12.13, 3.51)	−7.23 (−15.05, 0.58)	−9.40* (−17.22, −1.58)
LF/HF	2.03 (1.08, 2.98)	−0.37 (−1.34, 0.60)	0.29 (−0.67, 1.26)	0.13 (−0.84, 1.09)	0.14 (−0.83, 1.10)	0.98* (0.02, 1.95)
Respiration						
Respiratory rate (bpm)	14.49 (10.94, 18.04)	0.11 (−1.05, 1.27)	0.43 (−0.74, 1.59)	−0.21 (−1.37, 0.96)	0.22 (−0.94, 1.38)	−0.15 (−1.31, 1.02)
PPG signals						
Amplitude (V)	0.38 (0.29, 0.47)	−0.01 (−0.05, 0.03)	0.02 (−0.02, 0.06)	0.02 (−0.02, 0.06)	0.01 (−0.03, 0.05)	0.03 (−0.01, 0.07)
Systolic area (Vs)	94.50 (71.11, 117.90)	0.18 (−9.25, 9.61)	8.17 (−1.26, 17.60)	8.73 (−0.70, 18.16)	7.26 (−2.17, 116.69)	12.00** (2.57, 21.43)
ICG signals						
Cardiac output (ml/min)	7107.78 (2142.10,12,073.47)	−182.77 (−1218.29, 852.76)	−395.31 (−1430.84, 640.21)	−509.858 (−1545.39, 525.67)	−261.268 (−1296.80, 774.26)	−239.630 (−1275.16, 795.90)
Stroke volume (ml)	105.659 (16.99, 194.32)	−5.084 (−21.76, 11.60)	−8.855 (−25.54, 7.83)	−10.239 (−26.92, 6.44)	−11.781 (−28.46, 4.90)	−11.699 (−28.38, 4.98)

NN normal to normal interval, *SDNN* standard deviation of the NN interval, *RMSDD* square root of the mean squared differences of NN intervals, *TF* total frequency, *LF* low-frequency domain, *HF* high-frequency domain, *nLF* normalized low-frequency domain, *nHF* normalized high-frequency domain

**,*p* < 0.01; *,*p* < 0.05

[a]Values represent differences between the baseline and each assessment during the needling procedure (95% CI). The other details are identical to the footnote of Table 3 except for following abbreviations

Table 5 Results of assessments on the variables from radial artery ultrasonography

Variables	Assessment schedule					
	−5 min	0	+7 min	+14 min	+20 min	+27 min
	Baseline (Reference)[a]	Needle insertion[a]	During needle retention[a]		Needle removal[a]	Final[a]
Diameter of radial artery (mm)	2.01 (1.83, 2.19)	0.08 (−0.06, 0.21)	−0.00 (−0.14, 0.13)	0.06 (−0.08, 0.19)	0.00 (−0.13, 0.14)	−0.07 (−0.20, 0.07)
Maximum velocity of blood flow (cm/s)	5.29 (1.92, 8.65)	2.30*** (1.46, 3.15)	2.46*** (1.62, 3.31)	1.35** (0.50, 2.19)	0.54 (−0.30, 1.39)	0.19 (−0.66, 1.03)
Average velocity of blood flow (cm/s)	9.31 (3.50, 15.11)	4.09*** (2.60, 5.59)	4.52*** (3.02, 6.01)	2.45** (0.96, 3.95)	1.10 (−0.40, 2.59)	0.30 (−1.19, 1.80)

***,*p* < 0.001; **,*p* < 0.01;

[a]Values represent differences between the baseline and each assessment during the needling procedure (95% CI). The last details are identical to the footnote of Table 3

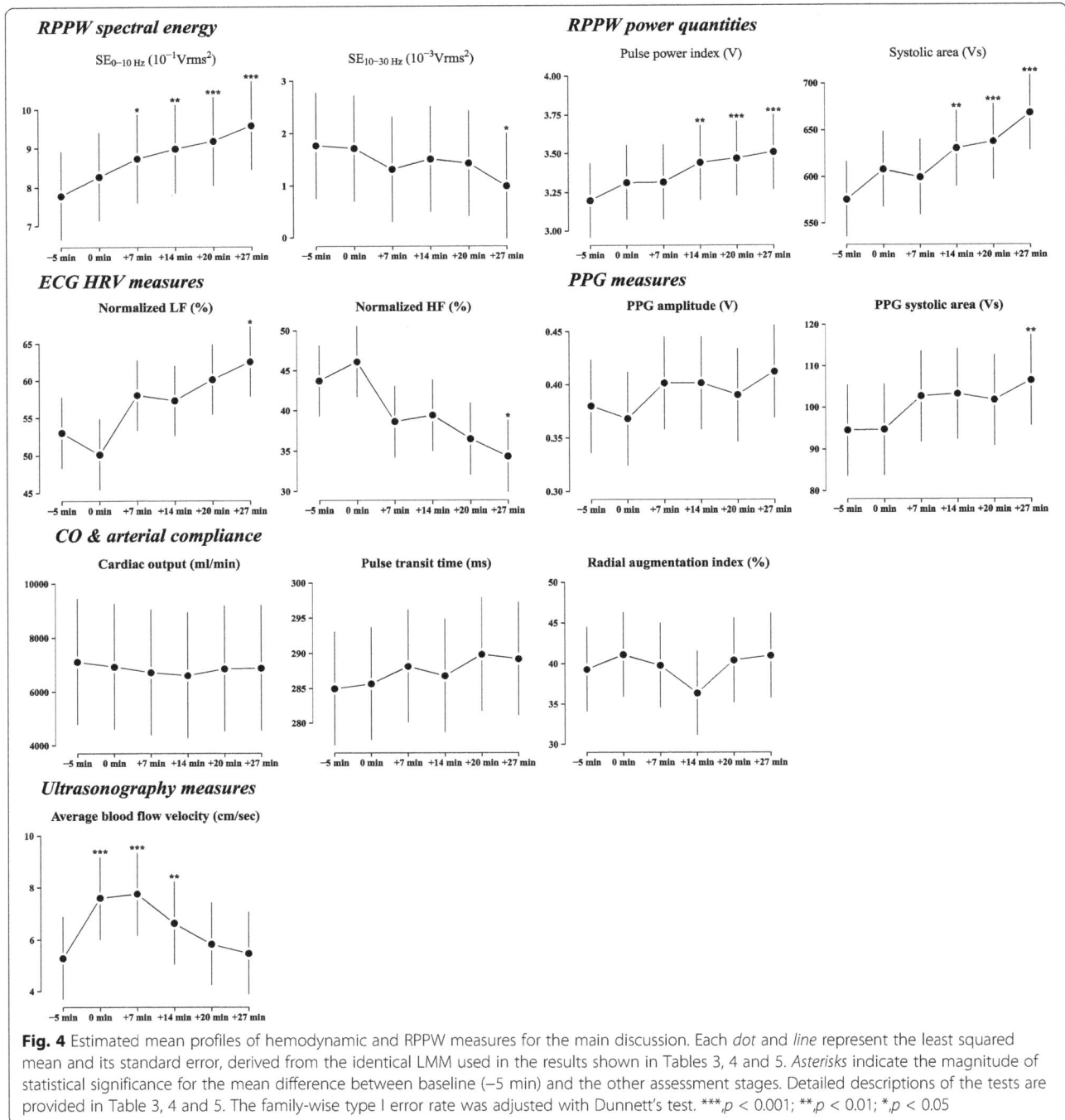

Fig. 4 Estimated mean profiles of hemodynamic and RPPW measures for the main discussion. Each *dot* and *line* represent the least squared mean and its standard error, derived from the identical LMM used in the results shown in Tables 3, 4 and 5. *Asterisks* indicate the magnitude of statistical significance for the mean difference between baseline (−5 min) and the other assessment stages. Detailed descriptions of the tests are provided in Table 3, 4 and 5. The family-wise type I error rate was adjusted with Dunnett's test. ***,$p < 0.001$; **,$p < 0.01$; *,$p < 0.05$

To investigate autonomic nerve activity, we acquired HRV data using ECG. From the ECG measurements, we found a tendency toward an increase in the low-frequency domain (0.04–0.15 Hz) of HRV and a decrease in the high-frequency domain (0.15–0.4 Hz) during the acupuncture session, although these changes did not reach statistical significance. These responses imply that the acupuncture treatment induced an increase in sympathetic activity and a decrease in parasympathetic activity. Typical physiological changes associated with increases in sympathetic tone are an increase in cardiac output (CO) and/or vascular constriction [22].

We assume that these hemodynamic changes are consequences of either increased CO and/or decreased arterial compliance. We calculated AIX and PTT from the RPPW and estimated the CO using an impedance cardiography module [23]. Previous studies have reported that acupuncture affected the blood flow in the peripheral arteries during the acupuncture session, and one possible mechanism was related to the regulation of systemic vascular resistance through the modulation of sympathetic tone without any changes in pulse rate, blood pressure or CO [9, 24]. Similarly, we found that CO did not change during the entire acupuncture session. We also found that AIX and PTT did not change during the entire acupuncture session. AIX and PTT can be used as surrogate indicators of arterial compliance (AIX and PTT) and peripheral resistance (AIX) [25]. Therefore, the lack of change in either AIX or PTT verifies that arterial compliance was not affected by the acupuncture stimulation. Hemodynamic changes, such as blood flow velocity or pulse pressure, should accompany changes in CO or arterial compliance, but our results revealed no changes in CO or in arterial compliance. These contradictory results can be understood with the following explanation. PPW and HRV measurements have been demonstrated to be accurate techniques, AIX and PTT are well defined, and their calculations are straightforward with minimal uncertainty [16, 26]. However, similar to other impedance-based bio-signal analyses [27], CO estimation is thought to have limited accuracy, and a subtle change that might have accompanied the acupuncture stimulation may not be traceable using the contemporary impedance cardiography technique [28]. Therefore, contrary to the conclusions of a previous, closely related work [24], we suggest that the increased blood flow velocity, pulse pressure, SEVR, and other hemodynamic variables indicating activated systemic circulation are possibly consequences of the elevated CO, especially in the systolic period, which was induced by the elevated sympathetic tone caused by acupuncture stimulation at ST36. The remaining variables that are not included in the above are provided as the Additional file 1: Figure S2

The most valuable feature of this study is that we simultaneously analyzed various hemodynamic variables during the acupuncture session. Previous studies assessed only one or two variables and could not draw comprehensive conclusions regarding the hemodynamic changes with acupuncture stimulation [8–10]. In this study, however, the simultaneous evaluation of diverse variables related to RPPW, PPG, peripheral arterial blood flow, autonomic nerve activity and cardiac function enabled us to generate an integrated picture of the hemodynamic changes that accompany acupuncture stimulation. Second, we included healthy young adults and strictly followed the predefined inclusion and exclusion criteria to reduce any confounding factors that might be related to the observed hemodynamic changes. On the day of study participation, excessive physical activity and the use of alcoholic or carbonated beverages were prohibited to control for possible influences on the bio-signals. The acupuncture stimulation and the assessment of hemodynamic variables

were conducted in an undisturbed room, where only the individual participant and research staff were present. We used a unified data acquisition system, which enabled the simultaneous processing of several hemodynamic variables. These efforts would have contributed to the internal validity of our study. Third, we tried to adopt a similar experimental design and acupuncture method, including acupuncture points and the same type of acupuncture needles, to ensure comparability with related studies [9, 20, 24, 29]. Different acupoints or stimulation types of may induce different changes on biosignals as there are some previous reports [9, 10, 30, 31]. Through this attempt, we could verify the previously reported hemodynamic effects of acupuncture and advance the knowledge in this area.

Our study has several limitations. Changes in the hemodynamic variables were observed for only a limited time around the acupuncture session. There is controversy over the effective duration related to acupuncture practice. Generally, studies on acupuncture treatment consider both short-term and long-term effects [7]. In this study, however, we focused on the short-term effects of acupuncture and observed hemodynamic changes before, during and directly after acupuncture treatment, which was maintained for 20 min. We found that many variables related to the RPPW, HRV and PPG signals showed significant changes at the last measurement session, implying that prolonged effects of acupuncture might be observed with a longer follow-up design. Second, this pilot study focused on the primary outcome variable with a minimal sample size. Many secondary outcome variables showed consistent patterns during the acupuncture stimulation, but the lack of statistically significant differences from the baseline value might be due to insufficient power. Third, for the assessment of RPPW, we read the pulse signal only at the left Guan. In the general practice of TEAM, practitioners use all three adjacent positions, Cun, Guan, and Chi, at both wrists to diagnose the pulse [32]. In this study, we measured many hemodynamic variables at several time points within a limited time schedule; this allowed only a single-point data acquisition for PPW, which may not reflect the current clinical practice of TEAM. Fourth, physicians typically select more than one acupuncture point for acupuncture treatments. To minimize the control parameters, we selected only ST36 at both legs for acupuncture stimulation. A previous study found that acupuncture stimulation at ST36 could change the bio-signals that are regulated by the cardiovascular system, such as baroreflex function and various hemodynamic variables [33, 34]. Thus, we chose only ST36. Even with this experimental evidence, stimulation at a single acupuncture point cannot appropriately reflect real clinical practice. All of these limitations were partially because of the use of repeated measurements with several devices within a limited time duration and the pioneering aspect of this study. Finally, stress is an important factor in the assessment of bio-signals. To avoid stress, all the participants rested for 20 min before the measurements and acupuncture treatments; nonetheless, we could not ensure that all possible confounding factors of stress were appropriately controlled in this study. In future studies, assessing basal stress levels would be necessary to prevent the inclusion of any participants in a generally stressful condition.

From the analysis of this study, several future research directions can be suggested. Several variables showed consistent trends but lacked statistically significant differences, probably due to the low power of this study. Therefore, a clinical study with a sufficiently large sample size is desired. Second, reflecting actual clinical practice, studies adopting acupuncture stimulations at multiple points are also necessary, and point-specific effects need to be investigated. Third, studies on actual patients need to be conducted. Compared to treatments of healthy subjects, appropriate acupuncture treatments on patients will improve body conditions that should be reflected more dramatically in pulse diagnosis and, thus, in PPW and other hemodynamic variables. In addition, studies with patients would allow disease-specific characteristics of pulse diagnosis to be more clearly identified, which will help elucidate the underlying mechanism of pulse diagnosis in diverse cases.

Conclusions

In conclusion, in an attempt to find scientific evidence and the mechanism underlying pulse diagnosis, we investigated the changes in RPPW and related bio-signals from PPG, ECG, and ultrasonography with a conventional acupuncture treatment in healthy subjects. The results indicated that ST36 acupuncture stimulations at both legs induced increases in the blood flow velocity in the radial artery and peripheral arterioles and induced a relaxation effect; the treatment increased the radial pulse pressure – especially the systolic pulse pressure and the power spectral density in the low-frequency domain (<10 Hz) – and increased the PPG systolic area and blood flow velocity at the radial artery. In addition, the treatment increased the high-frequency HRV and decreased the low-frequency HRV. Through further analysis, we showed that these increased blood flow velocity indicators were possibly the consequence of increased CO, especially during the systolic period. Using this integrative approach, the analysis of radial pulse pressure can be a predictive tool for the changes in hemodynamic variables during an acupuncture session. Studies with patients and diverse acupuncture point stimulations and more direct measurements of CO are needed to confirm our results and generate a deeper understanding of the mechanism of pulse diagnosis in various health conditions.

Additional file

Additional file 1: Figure S1. The estimated mean profiles of RPPW variables. The last details are identical with Fig. 4. **Figure S2.** The estimated mean profiles hemodynamic (HRV, PPG, and cardiac output) variables. The last details are identical with Fig. 4. **Figure S3.** The estimated mean profiles ultrasonography variables. The last details are identical with Fig. 4.

Abbreviations
AIX: Augmentation index; ASQ: Acupuncture Sensation Questionnaire; BMI: Body mass index; CEQ: Credibility/Expectancy Questionnaire; CI: Confidence interval; CO: Cardiac output; ECG: Electrocardiogram; GPAQ: Global Physical Activity Questionnaire; HF: High-frequency domain; HRV: Heart rate variability; KMD: Korean medicine doctor; LF/HF: Ratio of low to high frequency; LMM: Linear mixed model; MD: Mean difference; nHF: Normalized high-frequency domain; nLF: Normalized low-frequency domain; NN: Normal to normal interval; PDI: Pulse depth index; PPG: Photoplethysmogram; PPI: Pulse power index; PPW: Pressure pulse wave; PTT: Pulse transit time; PTT: Pulse transit time; PVI: Pulse volume index; RPPW: Radial pressure pulse wave; RSP: Respiration; SD: Standard deviation; SE_{0-10Hz}: Spectral energy from 0 to 10 Hz; $SE_{10-30Hz}$: Spectral energy from 10 to 30 Hz; SEVR: Subendocardial viability ratio; SIA: Sensations during insertion of the acupuncture needle; SM: Sensations during maintenance of the acupuncture needle; SMA: Sensations during manipulation of the acupuncture needle; SV: Stroke volume; TEAM: Traditional East Asian medicine

Acknowledgments
Not applicable.

Funding
This study was supported by the Korea Institute of Oriental Medicine (Grant no. K16021) which is funded by the Ministry of Science, ICT and Future Planning, Republic of Korea.

Authors' contributions
THK and BK contributed to designing the study and drafted the manuscript. BK performed the statistical analyses. JHB, and MHJ participated in the design of the study, provided expertise related to medical devices used in the study, and interpreted the study results. JYS participated in the development of the study protocol and performed monitoring. JWK administered the acupuncture stimulation. JK performed measurements of radial pressure pulse wave and other bio-signals using KIOM-PAS and relevant devices. JHL provided expertise regarding the study design and suggested the acupoints applied in this study. JUK conceived and supervised this study, acquired the funding and drafted the manuscript. All the authors read and approved the final manuscript.

Competing interests
The authors declare that they have no competing interests.

Consent for publication
The subjects in Fig. 2 were one of the authors. All the authors consent to publication.

Author details
[1]Korean Medicine Clinical Trial Center, Kyung Hee University Korean Medicine Hospital, #23 Kyungheedae-ro, Dongdaemun-gu, Seoul 02447, South Korea. [2]KM Fundamental Research Division, Korea Institute of Oriental Medicine, Daejeon 34054, South Korea. [3]Clinical Research Division, Korea Institute of Oriental Medicine, Daejeon 34054, South Korea. [4]Department of Acupuncture & Moxibustion, College of Korean Medicine, Kyung Hee University, Seoul 02447, South Korea.

References

1. Farquhar J. Knowing practice: the clinical encounter of Chinese medicine. Avalon Publishing; 1994.
2. Hall JE. Guyton and hall textbook of medical physiology. Philadelphia: Elsevier Health Sciences; 2015.
3. McEniery CM, Wallace S, Mackenzie IS, McDonnell B, Newby DE, Cockcroft JR, Wilkinson IB. Endothelial function is associated with pulse pressure, pulse wave velocity, and augmentation index in healthy humans. Hypertension. 2006;48(4):602–8.
4. Yamashina A, Tomiyama H, Arai T, Hirose K-i, Koji Y, Hirayama Y, Yamamoto Y, Hori S. Brachial-ankle pulse wave velocity as a marker of atherosclerotic vascular damage and cardiovascular risk. Hypertens Res. 2003;26(8):615–22.
5. Zebekakis PE, Nawrot T, Thijs L, Balkestein EJ, van der Heijden-Spek J, Van Bortel LM, Struijker-Boudier HA, Safar ME, Staessen JA. Obesity is associated with increased arterial stiffness from adolescence until old age. J Hypertens. 2005;23(10):1839–46.
6. Yeragani VK, Tancer M, Seema K, Josyulab K, Desai N. Increased pulse-wave velocity in patients with anxiety: implications for autonomic dysfunction. J Psychosom Res. 2006;61(1):25–31.
7. Bae S-C, Shin S-H, Kim K-W. Pulse diagnosis procedure before and after the acupuncture in Hwangjenaekyung. J Kor Med Class. 2011;24(3):15–25.
8. Anderson B, Nielsen A, McKee D, Jeffres A, Kligler B. Acupuncture and heart rate variability: a systems level approach to understanding mechanism. Explore (NY). 2012;8(2):99–106.
9. Takayama S, Watanabe M, Kusuyama H, Nagase S, Seki T, Nakazawa T, Yaegashi N. Evaluation of the effects of acupuncture on blood flow in humans with ultrasound color Doppler imaging. Evid Based Complement Alternat Med. 2012;2012:513638.
10. Boutouyrie P, Corvisier R, Azizi M, Lemoine D, Laloux B, Hallouin M-C, Laurent S. Effects of acupuncture on radial artery hemodynamics: controlled trials in sensitized and naive subjects. Am J Physiol Heart Circ Physiol. 2001;280(2):H628–33.
11. Shin JY, Lee JH, Ku, B, Bae JH, Jun MH, Kim TH, Kim JU. Effects of Acupuncture Stimulation on the Radial artery's Pressure Pulse Wave in Healthy Young Participants: Protocol for a prospective, single-Arm, Exploratory, Clinical Study. J Pharmacopuncture. 2016;19(3):197.
12. World Health Organization. WHO standard acupuncture point locations in the western Pacific region. Geneva: World Health Organization; 2008;(vol. 181).
13. Kim Y, Park J, Lee H, Bang H, Park H-J. Content validity of an acupuncture sensation questionnaire. J Altern Complement Med. 2008;14(8):957–63.
14. Natsume T, Okazumi S, Takayama W, Takeda A, Iwasaki K, Makino H, Sasagawa S, Cho A, Kouno T, Kondo S, et al. Evaluation of the hepatic blood flow increase in the cases with liver metastasis and prediction of patent cases of liver metastasis using dynamic CT. Hepato-Gastroenterology. 2007;54(78):1745–7.
15. Devilly GJ, Borkovec TD. Psychometric properties of the credibility/expectancy questionnaire. J Behav Ther Exp Psychiatry. 2000;31(2):73–86.
16. Bae JH, Jeon YJ, Kim JY, Kim JU. New assessment model of pulse depth based on sensor displacement in pulse diagnostic devices. Evid Based Complement Alternat Med. 2013;2013:938641.
17. World Health Organization. WHO draft guidelines for adverse event reporting and learning systems. Geneva: World Health Organization; 2005.
18. Spilker B: Quality of life and pharmacoeconomics in clinical trials. 1995.
19. R: A language and environment for statistical computing. R Foundation for Statistical Computing. https://www.r-project.org.
20. Huang CM, Chang HC, Li TC, Chen CC, Liao YT, Kao ST. Acupuncture effects on the pulse spectrum of radial pressure pulse in dyspepsia. Am J Chin Med. 2012;40(3):443–54.
21. Wei LY, Lee CT, Chow P. A new scientific method of pulse diagnosis. Am J Acupunct. 1984;12(3):205–18.
22. Gordan R, Gwathmey JK, Xie LH. Autonomic and endocrine control of cardiovascular function. World J Cardiol. 2015;7(4):204–14.
23. Yazdanian H, Mahnam A, Edrisi M, Esfahani MA. Design and implementation of a portable impedance cardiography system for noninvasive stroke volume monitoring. J Med Signals Sens. 2016;6(1):47–56.
24. Watanabe M, Takayama S, Hirano A, Seki T, Yaegashi N. Hemodynamic changes in the brachial artery induced by acupuncture stimulation on the lower limbs: a single-blind randomized controlled trial. Evid Based Complement Alternat Med. 2012;2012:958145.
25. Davies JI, Struthers AD. Beyond blood pressure: pulse wave analysis–a better way of assessing cardiovascular risk? Futur Cardiol. 2005;1(1):69–78.
26. Acharya UR, Faust O, Sree SV, Ghista DN, Dua S, Joseph P, Ahamed VI, Janarthanan N, Tamura T. An integrated diabetic index using heart rate variability signal features for diagnosis of diabetes. Comput Methods Biomech Biomed Engin. 2013;16(2):222–34.
27. Kyle UG, Bosaeus I, De Lorenzo AD, Deurenberg P, Elia M, Gomez JM, Heitmann BL, Kent-Smith L, Melchior JC, Pirlich M, et al. Bioelectrical impedance analysis–part I: review of principles and methods. Clin Nutr. 2004;23(5):1226–43.
28. Cybulski G, Strasz A, Niewiadomski W, Gasiorowska A. Impedance cardiography: recent advancements. Cardiol J. 2012;19(5):550–6.
29. Takayama S, Seki T, Sugita N, Konno S, Arai H, Saijo Y, Yambe T, Yaegashi N, Yoshizawa M, Nitta S. Radial artery hemodynamic changes related to acupuncture. Explore (NY). 2010;6(2):100–5.
30. Sandberg M, Lundeberg T, Lindberg LG, Gerdle B. Effects of acupuncture on skin and muscle blood flow in healthy subjects. Eur J Appl Physiol. 2003;90(1–2):114–9.
31. Boutouyrie P, Corvisier R, Ong KT, Vulser C, Lassalle C, Azizi M, et al. Acute and chronic effects of acupuncture on radial artery: a randomized double blind study in migraine. Artery Res. 2010;4(1):7–14.
32. Bilton K. Hammer L, Zaslawski C. Contemporary Chinese pulse diagnosis: a modern interpretation of an ancient and traditional method. J Acupunct Meridian Stud. 2013;6(5):227–33.
33. Hyun SH, Im JW, Jung WS, Cho KH, Kim YS, Ko CN, Park JM, Park SU, Cho SY, Moon SK. Effect of ST36 acupuncture on hyperventilation-induced CO 2 reactivity of the basilar and middle cerebral arteries and heart rate variability in normal subjects. Evid Based Complement Alternat Med. 2014;2014:574986
34. Lima J, Hentschke V, Rossato D, Quagliotto E, Pinheiro L, Almeida E, Dal Lago P, Lukrafka J. Chronic electroacupuncture of the ST36 point improves baroreflex function and haemodynamic parameters in heart failure rats. Auton Neurosci. 2015;193:31–7.

Permissions

All chapters in this book were first published in CAM, by BioMed Central; hereby published with permission under the Creative Commons Attribution License or equivalent. Every chapter published in this book has been scrutinized by our experts. Their significance has been extensively debated. The topics covered herein carry significant findings which will fuel the growth of the discipline. They may even be implemented as practical applications or may be referred to as a beginning point for another development.

The contributors of this book come from diverse backgrounds, making this book a truly international effort. This book will bring forth new frontiers with its revolutionizing research information and detailed analysis of the nascent developments around the world.

We would like to thank all the contributing authors for lending their expertise to make the book truly unique. They have played a crucial role in the development of this book. Without their invaluable contributions this book wouldn't have been possible. They have made vital efforts to compile up to date information on the varied aspects of this subject to make this book a valuable addition to the collection of many professionals and students.

This book was conceptualized with the vision of imparting up-to-date information and advanced data in this field. To ensure the same, a matchless editorial board was set up. Every individual on the board went through rigorous rounds of assessment to prove their worth. After which they invested a large part of their time researching and compiling the most relevant data for our readers.

The editorial board has been involved in producing this book since its inception. They have spent rigorous hours researching and exploring the diverse topics which have resulted in the successful publishing of this book. They have passed on their knowledge of decades through this book. To expedite this challenging task, the publisher supported the team at every step. A small team of assistant editors was also appointed to further simplify the editing procedure and attain best results for the readers.

Apart from the editorial board, the designing team has also invested a significant amount of their time in understanding the subject and creating the most relevant covers. They scrutinized every image to scout for the most suitable representation of the subject and create an appropriate cover for the book.

The publishing team has been an ardent support to the editorial, designing and production team. Their endless efforts to recruit the best for this project, has resulted in the accomplishment of this book. They are a veteran in the field of academics and their pool of knowledge is as vast as their experience in printing. Their expertise and guidance has proved useful at every step. Their uncompromising quality standards have made this book an exceptional effort. Their encouragement from time to time has been an inspiration for everyone.

The publisher and the editorial board hope that this book will prove to be a valuable piece of knowledge for researchers, students, practitioners and scholars across the globe.

List of Contributors

Lauren S. Penney
South Texas Veterans Health Care System, 7400 Merton Minter Blvd, San Antonio, TX 78229, USA

Cheryl Ritenbaugh
The University of Arizona-Department of Family and Community Medicine, 1450 N Cherry Ave, Tucson, AZ 85719, USA

Charles Elder, Jennifer Schneider and Lynn L. DeBar
Kaiser Permanente-Center for Health Research, 3800 N. Interstate Avenue, Portland, OR 97227-1098, USA

Richard A. Deyo
Oregon Health and Science University-Department of Family Medicine, Oregon Health and Science University, Mail Code FM, 3181 SW Sam Jackson Park Road, Portland, OR 97239, USA

Leonardo Yung dos Santos Maciel, Paula Michele dos Santos Leite, Mauricio Lima Poderoso Neto and Andreza Carvalho Rabelo Mendonça
Post Graduate Program in Health Sciences, Federal University of Sergipe, Rua Cláudio Batista, s/n, Santo Antônio, 49060-100 Aracaju, SE, Brasil

Carla Carolina Alves de Araujo and Jersica da Hora Santos Souza
Department of Physical Therapy, Federal University of Sergipe, Rua Cláudio Batista, s/n. Bairro Santo Antônio, CEP 49060-100 Aracaju, Sergipe, Brasil

Josimari Melo DeSantana
Professor of the Department of Physical Therapy and Post Graduate Programs in Health Sciences and Physiological Sciences, Federal University of Sergipe, Rua Cláudio Batista, s/n. Bairro Santo Antônio, CEP 49060-100 Aracaju, Sergipe, Brasil

Zhong Lin and Yuan Bo Liang
1The Eye Hospital, School of Ophthalmology and Optometry, Wenzhou Medical University, No. 270 West College Road, Wenzhou, Zhejiang 325027, China

Guang Yun Mao
The Eye Hospital, School of Ophthalmology and Optometry, Wenzhou Medical University, No. 270 West College Road, Wenzhou, Zhejiang 325027, China
School of Environmental Science &Public Health, Wenzhou Medical University, Wenzhou, Zhejiang, China

Balamurali Vasudevan
College of Optometry, Mid Western University, Glendale, AZ, USA

Su Jie Fang, Wei Han and Tie Ying Gao
Handan Eye Hospital, Handan, Hebei, China

Vishal Jhanji
Department of Ophthalmology and Visual Sciences, The Chinese University of Hong Kong, Hong Kong, China

Kenneth J. Ciuffreda
Department of Biological and Vision Sciences, SUNY College of Optometry, New York, NY, USA

Jeremy Y. Ng, Laurel Liang and Anna R. Gagliardi
Toronto General Hospital Research Institute, University Health Network, Toronto, Ontario, Canada

Tao Sha
College of Acupuncture and Massage, Tianjin University of Traditional Chinese Medicine, No. 312, Anshan West Road, Nankai District, Tianjin 300193, China

Lili Gao, Bo Chen, Qiwen Zhang, Tianyi Zhao, Bo Li, Jinxin Zou, Yongming Guo, Xingfang Pan and Yi Guo
College of Acupuncture and Massage, Tianjin University of Traditional Chinese Medicine, No. 312, Anshan West Road, Nankai District, Tianjin 300193, China
Acupuncture Research Center, Tianjin University of Traditional Chinese Medicine, No. 312, Anshan West Road,Tianjin 300193, China

Yi-Chun Ma
Graduate Institute of Chinese Medicine, College of Chinese Medicine, China Medical University, Taichung, Taiwan, ROC
Department of Pediatrics, Tai-An Hospital, Taichung, Taiwan

Ching-Tien Peng and Hung-Yi Lin
Children's Hospital of China Medical University, Taichung, Taiwan, ROC

Yu-Chuen Huang
School of Chinese Medicine, College of Chinese Medicine, China Medical University, Taichung, Taiwan, ROC
Department of Medical Research, China Medical University Hospital, Taichung, Taiwan, ROC

Jaung-Geng Lin
School of Chinese Medicine, College of Chinese Medicine, China Medical University, Taichung, Taiwan, ROC
China Medical University, No.91, Xueshi Rd., North Dist., Taichung City 40402, Taiwan, ROC

Chengwei Wang, Mengyue Liu and Ning Li
Department of Integrated Traditional and Western Medicine, West China Hospital, Sichuan University, Chengdu, China

Chao You, Lu Ma and Meng Tian
Neurosurgery, West China Hospital, Sichuan University, Chengdu, China

Horng-Sheng Shiue and Chi-Neu Tsai
Chang Gung Memorial Hospital and Chang Gung University College of Medicine, Taoyuan, Taiwan

Yun-Shien Lee
Department of Biotechnology, Ming Chuan University, Taoyuan, Taiwan

Hen-Hong Chang
School of Post-Baccalaureate Chinese Medicine, and Research Center for Chinese Medicine and Acupuncture, China Medical University, Taichung, Taiwan
Departments of Chinese Medicine, China Medical University Hospital, Taichung, Taiwan

Haebeom Lee
Department of Human Informatics of Korean Medicine, Interdisciplinary Programs, Kyung Hee University, Seoul, South Korea

Young-Jae Park and Young-Bae Park
Department of Human Informatics of Korean Medicine, Interdisciplinary Programs, Kyung Hee University, Seoul, South Korea
Department of Biofunctional Medicine & Diagnostics, College of Korean Medicine, Kyung Hee University, Seoul, South Korea

Hwan-Sup Oh
Department of Human Informatics of Korean Medicine, Interdisciplinary Programs, Kyung Hee University, Seoul, South Korea
Department of Mechanical Engineering, Kyung Hee University, Gyeonggi-do, South Korea

Hyunho Kim
Department of Biofunctional Medicine & Diagnostics, College of Korean Medicine, Kyung Hee University, Seoul, South Korea

Jungkuk Kim
Department of Electronics Engineering, Myongji University, Gyeonggi-do, South Korea

Xuhui Zhang, Yingzhou Song, Tuya Bao, Miao Yu, Mingmin Xu, Yu Guo, Yu Wang and Bingcong Zhao
Beijing University of Chinese Medicine, Beijing, Beijing 100029, China

Chuntao Zhang
Beijing University of Chinese Medicine, Beijing, Beijing 100029, China
Shanxi University of Chinese Medicine, Xianyang, Shanxi 712046, China

Xing Liu, Baoguo Wang, Qinglei Teng and Shuangyan Wang
Department of Anesthesiology, Beijing Sanbo Brain Hospital, Capital Medical University, Beijing 100093, China

Jing Wang
Department of Neurobiology, Capital Medical University, Beijing 100069, China

Ying Hua Wang
Center for Collaboration and Innovation in Brain and Learning Sciences, Beijing Normal University, Beijing 100875, China
State Key Laboratory of Cognitive Neuroscience and Learning & IDG/Mc Govern Institute for Brain Research, Beijing Normal University, Beijing 100875, China

Jiaqing Yan
Institute of Electrical Engineering, Yanshan University, Qinhuangdao 066004, China

You Wan
Neuroscience Research Institute, Key Lab for Neuroscience, Peking University Health Science Center, Beijing 100191, China

Wing-Fai Yeung and Yee-Man Yu
The Hong Kong Polytechnic University, Hunghom, Kowloon, Hong Kong SAR, China

Ka-Fai Chung and Wai-Chi Chan
Department of Psychiatry, University of Hong Kong, Pokfulam, Hong Kong SAR, China

Zhang-Jin Zhang and Li-Xing Lao
School of Chinese Medicine, University of Hong Kong, Pokfulam, Hong Kong SAR, China

Shi-Ping Zhang
School of Chinese Medicine, Hong Kong Baptist University, Kowloon Tong, Kowloon, Hong Kong SAR, China

Roger Man-Kin Ng
Department of Psychiatry, Kowloon Hospital, 147A Argyle Street, Kowloon, Hong Kong SAR, China

Connie Lai-Wah Chan
Department of Psychiatry, United Christian Hospital, 130 Hip Wo Street, Kwun Tong, Kowloon, Hong Kong SAR, China

Lai-Ming Ho
School of Public Health, University of Hong Kong, Pokfulam, Hong Kong SAR, China

Agnes Tiwari and Denise Shuk Ting Cheung
School of Nursing, Li Ka Shing Faculty of Medicine, The University of Hong Kong, 4/F, William M.W. Mong Block, 21 Sassoon Road, Pokfulam, Hong Kong

Lixing Lao, Jerry Wing Fai Yeung and Zhang-Jin Zhang
School of Chinese Medicine, Li Ka Shing Faculty of Medicine, The University of Hong Kong, 10 Sassoon Road, Pokfulam, Hong Kong

Amy Xiao-Min Wang
Department of Social Sciences, The University of Hong Kong, 11/F, The Jockey Club Tower, Centennial Campus, The University of Hong Kong, Pokfulam Road, Hong Kong, Hong Kong

Mike Ka Pui So
Department of Information Systems, Business Statistics and Operations Management, Hong Kong University of Science and Technology, Clear Water Bay, Kowloon, Hong Kong

Doris Sau Fung Yu
The Nethersole School of Nursing, The Chinese University of Hong Kong, 6/F, Esther Lee Building, The Chinese University of Hong Kong, Shatin, N.T., Hong Kong

Terry Yat Sang Lum
Department of Social Work and Social Administration, The University of Hong Kong, Room 534, Jockey Club Tower, The Centennial Campus, The University of Hong Kong, Pokfulam, Hong Kong

Helina Yin King Yuk Fung
HKSKH Lady MacLehose Centre, No.22, Wo Yi Hop Road, Kwai Chung, New Territories, Hong Kong

Byung-Kwan Seo†, Won-Suk Sung, Yeon-Cheol Park and Yong-Hyeon Baek
Department of Clinical Korean Medicine, Graduate School, Kyung Hee University, 26, Kyungheedae-ro, Dongdaemun-gu, Seoul 02447, Korea

Jiani Wu and Zhishun Liu
Department of Acupuncture, Guang'anmen Hospital, China Academy of Chinese Medical Sciences, Beijing 100053, China

Zongshi Qin and Jing Zhou
Department of Acupuncture, Guang'anmen Hospital, China Academy of Chinese Medical Sciences, Beijing 100053, China
Beijing University of Chinese Medicine, Beijing 100029, China

Zhiwei Zang
Department of Acupuncture, Yantai Hospital of Traditional Chinese Medicine, Yantai 265200, China

Shu-Wen Weng
Graduate Institute of Chinese Medicine, College of Chinese Medicine, China Medical University, Taichung 404, Taiwan
Department of Chinese Medicine, Taichung Hospital, Ministry of Health and Welfare, Taichung 403, Taiwan

Chien-Chang Liao
Graduate Institute of Chinese Medicine, College of Chinese Medicine, China Medical University, Taichung 404, Taiwan
Department of Anesthesiology, Taipei Medical University Hospital, Taipei 110, Taiwan
Department of Anesthesiology, School of Medicine, College of Medicine, Taipei Medical University, Taipei 110, Taiwan
Health Policy Research Center, Taipei Medical University Hospital, Taipei 110, Taiwan

Jaung-Geng Lin
Graduate Institute of Chinese Medicine, College of Chinese Medicine, China Medical University, Taichung 404, Taiwan
Department of Healthcare Administration, Asia University, Taichung 413, Taiwan

Ta-Liang Chen
Department of Anesthesiology, Taipei Medical University Hospital, Taipei 110, Taiwan
Department of Anesthesiology, School of Medicine, College of Medicine, Taipei Medical University, Taipei 110, Taiwan
Health Policy Research Center, Taipei Medical University Hospital, Taipei 110, Taiwan

Chun-Chieh Yeh
Department of Surgery, China Medical University Hospital, Taichung 110, Taiwan
Department of Surgery, University of Illinois, Chicago, Illinois, USA

Hsin-Long Lane
School of Chinese Medicine for Post-Baccalaureate, College of Medicine, I-Shou University, Kaohsiung City 824, Taiwan

Chun-Chuan Shih
School of Chinese Medicine for Post-Baccalaureate, College of Medicine, I-Shou University, Kaohsiung City 824, Taiwan
Ph.D. Program for the Clinical Drug Discovery from Botanical Herbs, College of Pharmacy, Taipei Medical University, Taipei 110, Taiwan

Chi Chen
Shanghai Qigong Research Institute, Shanghai, China

Wei Zhang and Jun Ji
Shanghai Qigong Research Institute, Shanghai, China
Graduate School, The Shanghai University of Traditional Chinese Medicine, Shanghai, China

Jian Ying
Shanghai Qigong Research Institute, Shanghai, China
The Longhua Hospital Shanghai University of Traditional Chinese Medicine, Shanghai, China

Minjie Zhou
Shanghai Qigong Research Institute, Shanghai, China
Shanghai TCM-INTEGRATED Hospital, Shanghai, Shanghai University of Traditional Chinese Medicine, Shanghai, China

Xueyong Shen
Graduate School, The Shanghai University of Traditional Chinese Medicine, Shanghai, China

Mingyue Yang
The Department of Pain Management, Luoyang Central Hospital, Luoyang, China

Lei Chen and Chao Yu
The Longhua Hospital Shanghai University of Traditional Chinese Medicine, Shanghai, China

Bong Hyun Kim, Se Hyun Kang and Hae Jeong Nam
Department of Ophthalmology and Otolaryngology of Korean Medicine, College of Korean Medicine, Kyung Hee University, 26, Kyungheedae-ro, Dongdaemun-gu, Seoul 02453, Republic of Korea

Department of Ophthalmology and Otolaryngology of Korean Medicine, Kyung Hee University Korean Medicine Hospital, 23, Kyungheedae-ro, Dongdaemun-gu, Seoul 02447, Republic of Korea

Min Hee Kim
Department of Ophthalmology and Otolaryngology of Korean Medicine, College of Korean Medicine, Kyung Hee University, 26, Kyungheedae-ro, Dongdaemun-gu, Seoul 02453, Republic of Korea
Department of Ophthalmology and Otolaryngology of Korean Medicine, Kyung Hee University Hospital at Gangdong, 892, Dongnam-ro, Gangdong-gu, Seoul, Republic of Korea

Yu-Kang Kim and Ju-Young Oh
Department of Science in Korean Medicine, Graduate School, Kyung Hee University, 26 Kyungheedae-ro, Dongdaemoon-gu, Seoul 02447, Republic of Korea
Acupuncture & Meridian Science Research Center, Kyung Hee University, 26 Kyungheedae-ro, Dongdaemoon-gu, Seoul 02447, Republic of Korea

Ji-Yeun Park
College of Korean Medicine, Daejeon University, 62 Daehak-ro, Dong-gu, Daejeon 34520, Republic of Korea

Seung-Nam Kim
College of Korean Medicine, Dongguk University. 32, Dongguk-ro, Ilsandong-gu, Goyang-si, Gyeonggi-do 10326, Republic of Korea

Mijung Yeom, Hyangsook Lee, Younbyoung Chae, Dae-Hyun Hahm and Hi-Joon Park
Acupuncture & Meridian Science Research Center, Kyung Hee University, 26 Kyungheedae-ro, Dongdaemoon-gu, Seoul 02447, Republic of Korea

Seungmin Lee
Department of Acupuncture and Moxibustion, College of Korean Medicine, Kyung Hee University, Seoul 130-701, Republic of Korea

Jing-Shan Wu, Hsin-Yi Lo, Chia-Cheng Li and Feng-Yuan Chen
Graduate Institute of Chinese Medicine, China Medical University, 91 Hsueh-Shih Road, Taichung 40402, Taiwan

Tin-Yun Ho
Graduate Institute of Chinese Medicine, China Medical University, 91 Hsueh-Shih Road, Taichung 40402, Taiwan
Department of Health and Nutrition Biotechnology, Asia University, Taichung 41354, Taiwan

Chien-Yun Hsiang
Department of Microbiology, China Medical University, 91 Hsueh-Shih Road, Taichung 40402, Taiwan

Zainab Assy and Henk S. Brand
Department of Oral Biochemistry, Academic Centre for Dentistry Amsterdam (ACTA), room 12N-37, Gustav Mahlerlaan 3004, 1081 LA Amsterdam, The Netherlands

Tae-Hun Kim
Korean Medicine Clinical Trial Center, Kyung Hee University Korean Medicine Hospital, #23 Kyungheedae-ro, Dongdaemun-gu, Seoul 02447, South Korea

Boncho Ku, Jang-Han Bae, Min-Ho Jun and Jaeuk U. Kim
KM Fundamental Research Division, Korea Institute of Oriental Medicine, Daejeon 34054, South Korea

Jae-Young Shin and Jun-Hwan Lee
Clinical Research Division, Korea Institute of Oriental Medicine, Daejeon 34054, South Korea

Jung Won Kang and Junghwan Kim
Department of Acupuncture & Moxibustion, College of Korean Medicine, Kyung Hee University, Seoul 02447, South Korea

Index

www.ingramcontent.com/pod-product-compliance
Lightning Source LLC
Chambersburg PA
CBHW061240190326
41458CB00011B/3541